URBAN HEALTH

URBAN HEALTH

Combating Disparities with Local Data

Steven Whitman

Ami M. Shah

Maureen R. Benjamins

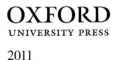

OXFORD
UNIVERSITY PRESS

2011

145.4.973

NOV 18 2011

OXFORD
UNIVERSITY PRESS

Oxford University Press, Inc., publishes works that further
Oxford University's objective of excellence
in research, scholarship, and education.

Oxford   New York
Auckland   Cape Town   Dar es Salaam   Hong Kong   Karachi
Kualsa Lumpur   Madrid   Melbourne   Mexico City   Nairobi
New Delhi   Shanghai   Taipei   Toronto

With offices in
Argentina   Austria   Brazil   Chile   Czech Republic   France   Greece
Guatemala   Hungary   Italy   Japan   Poland   Portugal   Singapore
South Korea   Switzerland   Thailand   Turkey   Ukraine   Vietnam

Published by Oxford University Press, Inc.
198 Madison Avenue, New York, New York 10016
www.oup.com

Library of Congress Cataloging-in-Publication Data

Whitman, Steven.
Urban health : combating disparities with local data /
Steven Whitman, Ami M. Shah, Maureen Benjamins.
p. ; cm.
Includes bibliographical references and index.
ISBN 978-0-19-973119-0   1. Urban health—Illinois—Chicago.
2. Health surveys—Illinois—Chicago.   I. Shah, Ami M.
II. Benjamins, Maureen.   III. Title.
[DNLM: 1. Healthcare Disparities—Chicago.
2. Urban Health Services—Chicago.   3. Community Health Services—Chicago.
4. Health Surveys—Chicago.   5. Models, Organizational—Chicago.
WA 380 W615u 2011]
RA566.4.I3W55 2011
362.1'04209773—dc22
2010003248

9 8 7 6 5 4 3
Printed in the United States of America
on acid-free paper

This book is dedicated to all those who struggle for what should be theirs by virtue of their humanity: The pursuit of a long, healthy, and productive life.

PREFACE

"For a successful technology, reality must take precedence over public relations, for Nature cannot be fooled."

—Richard P. Feynman

The near Westside of Chicago is home to a unique health delivery system, the Sinai Health System. Sinai's vision is to become the national model for the delivery of urban health care and our mission addresses our desire to make a difference in both the lives of individuals and the communities we serve. This commitment has been the seed of the Sinai Urban Health Institute (SUHI). SUHI works alongside Mount Sinai Hospital, a 325-bed teaching hospital with a Level 1 trauma program, 60,000 emergency visits, and 4,000 deliveries; Schwab Rehabilitation Hospital, a regional 90-bed rehabilitation center; Sinai Children's Hospital; and the Sinai Community Institute, which supports 25 ethnically diverse community-oriented programs starting with pregnant and parenting teens all the way to senior support programs and includes violence prevention and workforce development to name a few. Overall, Sinai supports a population base of 750,000 people including some of the most socio-economically challenged neighborhoods in Illinois. This makes Sinai Illinois' largest provider of Medicaid services and the source of specialty care not otherwise available to this diverse community.

The health-care status of a population is set by a variety of determinants. Repeatedly, it is acknowledged that throughout the world, public health measures, such as clean water and functioning sanitation systems, have extended life expectancy more than any other interventions. This is not news, but this learning has gotten lost in technological advances. Sinai recognizes that a micro-community (local level) understanding of health status and subsequent focused interventions are critical to eliminating health disparities. The goal of creating a healthier, more productive community is not dependent on sophisticated clinical interventions but on understanding the community and its needs.

It is clear that the United States has some of the best clinical services in the world as demonstrated by the amount of resources put into the health-care engine. With that investment, we have come to believe that end of life is optional, especially if we keep spending. We keep trying to fool nature.

This book is about reality. The reality of the community. The reality of making an investment that leads to understanding the strengths and needs of a community and creating interventions that are not designed to fool nature but designed to support her.

Today, we live with a delivery system that requires better understanding and actions based on the reality of the impact of housing, education, prevention, and discrimination. The current system is invested in technology that, although impressive and life-saving, is extraordinarily expensive and still ignores the basic determinants of health.

What the authors describe in clear terms is how understanding the nature of a community as a starting point can change the health status of a population dramatically. This does not remove the opportunity or the need to make the best use of medical technology, but it does demonstrate that it should be seen as part of an integrated model for creating healthier communities.

A return to recognizing the public health of a community—"pre-primary care"—will have an exciting and sustainable impact on a population's future health status.

Alan H. Channing
President and CEO
Sinai Health System

ACKNOWLEDGMENTS

All human activity is collective and based upon standing, however imperfectly, on the shoulders of those who have come before us. Many, many organizations and individuals have contributed to the various chapters in this book, and they are acknowledged as part of each chapter. In addition, we want to more generally thank those whose vision for improved health made this book possible.

The Robert Wood Johnson Foundation (RWJF) funded the initial community survey. This was proactive and courageous of them because we could only imagine at the beginning what might come out of such an effort. We thank Dr. James Knickman, then RWJF Vice President for Evaluation and Research, for initially understanding the potential of this work and Kimberly Lochner, our Program Officer, for her vision and guidance. When the survey was complete, the Chicago Community Trust generously funded the analysis and dissemination of this work for 3 years. We especially thank our Program Officer, Ada Mary Gugenheim, for her foresight regarding the survey data and its ability to improve the health of Chicago communities. In addition, we owe a special thanks to the leadership of the Michael Reese Health Trust, whose continued support of the Sinai Urban Health Institute enabled us to write this book.

Once the initial survey of six community areas was complete, the Jewish Federation of Metropolitan Chicago and the Asian Health Coalition of Illinois took on the responsibilities of obtaining resources and replicating the survey in four additional communities. We are indebted to them for taking this initiative and bringing the total to 10 Chicago communities with health survey data.

Many of our colleagues at the Sinai Urban Health Institute helped shape the survey, worked with the communities, and provided critical support throughout the entire process, and we offer our sincerest gratitude to them for everything. Most notable among them is Jade L. Dell, who not only authored one of the book chapters but also monitored the administration of the effort from beginning to end. We also thank the administration of the Sinai Health System, constantly beleaguered by the financial nature of the health care non-system in the United States. Despite this, the Sinai Health System has been heroic in supporting our work. We are grateful to Sinai's mission to serve the people of the communities in which we work, regardless of their ability to pay, and to Sinai's commitment to taking its services beyond the walls of its institution. We especially thank Benn Greenspan, who was CEO when this endeavor started, and Alan Channing our current CEO, who has bent over backward in multiple ways to help make this entire project a reality.

Finally, we would like to thank Oxford University Press editor William J. Lamsback, who supported this book from the beginning, and editor Regan Hoffman, who gave us the support and guidance necessary to bring it to fruition.

CONTENTS

CONTRIBUTORS

Leah H. Ansell, BA
Medical Student
Feinberg School of Medicine
Northwestern University
Chicago, IL

Maureen R. Benjamins, PhD
Senior Epidemiologist
Sinai Urban Health Institute
Sinai Health System
Chicago, IL

Adam B. Becker, PhD, MPH
Executive Director
Consortium to Lower Obesity in Chicago
    Children (CLOCC)
Children's Memorial Hospital
Chicago, IL

Juana Ballesteros, BSN, RN, MPH
Executive Director
Greater Humboldt Park Community of
    Wellness

Alan H. Channing, MHA, FACHE
President and CEO
Sinai Health System
Chicago, IL

**Katherine Kaufer Christoffel,
MD, MPH**
Professor of Pediatrics and Preventive
    Medicine
Feinberg School of Medicine
Northwestern University Medical School

Jaime Delgado, BA
Project Director
BLOCK-BY-BLOCK
The Greater Humboldt Park Community
    Campaign against Diabetes

Jade L. Dell, MRE
Coordinator of Research Programs
Sinai Urban Health Institute
Sinai Health System
Chicago, IL

Charlene J. Gamboa, MPH
Project Coordinator
Sinai Urban Health Institute
Chicago, IL

Lucy Guo, MPH
Epidemiologist
John H. Stroger, Jr. Hospital
Cook County

Melissa A. Gutierrez, MS
Epidemiologist
Sinai Urban Health Institute
Chicago, IL

Hong Liu, PhD
Former Executive Director
Asian Health Coalition of Illinois
Chicago, IL

Matt Longjohn, MD, MPH
Assistant Adjunct Professor
Department of Pediatrics
Feinberg School of Medicine
Northwestern University
Institute Fellow
Altarum Institute

José E. López, Executive Director
Juan Antonio Corretjer Puerto Rican
    Cultural Center
Instructor
Columbia College, University of Illinois
    and Northeastern Illinois University

Helen Margellos-Anast, MPH
Program Director and Senior
    Epidemiologist
Sinai Urban Health Institute
Sinai Health System
Chicago, IL

Molly Martin, MD, MAPP
Assistant Professor
Department of Preventive Medicine and
    Pediatrics
Section of Community and Social
    Medicine
Rush University Medical Center
Chicago, IL

Matthew J. Magee, MPH
Department of Epidemiology
Rollins School of Public Health
Emory University
Atlanta, GA

Miguel Angel Morales, BA
West Town Community Networker
Consortium to Lower Obesity in Chicago
    Children (CLOCC)
Chair
Active Lifestyles Task Force of the
    Greater Humboldt Park Community of
    Wellness

José Luis Rodríguez, BA
Program Director
Community Organizing for Obesity
    Prevention in Humboldt Park

Steven K. Rothschild, MD
Vice Chair of the Department of
    Preventive Medicine
Director of the Section of Community
    and Social Medicine
Rush University Medical Center
Chicago, IL

Ami M. Shah, MPH
Senior Epidemiologist
Sinai Urban Health Institute
Sinai Health System
Chicago, IL

Joseph F. West, ScD
Program Director and Senior
    Epidemiologist
Sinai Urban Health Institute
Sinai Health System
Chicago, IL

Steven Whitman, PhD
Founder and Director
Sinai Urban Health Institute
Sinai Health System
Chicago, IL

Section 1

Setting the Stage

1

INTRODUCING THE SINAI MODEL FOR REDUCING HEALTH DISPARITIES AND IMPROVING HEALTH

Steven Whitman, Ami M. Shah, and Maureen R. Benjamins

Much effort has been put forth to document health disparities at the national, state, and city levels. Despite this, disparities remain widespread and persistent. This book tells the story of how one research center in Chicago is attempting to improve on this inexcusable situation by collecting local data as a catalyst to developing and implementing effective, targeted interventions. The methods and experiences described in this book provide a useful model for how to systematically pursue health improvements in vulnerable communities and simultaneously achieve greater health equity. This book describes the data collection process and presents case studies of how the data were translated into action, information that is relevant for all urban communities throughout the United States.

The story begins in 2001. Members of the Sinai Urban Health Institute (SUHI), a research center based at Mount Sinai Hospital in Chicago, articulated a vision of how to begin reducing health disparities in Chicago by improving the health of individuals living in the poor communities of color served by the hospital. Specifically, it was believed that if survey data could be obtained to describe the health of people living in these communities, then effective interventions could be developed, and these interventions would eventually help to reduce health disparities in the city. In this context, the Director of SUHI (Steven Whitman) wrote a letter to The Robert

Wood Johnson Foundation in 2001. This resulted in an extended dialogue that eventually led to SUHI receiving a generous grant to implement such a survey. The process of implementing this survey and translating the findings into interventions is the focus of this book. In broad outline, the steps that were taken (and that are described in detail in the subsequent chapters) were as follows:

- The original survey was conducted in six of Chicago's officially designated 77 community areas. The six communities were selected to reflect the racial, ethnic, and socio-economic diversity of Chicago (the third largest city in the United States). They were also chosen based on their level of community organization and interest in such health data. The survey was substantial and would evolve into one of the largest door-to-door health surveys ever conducted in Chicago (Chapter 3).
- To construct the survey and select relevant topics and questions, a committee comprised of community residents and activists was assembled. This was not merely an "advisory committee." Rather it had full veto power over each and every question. The committee met frequently for many hours at a time. Its work is a vivification of much that is of value, and that is possible, when researchers truly work collaboratively with communities and the power often assumed by university and/or medical system affiliation is eliminated (Chapter 3).
- Even before data collection started, SUHI members made many presentations to introduce the survey and its potential to the communities in which the survey would be conducted. The nature of the survey was explained, as was the need for this type of local data and the importance of community participation throughout the process. At virtually every presentation, people would ask some variant of the following question: "Researchers like you come through here from time to time, ask us a bunch of questions, and then go away and we never hear from them again. What makes you different?" This prompted the investigators to reaffirm their goal that whatever was found, a touchstone of the work would be to report the findings back to the community, to help empower and mobilize them with data, and to help them improve the health of their communities. Although moving beyond documentation to action is still rather unique, authors of this book believe it to be a morally essential next step.
- After surveying the first six communities, which consisted of Black, White, Mexican, and Puerto Rican people, researchers made many presentations describing the findings. Following this, other organizations became interested in obtaining such data for their own communities. First, a representative from the Jewish Federation of Metropolitan

Chicago asked if the survey could be implemented in a Jewish community. He was told that the survey certainly could be replicated in other communities, if they could help to find funding for the data collection and assemble a community advisory team. Thus, a Jewish community became the seventh surveyed community (Chapter 4). Other communities followed suit. To date, this includes communities that are predominantly Chinese, Vietnamese, and Cambodian (Chapter 5). The data from these 10 communities present extraordinary insight into the unique problems faced by individuals living in each of these areas, as well as a greater understanding of how widely health can vary across different populations within the same city, even those within walking distance of each other (Chapter 6).

- Consistent with these events, SUHI's relationships with community-based organizations in the city intensified. There are many names and models for how to best achieve the difficult yet worthwhile goal of conducting research in partnership with community members and organizations, including community-based participatory research, translational research, and community engagement, to cite but a few. Although all of the existing models had some things in common with the community work described in this book, none seemed to satisfactorily define what was being done in the wake of the Sinai surveys. This led to an even greater effort to conceptualize this aspect of the work (Chapters 13 and 14).

- Based on the survey findings, engagement with communities, and the dissemination of results to lay and professional audiences, the study began to attract a great deal of attention. Literally hundreds of stories appeared in the mainstream press and on radio and television. As of this writing, SUHI members have made over 150 presentations describing survey-related findings. Audiences have included community-based organizations, medical centers, foundations, professional societies, and other groups.

- This dissemination provided a stimulus for funding interventions to improve health in the selected communities (Chapters 7–12). Such funding came from local foundations, the Illinois Department of Public Health, and several branches of the federal government including the National Institutes of Health (NIH) and the Centers for Disease Control and Prevention (CDC).

- Interventions were designed and implemented in cooperation with community organizations and individuals. A special effort was put forth to ensure that each intervention was carefully evaluated and that the results of these evaluations, both favorable and unfavorable, were transparently reported (Chapters 7–12).

- In addition, other agencies throughout the city, even those with whom SUHI had no contact, began to use the survey data to obtain grants and to guide their own work within vulnerable communities in Chicago. Several local foundations reported that many proposals submitted to them cited the SUHI survey data as the motivation for the proposed work.
- Finally, the desire to help eliminate racial and ethnic disparities in health intensified as the process continued. This ultimate goal of the data collection effort is being addressed as interventions continue to be implemented in underserved communities and communities of color. If these interventions are effective, they are not only improving the health of the individuals in those communities, they are also reducing disparities.

All of these events and lessons led to the development of the "Sinai Model for Reducing Health Disparities and Improving Health" (Box 1-1). As this model was discussed at various forums, people were excited by its potential to accomplish what its name implies and interested in its ability to be replicated in other cities. Although numerous community reports and articles describing this work have been published in peer-reviewed journals, none of these outlets afforded the space to detail the evolution of this model. The desire to tell this full story has led to the volume you are holding in your hands.

This book has been crafted in an effort to tell an interesting and coherent story, which it is hoped will be useful for public health practitioners, policymakers, students and professors at schools of public health, doctors, nurses, social workers, and others in related fields. It is especially anticipated that this book will be of use to communities wishing to improve their own health. With data that are most relevant to their communities, groups of individuals may use the information to set priorities, advocate for greater resources, and take meaningful action for change. It is also hoped that the book will be helpful to the professionals who work alongside these communities to achieve this common goal.

The purpose of this book is to describe the progress made along the path defined by the interactions of residents of Chicago with the survey. Along the way, of course, there have been successes and challenges. Because much can be learned from both of these, an effort is made to describe all aspects of the project in detail. It is hoped that this book will explain the motivation for gathering local data, the steps that were taken along the way, the extent to which such work has been effective here in Chicago, and, most importantly, how others might proceed to do similar work in their own communities.

BOX 1-1 Sinai Model for Reducing Health Disparities and Improving Health

- Implement a sound community survey in selected vulnerable communities.
- Meaningfully analyze the results and interpret them within the context of what is known about corresponding national and state-wide findings; locate community-level differences and describe their relevance.
- Disseminate the findings and analyses widely to communities, academic forums, peer-reviewed journals, and media.
- Partner with community organizations, empower them with information, and help organize and mobilize communities to prioritize key health concerns.
- Locate and/or develop potentially effective interventions to address the health issues.
- Work with community-based organizations to obtain funding for these interventions and bring greater resources to the community.
- Effectively implement community-driven interventions to improve health outcomes.
- Carefully, fully, and transparently evaluate the interventions to ensure success and replicate best practices.

Acknowledgments

We would like to thank those who authored the chapters, the people who designed the survey, the communities who welcomed us (and even those who criticized us), and the valiant people who have struggled for many years to improve their health, thus inspiring us to want to help them do that. We would also like to thank our colleagues at the Sinai Urban Health Institute for helping us conduct the survey, analyze the data, interpret the results, and plan, implement, and evaluate the interventions. None of this could have happened without each and every one of them.

We especially would like to thank Alan Channing, the CEO of Sinai Health System, for supporting our work, even while medical centers with far more resources are ignoring the issues raised by the research described throughout the book. Finally, we would like to thank Oxford University Press editors William J. Lamsback, who immediately understood our vision for this book, and Regan Hoffman, who gave us the support and guidance necessary to bring it to fruition.

2

A HISTORY OF THE MOVEMENT TO ADDRESS HEALTH DISPARITIES

Jade L. Dell and Steven Whitman

Introduction

Social epidemiologist Paula Braveman defined health disparities as "group differences in health that are unnecessary, preventable, and unjust" (Braveman, 2006). It is this constellation of attributes that moved the editors of this book to desire to help improve the health of people in general and people of color and low income people in particular. If this is accomplished, the health of the country as a whole will also be improved. This pursuit currently goes under the rubric of "reducing health disparities," a topic that will be discussed in much greater detail in the pages that follow.

Health Disparities: A Look Back and Overview

In the Time of Slavery

Going back to the 1840s, there was an expressed awareness that the health of Black persons in the United States was worse than the health of White persons. In the census of 1860, it was even predicted that because of the extremely low Black birth rate and the high rates of infant and maternal mortality, by the year 2000 Black people might be extinct (Byrd and Clayton, 2000; Washington, 2006).

During Reconstruction

Immediately after the Civil War, the Freedmen's Bureau, in the face of high Black mortality (Byrd and Clayton, 2000; Washington, 2006)[1] began to establish Black medical schools in the South (such as Meharry Medical College founded in 1876) and hospitals (such as Howard University Hospital chartered in 1867).[2] These institutions were important but faced heavy odds as Reconstruction era advances toward equal advantages and opportunities were lost in the reactionary White backlash of fear and racism.

Health disparities between Blacks and Whites were thus not addressed as the nation moved away from the institution of slavery but kept Black people segregated and bereft of most health-care infrastructure. Medical care for former slaves was still practiced by local Black healers, but White doctors who formerly treated slaves at the behest of their masters no longer did so. "Separate but equal" was legalized in the Plessy versus Ferguson[3] decision by the Supreme Court in 1896, and what followed was a codification of a separate social structure through Jim Crow laws. Separate drinking fountains, separate entrances, separate schools, separate hospitals—the list was long and in reality society was "separate and unequal"—including in the health arena.

Hoffman versus DuBois

The reasons for Black–White health disparities were argued from many points of view. In 1896, Frederick L. Hoffman, a Prudential Life Insurance statistician, suggested that "the American Negro" was racially inferior and thus more susceptible to disease (Hoffman, 1896). His analysis, based on vital and social statistics and population factors, concluded that the abolition of the institution of slavery did not improve the lives of African Americans. Hoffman's view lingers today in studies that predominately locate Black risk for ill health in genetics and behavior instead of acknowledging the role of social structural factors such as racism, dilapidated housing, inferior education, or lack of employment opportunities.

Opposing the "blame-the-victim" ideology, Atlanta University sponsored the "Eleventh Conference for the Study of Negro Problems" and adopted a resolution to form local Health Leagues instituted to provide health education to Black people. Further study of the problem was strongly suggested. At this 1906 Conference, W.E.B. DuBois, Harvard-educated intellect, sociologist, and civil rights activist, released a ground-breaking treatise entitled, "The Health and Physique of the Negro American" (DuBois, 1906). Using census data, U.S. Surgeon General Reports, vital statistics, insurance company records, reports from Black hospitals and drug stores, reports from medical schools, letters from physicians, voluminous references, and the measurement of 1,000 students, DuBois and his colleagues concluded that disparities in health between Black and White people were "not a racial disease but a social disease" (DuBois, 1906, p. 89). The book was called a sociological study (although it might now be called an epidemiological study) of the well-being of the Negro American whose poor health was judged a direct result of racism and poverty.

The National Medical Association versus the American Medical Association

There were many other attempts to address the health-care needs of Black people in the United States. The National Medical Association (NMA) was established in Atlanta, Georgia, in 1895 to afford a place for Black physicians to gather for support, education, and conferencing. The NMA established clinics and hospitals as well as medical schools for Black people to become doctors, nurses, and dentists (Byrd and Clayton, 2000). This was a crucial move because Black doctors and other health professionals were historically excluded from the American Medical Association (AMA) and other professional societies. Until the late 1960s, the AMA rejected the membership of Black professionals using the excuse that "membership matters are controlled by constituent societies" (AMA, 2009, p. 4). This decision, reminiscent of the "states rights" argument around slavery, was voted on and affirmed by the AMA House of Delegates every time it was challenged: in 1939, 1944, 1948, 1950, 1951, 1963, and finally in 1965.

Negro Health Week

Around 1915, the National Negro Business League of Virginia established a Negro Health Week using churches and schools to mobilize people for neighborhood clean-up and education about health and hygiene (Gamble and Stone, 2006). Booker T. Washington, who was then the President of the National Negro Business League, adopted the Virginia program idea and suggested it to other local leagues (Gamble and Stone, 2006). In the following two decades, 32 states participated in this endeavor with 2,200 communities involved in 1935 at the height of the movement. Following this success, the U.S. Public Health Service took over organizing National Negro Health Week under the Office of Negro Health Work and provided administration and funding for educational materials and a journal, *National Negro Health News* (Gamble and Stone, 2006). Communal activism seemed to have played a part in affecting these improvements.

The Desegregation of Health Care

The Hill-Burton Act

During all of this activity, Black doctors and patients were not welcome in White hospitals. In 1946 Congress passed a law, the "Hospital Survey and Construction Act"—commonly known as the Hill-Burton Act. This law prohibited discrimination on the basis of race, creed, or color in hospital facilities constructed with federal monies. This was a move in the direction of health-care equity. Yet, surreptitiously embedded in the law was an exception carefully worded by Alabama Senator Lister Hill encoding a provision that would maintain the "separate but equal" status quo: "... an exception shall be made in cases where separate hospital facilities are provided for separate population groups, if the plan makes equitable provision on the basis of need for facilities and services of like quality for each such group ..." (Smith, 1999, p. 47). The Hill-Burton Act was the law of the land, but provisions like this inhibited its full impact until the 1960s.

Brown versus Topeka Board of Education and Simkins versus Cone

Societal movement toward racial integration was beginning to take hold in the 1950s, and separate programs for Black people were shut down along with the Office of Negro Health Work (Gamble and Stone, 2006). Activists, both Black and White, argued that separate facilities almost always meant that Black facilities—whether they were schools, hospitals, or something else— were inferior to White facilities. The landmark Supreme Court ruling of 1954, Brown v. Topeka Board of Education, made segregation in public schools illegal. Health activists, encouraged by this victory, began working to end the segregation of medical facilities. In 1963, the Simkins v. Moses H. Cone Memorial Hospital case was settled against two North Carolina hospitals that had taken $1,269,950 in federal money for building programs while refusing to accept Black patients (JNMA, 1963; Smith, 1999). This case is sometimes called "The Brown case for hospitals" (Reynolds, 1997b). After Simkins v. Cone, any hospital applying for federal money had to guarantee open admission to all races, had to allow all qualified physicians to have staff privileges, and could not segregate patients by race (Terry, 1965; Reynolds, 1997b).

The Civil Rights Act, 1964, and the Revision of Hill-Burton, 1964

The Civil Rights Act was passed on July 2, 1964 after the longest debate in the Senate's history, lasting more than 534 hours (Smith, 1999). It stipulated that any program that received federal assistance could not practice racial segregation or it would lose its funding. The repercussions of this Act reached far and wide. For example, the Hill-Burton Act was revised on August 18, 1964 (Smith, 1999) to eliminate the "separate-but-equal" clause (discussed on the previous page). President Lyndon Baines Johnson signed it.

Moving in the Right Direction on the Back of Federal Policies

The Great Society and National Programs

On July 30, 1965, as part of what has been called the "Great Society Movement," President Johnson pushed and Congress finally approved the establishment of two new national programs, Medicare (to provide health care for those aged 65 and over) and Medicaid (for those unable to afford health care at any age). Part of the stipulation in these new programs was that no federal funds would be awarded to any entity that did not allow all citizens to participate. This was another incentive in the difficult process to desegregate U.S. health-care systems. Hospitals, medical schools, and clinics that had previously refused entry to Black persons now had to admit them or face the possibility that federal funding would be withdrawn (Reynolds, 1997a; Eichner and Vladeck, 2005). In addition, Black physicians were slowly and reluctantly admitted to practice at formerly all White hospitals. As noted in "Achieving Health Equity: an Incremental Journey," "…it took the passage of the Medicare/Medicaid Act in 1965, along with the social justice victories of the civil rights movement, before Americans from racial and ethnic minority populations, most notably African Americans, were free to enter the nation's medical care institutions" (Ibrahim, Thomas and Fine, 2003, p. 2).

According to the National Medical Association (NMA), many Black people were able to access health care for the first time in the years after 1965, and some Black doctors were even invited to serve on hospital staffs. Dr. Rodney G. Hood of the NMA notes that as a result, "African American health improved dramatically in virtually every measurable health status, utilization, and outcome parameter for ten years" (Hood, 2001, p. 2). It is reported that 1,000 hospitals desegregated their staffs and facilities in a 4-month period in 1965 (Eichner and Vladeck, 2005). The federal government was firm in its requirement that health-care facilities be compliant with this new federal law.

Sadly, by 1980 a puzzling deterioration in the health outcomes for Black Americans was observed (Hood, 2001). In 1999 the CDC reviewed health data from 1980 to 1997 and concluded that "the slave health deficit has never been corrected" (Hood, 2001, p. 584). It seemed that merely desegregating health-care facilities did not result in a correction of the underlying racism in the health-care structure. As Eichner and Vladeck noted: "...Medicare and its providers are part of the U.S. health care system, not a distinct health system unto themselves. So to the extent that biases pervade the system, they affect minority Medicare beneficiaries as well" (Eichner and Vladeck, 2005, p. 2).

NMA/NAACP versus USDHEW

In addition, it is well-documented that opposition to the Medicare Act was essentially opposition to the desegregation of health services related to "race-loaded implications" (Boychuk, 2005). These implications can be traced to the intimacy in the hospital setting where persons of different races might be lying next to each other in adjacent beds, White people might get treated by a Black physician, or the supply of blood products might be mixed up without regard to who receives whose blood. There were also many strong words exchanged between the NMA and the National Association for the Advancement of Colored People (NAACP) on one side and the U.S. Department of Health, Education and Welfare (USDHEW) on the other side. The Black organizations charged that the USDHEW did not make clear enough the mandate that only desegregated hospitals would receive Medicare funds (New York Times, 1965).

It seems that the attempt of "The Great Society" to address segregated health services was just a beginning. More efforts would be required.

The Next Steps: Establishing the Foundation for the Healthy People Goals

Public Health Service Reports

Progressive forces such as Medicare, Medicaid, the NMA, and the NAACP had as their intent improving the health and well-being of all citizens with an emphasis on minority citizens. Despite their desire and efforts to level the health playing field, racism and disparities persisted (Smith, 1999). It thus became important to track improvements and failures. For a first step, the Public Health Service Act Section 308 called for an annual report to the President and to the Congress on the health status of the nation. These reports were dispensed through the 1970s. In January 1977, with the appointment of Joseph A. Califano, Jr. to the position of Secretary of the USDHEW by newly elected President Jimmy Carter, there was a dramatic change in the force and essence of these routine health status reports.

TABLE 2-1   Programs of "The Great Society" Selected to Show Improvements in Health for All

Poverty
    War on Poverty Programs (40 Programs)
    The Food Stamp Act of 1964
Education
    Bills to provide classroom equipment and minority scholarships (60 Bills)
    The Vocational Education Act of 1963
Children's Health and Welfare
    Head Start, a program for preschoolers from low-income families
    The Child Nutrition Act of 1966
    The Child Protection Act of 1966
    The National School Lunch Act of 1968
Racism
    The Civil Rights Act of 1964
    The Voting Rights Act of 1965
    Amendment to the Immigration and Nationality Act, 1965
Aging and the Elderly
    The Older Americans Act of 1965
    Social Security Amendments of 1965
    Establishment of Medicare, 1965

Source: http://www.colorado.edu/AmStudies/lewis/2010/gresoc.htm

Joseph A. Califano's Contribution

Joseph Califano (a lawyer by trade) had, as Special Presidential Assistant, helped to create the Great Society programs of the 1960s during the presidency of Lyndon B. Johnson. As Califano notes in his book, *Governing America: An Insider's Report from the White House and the Cabinet,* "My years with Lyndon Johnson greatly influenced my work at HEW" (Califano, 1981, p. 11). In his words, "... what put HEW at the cutting edge of social policy were the Great Society programs of the Johnson years," including, as already noted, the establishment of Medicare, which desegregated hospitals and clinics (Califano, 1981, p 24). The Great Society programs encompassed some of the most radical initiatives and addressed many pressing domestic issues related to child welfare, poverty, civil rights, and elder issues. Examples of some of these initiatives are provided in Table 2-1.[4]

Reorganization of USDHEW

On March 8, 1977, just months after his appointment by President Carter, Califano reorganized USDHEW into five operating divisions, one of which created a brand new "Office for Disease Prevention and Health Promotion" (Califano, 1981). He personally recruited staff, began to measure performance, and started assessing delivery of services. Califano was eager to demonstrate that "…the programs of the New Deal and Great Society and the enormous social commitment of the American people could be executed efficiently, as well as compassionately" (Califano, 1981, p. 48).

National Health Insurance

Another of Califano's passions was the establishment of National Health Insurance (NHI), and in April 1977 he set up the Advisory Committee on National Health Insurance Issues. Califano designed four prototype plans and worked diligently to bring all sides on board. This initiative was beset with disagreements and heated internal arguments between Massachusetts Senator Edward Kennedy (a strong proponent of NHI) and President Carter. In the end, Carter decided that because of pressing budget issues, high inflation, disagreements on implementation, and the conflicting demands of labor unions, the AMA, hospital associations, physicians, and other special interest groups, it was not possible to pass legislation on NHI during his presidency.

Major Initiatives

During Califano's 2.5 years as head of USDHEW, his major initiatives included: childhood immunizations; monetary aid to elementary, secondary, and higher education; equal opportunity for women athletes in collegiate sports; civil rights for minorities (particularly for women, non-White racial/ ethnic groups, and persons with handicapping conditions); improving access to health care; an alcoholism program; and a national anti-smoking campaign. In fact, it is well-known that it was his anti-tobacco stance that essentially led to his being fired.[5] He often called smoking "slow motion suicide" and "Public Health Enemy Number One" (Califano, 1981, p. 185). For that he was strongly opposed by southern tobacco growers and those legislators and lobbyists who represented them (Southern Oral History Program Collection, 1991). It was also relevant that President Carter hailed from Georgia, a major tobacco growing state.

Healthy People—a Call for Public Health Goals

It was suggested that USDHEW set up "health initiatives" with targets or goals (Califano, 1981). This alternative to merely reporting health statistics is what Califano would pursue as he served the remainder of his tenure, which ended in July 1979 when he was fired by the Carter Administration.

In the meantime, Califano issued and wrote the foreword to a publication entitled *Healthy People: The Surgeon General's Report on Health Promotion and Disease Prevention,* which for the first time set health goals for the people of the United States. In the foreword to that publication, Califano noted a need for dramatic change and called for "a second public health revolution in the history of the United States" (USDHEW, 1979, p. vii).

Secretary Califano noted that the first public health revolution in the United States, spanning the late 19th century, involved battling a host of infectious diseases such as influenza, pneumonia, diphtheria, tuberculosis, and gastrointestinal infection through improving sanitation and instituting the use of vaccines. His view of a health revolution for the late 20th century was based on the principle of disease prevention rather than treatment of already acquired disease. Califano wrote, "We are killing ourselves by our own careless habits. We are killing ourselves by carelessly polluting the environment. We are killing ourselves by permitting harmful social conditions to persist—conditions like poverty, hunger and ignorance—which destroy health, especially for infants and children" (USDHEW, 1979, p. viii). He expressed concern that citizens of the United States would need to mobilize both their personal discipline and their political will to address the health problems confronting the nation.

This precursor to the Healthy People reports was the impetus for the development of a national program of setting goals and objectives for improving the health of the people by stressing an "ounce of prevention" rather than a "pound of cure." Responding to the challenge put forth by the report, individuals in the USDHEW strategized to set goals for public health, especially for the 21st century, which was fast approaching.

Promoting Health/Preventing Disease: Objectives for the Nation, 1980

USDHEW becomes USDHHS

When Califano abruptly left his government office in August 1979, USDHEW was soon subsumed into a cabinet-level entity called the Department of Education; "Health and Welfare" was renamed the U.S. Department of Health and Human Services (USDHHS).[6] USDHHS assumed leadership and gathered together professionals, citizens, private organizations, and public agencies from all over the country to establish a set of health promotion and disease prevention objectives.

Promoting Health/Preventing Disease

These objectives became the first "Healthy People" document and were published in 1980 as *Promoting Health/Preventing Disease: Objectives for the Nation* (USDHHS, 1980). That volume was followed by annual reports on the health status of the people of the United States. Each year, goals for additional measures were added and old goals were refined. These reports, entitled *Health, United States*, featured data from hundreds of sources, including the National Center for Health Statistics (NCHS), the Health Resources and Services Administration (HRSA), the National Institutes of Health (NIH), and the Public Health Foundation (National Center for Health Statistics, 1993).

The Health Status of Minority People—Front and Center

The Malone-Heckler Report

In 1983, Margaret M. Heckler, a Republican appointed by President Ronald Reagan, became USDHHS Secretary. Heckler continued the practice of publishing the *Health, United States* reports. After releasing the 1983 edition, she noted that "... there was a continuing disparity in the burden of death and illness experienced by Blacks and other minority Americans as compared with our nation's population as a whole" (USDHHS, 1985, p. 9; Gamble and Stone, 2006, p. 9). In January of 1984, Heckler established a Task Force, and less than 2 years later under her watch, USDHHS produced a ground-breaking 10-volume report, "Black & Minority Health. Report of the Secretary's Task Force," often called the "Malone-Heckler Report" (Byrd and Clayton, 2000). In February of 1986, *Morbidity and Mortality Weekly Report* characterized Heckler's initiative as a "... response to the national paradox of steady improvement in overall health, with substantial inequities in the health of U.S. minorities" (CDC, 1986, p. 109).

In the introduction to that document, the Chair of the Task Force, Dr. Thomas E. Malone, wrote:

> "This report should serve not only as a standard resource for department wide strategy, but as the generating force for an accelerated national assault on the persistent health disparities which led you [Heckler] to establish the Task Force a little more than a year ago." (USDHHS, 1985, p. 7)

Expanding Data by Race/Ethnicity

Uniquely, this report provided data on the health of Asian and Pacific Islanders, Native American and Alaskan Natives, and Hispanic people in addition to Black and White people (Nickens, 1996). The Secretary's Task Force spent a year reviewing data sources and analyzing the morbidity and mortality rates of more than 40 diseases.

Calculating Excess Deaths

To define disparities in mortality among minority persons, the Task Force employed the statistical technique of calculating "excess deaths," which estimates how many deaths would not have occurred if a minority person had experienced the same mortality rate as a non-minority person (Gamble and Stone, 2006). Black Americans were reported to suffer an excess of 60,000 deaths per year (USDHHS, 1985; CDC, 1986; Gamble and Stone, 2006). This estimate, by the way, was recently updated to 84,000 by Satcher and his colleagues using 2002 data (Satcher et al., 2005).

Using health status indicators (HSIs) such as years of life lost, life expectancy, prevalence rates of chronic diseases, hospital admissions, physician visits, and relative risk, researchers identified six causes of death—heart disease/stroke, homicide/accidents, cancer, infant mortality, cirrhosis of the liver, and diabetes—which were responsible for over 80% of the excess mortality experienced by minority persons (CDC, 1986).

The process from inception to publication of the Malone-Heckler Report took just over 17 months. The *MMWR* stated that the report "represents a significant step in the process of establishing a consensus on the major health problems affecting minority Americans" (CDC, 1986, p. 111).

The Office of Minority Health, 1986

As a direct response to these publications, in 1986 USDHHS set up the Office of Minority Health, the first such federal office since the Office of Negro Health Work, which was closed in 1951. In addition, subcommittees were established to study nonhealth factors that might contribute to health disparities, to propose interventions, and to carry out the eight recommendations that the Office of Minority Health developed as listed in Table 2-2 (CDC, 1986).

Mixed Response to the Malone-Heckler Report

The response of the NMA and others to the Malone-Heckler report was mixed (Jones, 1985; Gamble and Stone, 2006). Although the report moved the discussion of disparities to a new level, the recommendations emphasized the importance of health education, research, and encouraging lifestyle changes for people with poor health. Critics noted that the report blamed the victim's lack of knowledge about health, instead of questioning whether the nation really had the will to address the systemic issues that limit health equity, such as unequal access, limited economic opportunity, racial discrimination, and cultural incompetency. Research on the topic of disparities has continued apace, but actually moving beyond research to action has mostly idled (Gamble and Stone, 2006).

TABLE 2-2   Eight Recommendations of the Task Force of the Office of Minority Health Designed to Carry Out the Mandates of the Malone-Heckler Report (CDC, 1986)

1. Implement an outreach campaign, specifically designed for minority populations, to disseminate targeted health information, educational materials, and program strategies.
2. Increase patient education by developing materials and programs responsive to minority needs and by improving provider awareness of minority cultural and language needs.
3. Improve the access, delivery, and financing of health services to minority populations through increased efficiency and acceptability.
4. Develop strategies to improve the availability and accessibility of health professionals to minority communities through communication and coordination with nonfederal entities.
5. Promote and improve communications among federal agencies in administering existing programs for improving the health status and availability of health professionals to minorities.
6. Provide technical assistance and encourage efforts by local and community agencies to meet minority health needs.
7. Improve the quality, availability, and use of health data pertaining to minority populations.
8. Adopt and support research to investigate factors affecting minority health, including risk-factor identification, education interventions, and prevention and treatment services.

Source: Centers for Disease Control and Prevention (CDC). 1986. Perspectives in disease prevention and health promotion, Report of the Secretary's Task Force on Black and minority health. *Morbidity and Mortality Weekly Report* 35(8):109–112.

The Healthy People Movement Gains Momentum

Healthy People, 2000

USDHHS continued to track health data through the 1980s and released a new document in 1990 entitled *Healthy People 2000: National Health Promotion and Disease Prevention Objectives* (HP 2000), that set standards to be met by the year 2000 (USDHHS, 1990). Its introduction paints a picture of a hopeful future: "*Healthy People 2000* offers a vision for the new century, characterized by significant reductions in preventable death and disability, enhanced quality of life, and greatly reduced disparities in the health status of populations within our society" (USDHHS, 1990, p. 1). Describing the goal of reducing health disparities, *HP 2000* states: "The greatest opportunities for improvement and the greatest threats to the future health status of the nation reside in population groups that have historically been disadvantaged economically, educationally, and politically. These must be our first priority" (USDHHS, 1990, p. 46). In fact, building on the 1985 *Black and Minority Health Report*, many health objectives were set for special population groups—for example, low-income persons, racial/ethnic minorities, adolescents, women, older persons, and persons with disabilities.

Three overarching goals summarized the vision of the authors in this iteration:

1. Increase the span of healthy life for Americans;
2. reduce health disparities among Americans; and
3. achieve access to preventive services for all Americans (USDHHS, 1990, p. 6).

Healthy People Reviews, 1991–1999

Using *Healthy People 2000* as its standard, USDHHS monitored progress in the 1990s toward these goals and more than 300 subobjectives. Annual *Healthy People 2000 Reviews* were published between 1991 and 1999 as well as Fact Sheets and a consensus of HSIs for the Nation (USDHHS, 1999).

On February 21, 1998, President Bill Clinton made public an initiative to eliminate health disparities (Ibrahim, Thomas, and Fine, 2003), moving the nation from "reducing" to "eliminating" health disparities and repudiating separate, less ambitious goals for racial and ethnic minorities. Six areas were targeted: infant mortality, cancer screening and management, diabetes, cardiovascular disease, HIV/AIDS, and immunization. Four hundred million dollars was pledged for this effort (APHA Policy Statement, 2000).[7]

Healthy People 2010

As ambitious plans were made to develop and publish *Healthy People 2010*, U.S. Surgeon General Dr. David Satcher summoned national leaders in a "Call to the Nation" to establish a methodology to eliminate racial and ethnic health disparities. Satcher was instrumental in getting the issue of health disparities back on track, pushing to eliminate disparities as the goal (Gamble and Stone, 2006). After meeting, the American Public Health Association, the NMA, the National Center for Vital and Health Statistics, the Office for Civil Rights, NIH, and 35 other leading health organizations, both federal and private, supported the plan but concluded that this goal was reachable only with the collaboration of the federal government and the American people, along with the muscle of a national coalition (Kanaan, 2000; APHA Policy Statement, 2000; Hood, 2001).

In January 2000, the *Healthy People 2010* initiative was officially launched and in November 2000, USDHHS published *Healthy People 2010: Understanding and Improving Health* (USDHHS, 2000), the third attempt to elucidate comprehensive national health objectives. Established for the first time was the goal of *eliminating* health disparities among subgroups (as urged by Satcher), in addition to a goal to "increase quality and years of healthy life." The following statement captures the guiding principle of *HP 2010*:

> ... regardless of age, gender, race or ethnicity, income, education, geographic location, disability, and sexual orientation – every person in every community across the Nation deserves equal access to comprehensive, culturally competent, community-based health care systems that are committed to serving the needs of the individual and promoting community health. (USDHHS, 2000, p. 16)

Progress toward meeting these goals will be measured by analyzing data collected on 498 population-based objectives. One expert in the field of health disparity research, Kenneth Keppel, maintains that the *Healthy People 2010* analysis will result in the most complete and extensive measurement of health disparities to date (Keppel, 2007).

The Healthy People Consortium Established and Citizen Participation Encouraged

In an effort to involve a greater cross-section of ideas and expertise, USDHHS established The Healthy People Consortium, an alliance of national and state agencies, experts in public and environmental health, and individuals and local organizations who shared testimonies and comments that were considered as this new set of objectives was formulated. Three national meetings and five regional meetings occurred in 1998 (USDHHS, 2000). And for the first time, individual citizens were asked for their contributions, of which over 11,000 were received and examined by the Consortium (USDHHS, 2000).

The National Healthcare Disparities Reports

Analyzing health disparities in the Year 2010 publication included addressing differences in education, sexual orientation, and rural–urban living in addition to the special population groups included in the Healthy People 2000 publication: low income, racial/ethnic minority, and disabled.

Because the issue of disparities was now front and center, Congress requested that the Agency for Healthcare Research and Quality also begin producing an annual report, the "National Healthcare Disparities Report" (NHDR). This was initiated with the 2003 issue. When the 2007 report was published, the authors noted a distinct lack of improvement:

> Based on 2000 and 2001 data ..., the number of measures on which disparities have gotten significantly worse or have remained unchanged since the first NHDR is

TABLE 2-3   Ten National Medical Association Recommendations for Health Equity, Paraphrased (Hood, 2001)

---

1. Create a Health Policy and Research Institute to document racial bias
2. Accept racial bias and racism as risk factors for health disparities
3. Address the impact of racial bias and racism in the medical arena
4. Legislate tax incentives for small businesses to enable them to provide insurance for low-wage workers
5. Restructure Medicaid and Medicare eligibility to respond to medical necessity not income, especially for elderly and disabled persons
6. Reform Medicaid and Medicare so provider compensation is tied to severity of illness and comorbidity
7. Hold Congressional hearings on the impact of racism on health care
8. Establish a national committee on racial bias and ethnic health disparities
9. Adopt uniform standards to collect health care outcome data by race/ethnicity
10. Increase funding for NIH Center for Minority Health Disparities

---

Source: Hood, Rodney G. 2001. Confronting racial and ethnic disparities in health care. *Academic Medicine* 76(6):584–585.

higher than the number of measures on which they have gotten significantly better for Blacks, Hispanics, American Indians and Alaskan Natives, Asians and poor populations. (2007 National Healthcare Disparities Report, 2008, p. 1)

The NMA, responding to the call for the elimination of health disparities, established the "Commission for Health Parity for African Americans" in 2001 and published 10 recommendations (Table 2-3) of their own toward achieving health equity (Hood, 2001, pp. 584–585). Clearly, the NMA was interested in an overhaul of the system to address the root causes of racial health disparities. In their recommendations, they steer away from blaming the victim, urging behavioral change, or calling for more research. Instead the emphasis is on moving toward re-orienting the focus of health disparities away from the sufferer and toward what the powerful need to do to correct the injustice.

Using the Healthy People Paradigm to Measure Health Disparities in Real Time

Dr. Walter Tsou, past president of the American Public Health Association, says of health disparities that "... we value what we measure and we measure what we value. This is why we can find the price of any stock instantaneously at any minute of the day and also why, until recently, we have not had very many measures of health disparities" (Tsou, 2004). The field of disparities research is now beginning to respond to Tsou's observation.

Measuring disparities to measure our progress in eliminating them is a comparatively new endeavor in public health and epidemiology. Although some researchers, like W.E.B. DuBois (*see* pages 9–10 of this chapter), had such matters on their minds many decades ago, a process like the one that is under construction now is growing every day. This process has substantial potential to guide us in the direction of eliminating health disparities.

Health Status Indicators (HSIs)

There is a substantial literature on the various methodologies one could use to measure a disparity in health, and this topic is receiving illuminating but limited attention in the literature (Pearcy and Keppel, 2002; Keppel et al., 2005; Harper et al., 2008). At the same time, it is worth noting that most studies of disparities have proceeded by looking at one disease or condition at a time, with only very few efforts to analyze several at once (Geronimus, Bound, Waidmann, 1999; Williams 1999). In an effort to overcome this shortcoming and in an implicit effort to establish a paradigm for the measurement of several health disparities at once, a study was published on 22 HSIs in Chicago comparing outcomes for Black and White people between 1980 and 1998 (Silva et al., 2001). Using measures of mortality, birth outcomes, and infectious diseases, they found no progress in reducing racial disparities during this 18-year period.

Another important contribution in this area came in 2002 and evaluated the HP 2000 goal of reducing health disparities at the national level by examining progress in reducing disparities among the five largest racial/ethnic groups in the United States for 17 HSIs between 1990 and 1998 (Keppel, Pearcy, and Wagener, 2002). The analysis revealed that for the majority of indicators, racial/ethnic disparities had declined on a national level over the period, but mostly by only small amounts. However, a comparable Chicago-specific analysis focusing on non-Hispanic Black/non-Hispanic White disparities found that although the majority of racial disparities narrowed between 1990 and 1998 nationally, the opposite was true in Chicago where the majority widened over the same interval (Margellos, Silva, Whitman, 2004).

Recently, these analyses of Keppel et al. and Margellos et al. have been updated through 2005 (Orsi, Margellos-Anast, Whitman, 2010). The results are disappointing: the United States as a whole is making little progress in reducing Black–White health disparities, and Chicago continues to get worse over time, a process that the authors refer to as "backwards propulsion." For example, in 1990 the Black all-cause mortality rate in Chicago was 36% higher than the White rate; in 2005 it was 42% higher. In 1990 the breast cancer mortality rate was 20% higher in Black women; in 2005 it was

99% higher. As the authors comment, "Overall, progress toward meeting the Healthy People 2010 goal of eliminating health disparities in the U.S. and in Chicago remains bleak. With over 15 years of time and effort spent at the national and local level to reduce disparities, the impact remains negligible" (Orsi, Margellos, and Whitman, 2010, p. 1).

Eliminating Disparities

These research analyses, taken together and built on the foundation of the Healthy People initiatives, suggest a model or paradigm (Kuhn, 1962) for investigating how a society's (community, city, state, country) progress toward the elimination of health disparities might be evaluated beyond analyzing just one health measure at a time. This matter is far from settled but it is best to make this consideration explicit, as has been attempted here, to call for more research in this area.

National data show that health disparities among Americans—especially among the poor and among racial/ethnic minorities—are increasing. How does one understand the goal of eliminating such disparities in this context? Is the goal an impossible one? One article notes, "These disparities are historically rooted in inequities from the past that persist today" (Ibrahim, 2003, p. 1621). In 2008, the *American Journal of Public Health* reprinted an editorial from 2000 which noted that "... long established and growing health disparities are rooted in fundamental social structure inequalities, which are inextricably bound up with the racism that continues to pervade U.S. society" (Cohen and Northridge, 2008, p. S17). Can a society legislate that disparities disappear or does it need to address the underlying issue of racism?

Healthy People 2020 and the Future

As this book is being written, conversations are taking place about the development of *Healthy People 2020 (HP 2020)*, and embedded in those conversations are the issues of health disparities, health equity, and differences in these concepts (USDHHS, Phase I Report). Announcements have gone out inviting members of the public to submit written comments and to attend the meetings of the Secretary's Advisory Committee on National Health Promotion and Disease Prevention Objectives for 2020.[8]

Four key values have been crafted by the Advisory Committee for *HP 2020* that will guide how the elimination of health disparities may lead to health equity:

1. We must value all people equally;
2. health is a high value both personally and societally;

3. everyone should be able to achieve the highest health level possible;
4. health resources should be distributed fairly (USDHHS. Phase I Report).

By the year 2050, non-White people will comprise fully 54% of the U.S. population.[9] Can a society prosper if one-half of its members suffer ill health because of discrimination and racism? Will the United States have the social and political will to eliminate disparities and foster equity? As epidemiologist Camara Phyllis Jones says, "We will need to understand that these racial disparities represent opportunities to increase our scientific understanding of many disease processes, to succeed in primary prevention rather than just screening and treating vulnerable populations, and to combat ideas of biologic determinism that shape public attitudes about the possibility of change" (Jones, 2001, p 304).

Some headway has been made in the last century and a half. Table 2-4 highlights some of the milestones discussed in this chapter.

TABLE 2-4   List of Important Dates in the History of Racial/Ethnic Health Disparities, United States, 1847–2010

1847	American Medical Association is founded; closed to all non-White persons
1862	Freedmen's Hospital (Washington, DC) founded to provide medical care to freed slaves and displaced White people; later became Howard University Hospital (American Medical Association, 2009)
1867	Howard University Hospital established
1876	Meharry Medical College founded, the first Medical school open to Black persons seeking to become Doctors or Nurses
1895	National Medical Association founded in Atlanta, GA
1896	Plessy v. Ferguson Supreme court Decision rules that segregating railroad passenger cars was not a violation of the 14th amendment.
1896	Frederick L. Hoffman publishes *Race Traits and Tendencies of the American Negro*
1906	Atlanta University Sponsors Conference for the Study of Negro Problems, Atlanta, GA
1906	W.E.B. DuBois publishes *The Health and Physique of the Negro American*
1915	First Negro Health Week held
1946	The Hospital Survey and Construction Act (Hill-Burton) passed
1951	Office of Negro Health Work closed
1954	Brown v. Topeka Board of Education: Supreme Court ruling against segregation in U.S. schools
1963	Simkins v. Moses Cone Memorial Hospital case lays groundwork for desegregation of health facilities

(continued)

TABLE 2-4 *(continued)*

1964	Civil Rights Act passed, ending federal assistance for any program that practiced racial segregation
1964	Hill-Burton Act revised to eliminate "separate but equal" clauses
1965	"The Great Society Movement" initiated under President Lyndon Johnson
1965	Medicare/Medicaid Act starts the push for complete desegregation of Health Care facilities
1977	Reorganization of U.S. Dept. of Health Education and Welfare
1979	Healthy People Report from Surgeon General published with Califano foreword
1979	U.S. Dept. of Health Education and Welfare becomes U.S. Dept. of Health and Human Services (USDHHS)
1980	First Healthy People document published: *Promoting Health/ Preventing Disease: Objectives for the Nation*
1985	The Malone-Heckler Report, *Black & Minority Health,* published
1986	USDHHS Establishes Office of Minority Health
1990	*Healthy People 2000: National Health Promotion and Disease Prevention Objectives* published
1991–1999	*Healthy People Reviews* published
1998	Mandate to Eliminate Health Disparities, made by President Bill Clinton
2000	*Healthy People 2010: Understanding and Improving Health* published
2003	National Healthcare Disparities Reports begun
2010	*Healthy People 2020,* yet to be published

Source: Compiled from information discussed in this chapter.

Conclusion

John Ayanian, one of the most prolific analyzers of health-care disparities in the United States (Ayanian et al., 2005; Trivedi and Ayanian, 2006; Sequist et al., 2008), writes that "…the field of healthcare disparities research has developed in three phases." He notes that Phase 1 started with the 1985 *Black & Minority Health Report* (as discussed above). The purpose of that report was to demonstrate the existence and magnitude of health-care disparities. Phase 2, he continues, started in the mid-1990s when we tried to delineate "the mediators of racial, ethnic, and socio-economic disparities in care and their impact on health outcomes." Phase 3, which started about 2000, follows directly from the previous two phases and is concerned with what interventions and programs are implemented to ameliorate health-care disparities (Ayanian, 2008).

Although the *health-care disparities* that Ayanian discusses are not the same as *health disparities,* his model is applicable to the latter as well. One can always know more about the magnitude and causes of health disparities, and such research is welcomed. However, the time has come now to act: to reduce and then eliminate them, as called for by *Healthy People 2000* and *Healthy People 2010.*

To do less is not an option. Karl Marx suggested more than 150 years ago, "The philosophers have only interpreted the world in various ways; the point, however, is to change it" (Marx, 1845). This book is an attempt to help move such a process ahead with respect to public health practitioners and health disparities.

Notes

1. Harriet Washington reports that one quarter of all Black slaves who fled north when the Civil War began died in make-shift camps set up by the Union Army (Washington, 2006).
2. The Howard and Meharry medical schools were the only ones still in operation by 1920 (Smith, 1999).
3. In Plessy v Ferguson, the Supreme Court ruled that segregating railroad passenger cars was not a violation of the 14th amendment.
4. Go to the URL below to see the full list of "Great Society" programs. Online. Available: http://www.colorado.edu/AmStudies/lewis/2010/gresoc.htm. Accessed: October 15, 2009.
5. Go to the URLs below to read the story of Califano's tenure under President Carter and the smoking issue. Online. Available: http://docsouth.unc.edu/sohp/L-0125/menu.html. Accessed: March 30, 2009. www.protectthetruth.org/josephcalifano.htm. Accessed March 30, 2009.
6. Go to the URL below to read the history of the United States Department of Health and Human Services. Online. Available: http://en.wikipedia.org/wiki/United_States_Department_of_Health,_Education,_and_Welfare. Accessed: April 23, 2009.
7. To access all Advocacy and Policy Statements by the American Public Health Association beginning in 1948 through the present, see the following URL; to access policies related to *Healthy People 2010*, search for Policy # 20005, dated 1/1/2000. Online. Available: www.apha.org/advocacy/policy/policysearch/default.htm?NRMODE=Published. Accessed: October 15, 2009.
8. Interested persons are encouraged to register or submit comments. Online. Available: www.healthypeople.gov/hp2020/advisory/default.asp. Accessed: October 15, 2009.
9. Go to the following URL to access the U.S. Census website. Online. Available: http://www.census.gov/Press-Release/www/releases/archives/population/001720.html. Google: "Population percent US 2050." Accessed: October 15, 2009.

References

2007 National Healthcare Disparities Report (NHDR). 2008. Rockville, MD: Agency for Healthcare Research and Quality. AHRQ Pub. No. 08-0041. Online. Available: www.ahrq.gov/qual/nhdr07/Glance.htm. Accessed: September 17, 2009.

American Medical Association. 2009. African American Physicians and Organized Medicine, 1846–1968. Online. Available: www.ama-assn.org/ama1/pub/upload/mm/369/afamtimeline.pdf, p. 1–16. Accessed: September 15, 2009.

APHA Policy Statement Number 20005: Effective interventions for Reducing Racial and Ethnic Disparities in Health. 2000. APHA Public Policy Statements, 1948-present, cumulative. Washington, DC: American Public Health Association. Online. Available: www.apha.org/advocacy/policy/policysearch/default.htm?NRMODE=Published. Accessed: June 23, 2009.

Ayanian, John Z. 2008. Determinants of racial and ethnic disparities in surgical care. *World Journal of Surgery* 32:509–515.

Ayanian, John Z., Alan M. Zaslavsky, Edward Guadagnoli, Charles S. Fuchs, Kathleen J. Yost, Cynthia M. Creech, et al. 2005. Patients' perceptions of quality of care for colorectal cancer by race, ethnicity and language. *Journal of Clinical Oncology* 23(27):6576–6586. Epub 2005 August 22.

Boychuk, Gerard. 2005. Medicare and the politics of race, 1957–1965. Presented at the 2005 Annual Meeting of the American Political Science Association, Washington, DC, September 1–6, 2005.

Braveman, Paula. 2006. Health disparities and health equity: Concepts and measurement. *Annual Review of Public Health* 27:167–194.

Byrd, W. Michael and Linda A. Clayton. 2000. *An American Health Dilemma: A Medical History of African Americans and the Problem of Race, Beginnings to 1900.* New York, NY: Routledge.

Califano, Joseph A., Jr. 1981. *Governing America: An Insider's Report from the White House and the Cabinet.* New York, NY: Simon and Schuster.

Centers for Disease Control and Prevention (CDC). 1986. Perspectives in disease prevention and health promotion, Report of the Secretary's Task Force on Black and minority health. *MMWR* 35(8):109–112.

Cohen, Hillel W. and Mary E. Northridge. 2008. Getting political: Racism and urban health. *American Journal of Public Health* 98:S17-S19. Originally published as Hillel W. Cohen and Mary E. Northridge. 2000. Getting political: Racism and urban health. *American Journal of Public Health* 90:841–842.

DuBois, W. E. Burghardt. ed. 1906. *The Health and Physique of the Negro American.* Atlanta, GA: The Atlanta University Press.

Eichner, June and Bruce C. Vladeck. 2005. Medicare as a catalyst for reducing health disparities. *Health Affairs* 24(2):365–375.

Gamble, Vanessa N. and Deborah Stone. 2006. U.S. policy on health inequities: The interplay of politics and research. *Journal of Health Politics, Policy and Law* 31:93–126.

Geronimus, Arline T., John Bound, and Timothy A. Waidmann. 1999. Poverty, time, and place: Variation in excess mortality across selected US populations, 1980–1990. *Journal of Epidemiology and Community Health* 53(6):325–334.

Harper, Sam, John Lynch, Stephen C. Meersman, Nancy Breen, William W. Davis, and Marsha E. Reichman. 2008. An overview of methods for monitoring social disparities in cancer with an example using trends in lung cancer incidence by area-socioeconomic position and race-ethnicity, 1992–2004. *American Journal of Epidemiology* 167:889–907.

Hoffman, Frederick L. 1896. Race traits and tendencies of the American Negro. *The American Economic Association* 11(1–3):1–329.

Hood, Rodney G. 2001. Confronting racial and ethnic disparities in health care. *Academic Medicine* 76(6):584–585.

Ibrahim, Said A., Stephen B. Thomas, and Michael J. Fine. 2003, Achieving health equity: An incremental journey. *American Journal of Public Health* 93(10):1619–1621.

Jones, Camara Phyllis. 2001. Invited commentary: Race, racism, and the practice of epidemiology. *American Journal of Epidemiology* 154(4):299–304.

Jones, Edith Irby. 1985. Closing the health status gap for Blacks and other minorities. *Journal of the National Medical Association* 78:485–486.

Journal of the National Medical Association (JNMA). 1963. Federal court rules bias in federally aided hospitals unconstitutional. 55:558. Online. Available: www.ncbi.nlm. nih.gov/pmc/articles/PMC2642433/pdf/jnma00682-0090a.pdf

Kanaan, Susan Baird. 2000. National Committee on Vital and Health Statistics—1949–1999—a History. U.S. Department of Health and Human Services. Online. Available: www.ncvhs.hhs.gov/50history.htm. Accessed September 23, 2009.

Keppel, Kenneth G. 2007. Ten largest racial and ethnic health disparities in the United States based on Healthy People 2010 objectives. *American Journal of Epidemiology* 166(1):97–103.

Keppel, Kenneth G., Elsie Pamuk, John Lynch, Olivia Carter-Pokras, Insun Kim, and Vickie M. Mays. 2005. Methodological issues in measuring health disparities. *Vital Health Statistics* 2:141.

Keppel, Kenneth G., Jeffrey N. Pearcy, and Diane K. Wagener. 2002. Trends in racial and ethnic-specific rates for the Health Status Indicators: United States, 1990-98. In: *Healthy People Statistical Notes.* No.23. Hyattsville, MD: National Center for Health Statistics, pp. 1–16.

Kuhn, Thomas. 1962. *The Structure of Scientific Revolutions.* Chicago, IL: The University of Chicago Press.

Margellos, Helen, Abigail Silva, and Steven Whitman. 2004. Comparison of health status indicators in Chicago: Are Black-White disparities worsening? *American Journal of Public Health* 94(1):116–121.

Marx, Karl. 1969. Theses on Feuerbach, 1845. In: *Collected Works*, Volume 1, pp. 13–15. Marx K and Engels F. Moscow, USSR: Progress Publishers.

National Center for Health Statistics (NCHS). 1993. *Health United States, 1992.* Hyattsville, MD: Public Health Service.

New York Times. 1965. Medicare drive on rights urged. *New York Times*, December 17, p. 23.

Nickens, Herbert W. 1996. A compelling research agenda. *Annals of Internal Medicine* 125(3):237–239.

Orsi, Jennifer M., Helen Margellos-Anast, and Steven Whitman. 2010. Black: White health disparities in the United States and Chicago: Any progress? *American Journal of Public Health* 100(2):349–356.

Pearcy, Jeffrey N. and Kenneth G. Keppel. 2002. A summary measure of health disparity. *Public Health Reports* 117(3):273–280.

Reynolds, P. Preston. 1997a. The Federal Government's use of Title VI and Medicare to racially integrate hospitals in the United States, 1963 through 1967. *American Journal of Public Health* 87(11):1850–1858.

Reynolds, P. Preston. 1997b. Hospitals and civil rights, 1945–1963: The case of Simkins v. Moses H. Cone Memorial Hospital. *Annals of Internal Medicine* 126(11):898–906.

Satcher, David, George E. Fryer, Jr., Jessica McCann, Adewale Troutman, Steven H. Woolf, and George Rust. 2005. What if we were equal? A comparison of the Black-White mortality gap in 1960 and 2000. *Health Affairs* 24(2):459–464.

Sequist, Thomas D., John. Z. Ayanian, Richard Marshall, Garrett M. Fitzmaurice, and Dana G. Safran. 2008. Primary-care clinician perceptions of racial disparities in diabetes care. *Journal of Gen Internal Medicine* 23(5):678–684. Epub 2008 January 24.

Silva, Abigail, Steven Whitman, Helen Margellos, and David Ansell. 2001. Evaluating Chicago's success in reaching the Healthy People 2000 goal of reducing health disparities. *Public Health Reports* 116:484–494.

Smith, David Barton. 1999. *Health Care Divided: Race and Healing a Nation.* Ann Arbor, MI: The University of Michigan Press.

Southern Oral History Program Collection. 1991. Oral History Interview with Joseph Califano, April 5, 1991. Interview L-0125. Chapel Hill, NC: The University Library, The University of North Carolina. Online. Available: http://docsouth.unc.edu/sohp/L-0125/menu.html. Accessed March 30, 2009.

Terry, Luther L. 1965. Hospitals and Title VI of the Civil Rights Act. *Journal of the American Hospital Association* 39(1):34–37.

Trivedi, Amal N., and John. Z. Ayanian. 2006. Perceived discrimination and use of preventive health services. *Journal of General Internal Medicine* 21(6):553–558.

Tsou, Walter. 2004. Personal Communication.

U.S. Department of Health and Human Services (USDHHS). Phase I Report. Recommendations for the framework and format of Healthy People 2020, Appendix 10. Clarification and examples of health disparities and health equity. Online. Available: www.healthypeople.gov/hp2020/advisory/PhaseI/appendix10.htm. Accessed June 18, 2009.

U.S. Department of Health and Human Services (USDHHS). 1985. *Black & Minority Health. Report of the Secretary's Task Force. Volume 1: Executive Summary.* Washington, DC: U.S. Government Printing Office.

U.S. Department of Health and Human Services (USDHHS). Public Health Service. 1990. *Healthy People 2000: National Health Promotion and Disease Prevention Objectives.* DHHS Publication No. (PHS) 91-50212. Washington, DC: U.S. Government Printing Office.

U.S. Department of Health, Education, and Welfare (USDHEW). Public Health Service. 1979. Healthy People: The Surgeon General's Report on Health Promotion and Disease Prevention. DHHS Publication No. (PHS) 79-55071. Washington, DC: U.S. Government Printing Office.

U.S. Department of Health and Human Services (USDHHS). Public Health Service. 1980. *Promoting Health/Preventing Disease: Objectives for the Nation.* Washington, DC: U.S. Government Printing Office.

U.S. Department of Health and Human Services (USDHHS). Public Health Service. 1999. An Invitation to Celebrate the Launch of *Healthy People 2010.* Washington, DC: U.S. Government Printing Office.

U.S. Department of Health and Human Services (USDHHS). 2000. *Healthy People 2010: Understanding and Improving Health,* 2nd ed. Washington, DC: U.S. Government Printing Office.

Washington, Harriet A. 2006. *Medical Apartheid: The Dark History of Medical Experimentation on Black Americans from Colonial Times to the Present.* New York, NY: Harlem Moon/Broadway Books.

Williams, David. R. 1999. Race, socioeconomic status, and health. The added effects of racism and discrimination. *Annals New York Academy of Science* 896:173–188.

Section 2

The Importance of Local Data

Ami M. Shah, Steven Whitman, and
Maureen R. Benjamins

Introduction

The Sinai Model is designed to reduce disparities and improve health. The first step to achieving this goal is to obtain meaningful health data. It has become increasingly evident that existing health data for large geographic areas mask important differences in how groups within a heterogeneous population experience health (Northridge et al., 1998). Local-level data collection is one possible solution to this problem. It allows for the examination of health problems for specific groups at the community level, which is particularly relevant for large, diverse urban centers. The study of populations in smaller geographic areas can help to uncover the nature of health disparities and offer insight to shape targeted community-based interventions. This is especially noteworthy because one of the overarching goals for the "Healthy People" Initiative has been to reduce and eliminate disparities over the last two decades (United States Public Health Service, 1991; United States Department of Health and Human Services, 2000).

Small-area studies have slowly gained prominence in health research beginning with Wennberg and his colleagues in their examination of variations in health-care service utilization (Wennberg and Gittelsohn, 1973; McPherson et al., 1982; Skinner et al., 2003). This approach has since been used to facilitate many public health efforts such as: to contest the placement of tobacco and alcohol advertising in certain minority neighborhoods (Hackbarth et al., 2001); to study the relationship between neighborhood socio-economic factors and birth weight in California (Pearl, Braveman, and Abrams, 2001); and to track the movement of the AIDS epidemic (Zierler et al., 2000; Needle et al., 2003). In addition, it has been used more generally to examine the relationship between neighborhood and health (Diez-Roux, 2001; Kawachi and Berkman, 2003; Whitman et al, 2004; Shah, Whitman, and Silva, 2006; Cummins, Curtis, and Diez-Roux, 2007).

Some health data are available at the local level. For example, existing data that can be geocoded to the county, city, zip code, or community level may be derived from traditional surveillance systems (e.g., vital records and communicable disease registries). These data provide information on small-area trends and variances in mortality (Fang et al., 1995; Whitman et al., 2004) or measure issues related to birth outcomes (Krieger et al., 2003) and infectious diseases (Krieger et al., 2003). Information for other health measures, such as the prevalence of chronic diseases, health behaviors, and other risk factors, come from health surveys and are not available at the local level. Existing surveys are routinely conducted at the national (e.g., National Health Interview Survey) and state (e.g., Behavioral Risk Factor Surveillance System [BRFSS], California Health Interview Survey) levels, sometimes at the county level (e.g., Community Health Indicator Project [Metzler et al., 2008]; The Health of King County Report [Public Health Seattle & King County, 2008]) but rarely at the city level (e.g., New York City Community Health Survey). For some counties and cities, such information can be derived from state surveys (e.g., Chicago BRFSS), but rarely are health survey data available at the community level (however this may be defined). These health data are most valuable because they describe modifiable health behaviors or practices that are relevant to guiding planning, programs, and policies, and yet, they are almost never known. For example, there are limited data or surveillance systems that measure the proportion of people who smoke or who are overweight at a community or neighborhood level.

One response to these problems is to conduct a local area health survey. This type of survey can not only uncover important variations in health but also has the potential to inspire communities and public health professionals in pursuit of solutions to the health problems detected. For example, there may be some impact from telling a community that 20% of adults in the United States smoke. However, telling people that a local survey found that 20% of adults *in their community* smoked is far more likely to catalyze collective action around the problem of smoking.

The city of Chicago is an excellent place for a study of small areas. After all, it is the "city of neighborhoods" (Pacyga and Skerrett, 1986). In 2000, Chicago was the third largest city in the United States with a population of almost 3,000,000 that was 36% non-Hispanic Black, 31% non-Hispanic

White, and 26% Hispanic. Chicago is also one of the most segregated cities in the United States (Massey and Denton, 1993), well-known for its racial and ethnic enclaves (Holli and Jones, 1995). Existing health data for Chicago are typically presented by its 77 officially designated community areas (CAs), most of which are racially and ethnically homogenous (The Chicago Fact Book Consortium, 1995). The CAs are aligned with census tracts, making sociodemographic data about the CA available. Health data from vital records and communicable disease registries are also available at this level, but health survey data, which are the primary source for chronic disease surveillance, health behaviors, and associated risk factors, are not, as described earlier.

According to the Sinai Model, local is defined at the community or neighborhood level, often based on shared experiences and common background. This book describes exactly how this type of local data was collected in Chicago. Section 2 of this book contains four chapters that describe how local level survey data were collected to measure the health status of 10 culturally diverse Chicago communities. Specifically, Chapter 3 describes the methods used by the Sinai Urban Health Institute to examine the health of six racially and ethnically diverse community areas, presenting data from *Sinai's Improving Community Health Survey*. Four of the communities selected are predominantly homogenous and represent the primary racial and ethnic groups in Chicago (e.g., White, Black, and Mexican). For the first time, data from the other two communities capture the health of the largest Puerto Rican population in Chicago and respond to demands from active community groups for such information. Chapter 4 describes the methods and key findings from a Jewish community that recognized the significance of having local health data. The survey was conducted in the most densely populated Jewish community in Chicago (with borders defined by community leaders). Chapter 5 describes how three Asian surveys were conducted to capture the health of Chinese, Vietnamese, and Cambodian populations within three communities. The Chinese community was surveyed in Chicago's Armour Square (also known as Chinatown), an area with the highest concentration of Asians. The Vietnamese and Cambodian populations were more dispersed but located based on collaboration with community partners, who again saw value in having specific health data about the community they serve. The final chapter synthesizes survey data relevant to five major health outcomes for all 10 of these communities to illustrate the importance of small area studies in identifying meaningful variations. The data gathered from all 10 communities represent the first step of the Sinai Model toward eliminating disparities and can ultimately be used to motivate communities, direct health interventions, and improve health.

References

Cummins, Steven, Sarah Curtis, Ana V. Diez-Roux, and Sally Macintyre. 2007. Understanding and representing place in health research: A relational approach. *Social Science and Medicine* 65(9):1825–1838.

Diez-Roux, Ana V. 2001. Investigating neighborhood and area effects on health. *American Journal of Public Health* 91(11):1783–1789.

Fang, Jing, William Bosworth, Shantha Madhavan, Hillel Cohen, Michael H. Alderman. 1995. Differential mortality in New York City (1988-1992), part two: Excess mortality in the South Bronx. *Bull N Y Academy Medicine* 72(2):483–499.

Hackbarth, Diana P., Daniel Schnopp-Wyatt, David Katz, Janet Williams, Barbara Silvestri, and Rev. Michael Pfleger. 2001. Collaborative research and action to control the geographic placement of outdoor advertising of alcohol and tobacco products in Chicago. *Public Health Reports* 116(6):558–567.

Holli, Melvin G. and Peter d'A. Jones, eds. 1995. *Ethnic Chicago: A Multicultural Portrait,* 4th ed. Grand Rapids, MI: William B. Eerdmans Publishing Company.

Kawachi, Ichiro, and Lisa F. Berkman, eds. 2003. *Neighborhoods and Health.* New York: Oxford University Press.

Krieger, Nancy, Jarvis T. Chen, Pamela D. Waterman, Mah-Jabeen Soobader, S. V. Subramanian, and Rosa Carson. 2003. Choosing area based socioeconomic measures to monitor social inequalities in low birthweight and childhood lead poisoning: The Public Health Disparities Geocoding Project (US). *Journal of Epidemiology and Community Health* 57:186–199.

Krieger, Nancy, Pamela D. Waterman, Jarvis T. Chen, Mah-Jabeen Soobader, and S. V. Subramanian. 2003. Monitoring socioeconomic inequalities in sexually transmitted infections, tuberculosis, and violence: Geocoding and choice of area-based socio-economic measures—the Public Health Disparities Geocoding Project (US). *Public Health Reports* 118:240–260.

Massey, Douglas S. and Nancy A. Denton. 1993. *American Apartheid: Segregation and the Making of the Underclass.* Cambridge, MA: Harvard University Press.

McPherson Klim, John E. Wennberg, O. B. Hovind, and Peter Clifford. 1982. Small-area variations in the use of common surgical procedures: An international comparison of New England, England and Norway. *New England Journal of Medicine* 307:1310–1314.

Metzler, Marilyn, Norma Kanarek, Keisher Highsmith, Ron Bialek, Roger Straw, Ione Auston, et al. 2008. Community Health Status Indicators Project: The development of a national approach to community health. *Preventing Chronic Disease* 5(3). Online. Available: http://www.cdc.gov/pcd/issues/2008/jul/07_0225.htm. Accessed December 15, 2009.

Needle, Richard H., Robert T. Trotter, II, Merrill Singer, Christopher Bates, J. Bryan Page, David Metzger, et al. 2003. Rapid assessment of the HIV/AIDS crisis in racial and ethnic minority communities: An approach for timely community interventions. *American Journal of Public Health* 93(6):970–979.

Northridge, Mary E., A. Morabia, M. L. Ganz, M. T. Bassett, D. Gemson, H. Andrews and C. McCord. 1998. Contribution of smoking to excess mortality in Harlem. *American Journal of Epidemiology* 147(3) 250–258.

Pacyga, Dominic A. and Ellen Skerrett. 1986. *Chicago City of Neighborhoods: Histories and Tours.* Chicago: Loyola University Press.

Pearl, Michelle P., Paula Braveman, and Barbara Abrams. 2001. The relationship of neighborhood socioeconomic characteristics to birthweight among 5 ethnic groups in California. *American Journal of Public Health* 91(11):1808–1814.

Public Health Seattle & King County. 2008. *The Health of King County 2006 Report.* Online. Available: http://www.kingcounty.gov/healthservices/health/data/hokc.aspx. Accessed December 16, 2009.

Shah, Ami M., Steven Whitman, and Abigail Silva. 2006. Variations in the health conditions of 6 Chicago community areas: A case for local-level data. *American Journal of Public Health* 96(8):1485–1491.

Skinner, Jonathan, James N. Weinstein, Scott M. Sporer, and John E. Wennberg. 2003. Racial, ethnic, and geographic disparities in rates of knew arthroplasty among medicare patients. *New England Journal of Medicine* 349:1350–1359.

The Chicago Fact Book Consortium. 1995. *Local Community Fact Book: Chicago Metropolitan Area, 1990.* Chicago, IL: Academy Chicago Publishers.

United States Department of Health and Human Services (USDHHS). 2000. *Healthy People 2010: Understanding and Improving Health,* 2nd ed. Washington, D.C.: U.S. Government Printing Office.

United States Public Health Service. 1991. *Healthy People 2000: National Health Promotion and Disease Prevention Objectives.* Department of Health and Human Services Publication No. (PHS) 91-50212. Washington, D.C.: U.S. Government Printing Office.

Wennberg, John and Alan Gittelsohn. 1973. Small area variations in health care delivery. *Science* 182:1102–1108.

Whitman, Steve, Abigail Silva, Ami M. Shah, and David Ansell. 2004. Diversity and disparity: GIS and small area analysis in six Chicago neighborhoods. *Journal of Medical Systems* 28(4):397–411.

Zierler, Sally, Nancy Krieger, Yuren Tang, William Coady, Erika Siegfried, Alfred DeMaria, et al. 2000. Economic deprivation and AIDS incidence in Massachusetts. *American Journal of Public Health* 90(7):1064–1073.

3

SINAI'S IMPROVING COMMUNITY HEALTH SURVEY: METHODOLOGY AND KEY FINDINGS

Ami M. Shah and Steven Whitman

In fond memory of Ingrid Graf and Charles Ward

Introduction

In response to growing inequities in health, the Sinai Health System conducted a survey that has altered the way public health data are used in Chicago. The Sinai Urban Health Institute (SUHI), a member of the Sinai Health System, partnered with several community organizations, residents, and local leaders to complete one of the largest, most comprehensive door-to-door health surveys in Chicago, titled *Sinai's Improving Community Health Survey* (Sinai Survey). For the first time, meaningful, local data were available to delineate major health problems facing Chicago neighborhoods. Findings were shared with policymakers, residents, and others who needed to know how to influence change toward improved health. Specifically, this chapter describes how the survey was conducted, presents selected key findings, and describes how these results were disseminated. Overall, it exemplifies how public health surveillance can be political and consequential.

Rationale for a Local Health Survey

Sinai sits on the near west side of Chicago amid poor communities with poor health. It was believed that if more were understood about this situation, then steps could be taken to improve matters. Existing data sources are not adequate for this task. Although birth and death data are available from accessible vital records files and can be tabulated at a local level, little other health information is similarly available. It is not possible to calculate the proportion of the population affected by a particular disease (prevalence) or the *"actual causes"* of death and disability, as described in a seminal article by McGinnis and Foege (1993). Without fully understanding these underlying or root causes of poor health, developing long term and sustainable interventions for improvement becomes a serious challenge.

Information on such root causes traditionally comes from risk factor data that may be gathered by existing health surveys like the Behavioral Risk Factor Surveillance System (BRFSS) survey and the National Health Interview Survey (NHIS). These surveys reflect the overall health of the nation, a state, or sometimes a city but rarely have sample sizes that are adequate to describe communities (or neighborhoods) and smaller racial and ethnic groups of a diverse city like Chicago. For example, most survey data are limited to non-Hispanic (NH) Blacks, NH Whites, and sometimes Hispanics, but seldom are they available for Hispanic subgroups, Asians, or any of their many subgroups. Existing health survey data are thus not local enough. The need for such information was the rationale for the Sinai Survey.

Partnerships and Funding

The inception of the Sinai Survey began in 2000 with a letter of inquiry to The Robert Wood Johnson Foundation, one of the nation's leading foundations working to improve health and health care for all Americans. The letter expressed SUHI's idea to gather and utilize local health data as a catalyst for improved public health programs and policies. It described the gaps in existing health data (Benbow, Wang, and Whitman, 1998), the importance of small area studies in improving health (Wennberg and Gittelsohn, 1973), and the commitment and ability of the Sinai Health System to improve health. Following the initial letter, an invitation to write a full proposal was made, and a 2-year grant (starting January 2002) was eventually awarded.

The Sinai Health System received funding to implement this grant because of its unique commitment to improving the health of the communities it serves. The grant proposal emphasized the importance of local health

TABLE 3-1   Prominent Individuals Who Wrote Support Letters on behalf of Sinai Health System's Proposal to The Robert Wood Johnson Foundation, 2001

Danny K. Davis, Member of Congress

Emil Jones, Jr., Illinois Senate Democratic Leader

Susana A. Mendoza, Illinois State Representative, 1st District

William Delgado, Illinois State Representative, 3rd District

Cynthia Soto, Illinois State Representative, 4th District

Arthur L. Turner, Illinois State Representative, 9th District

Roberto Maldonado, Cook County Commissioner, 8th District

Dorothy H. Gardner, President, Michael Reese Health Trust

Greg Darnieder, Executive Director, Steans Family Foundation

Debra Wesley Freeman, President and CEO, Sinai Community Institute

Anne M. Meegan, Program Director, Seattle STD/HIV Prevention Training Center

data and its potential in informing new programs, bringing in resources, and galvanizing communities. It also described how the Sinai Health System is comprised of a research arm (SUHI) and a community arm, the Sinai Community Institute, which enables them to effectively drive change at the community level. Thus, although SUHI led this initiative, it could not have been possible without support from the Sinai Health System's administration and the Sinai Community Institute, along with their community partners. Table 3-1 presents a list of prominent individuals who wrote support letters on behalf of Sinai's pursuit of the grant.

Methodology

From the beginning, SUHI researchers understood that the value of a local survey would be maximized if it were conducted with the greatest scientific precision, pursuing the highest possible standards. The Survey Research Laboratory (SRL) of the University of Illinois at Chicago was thus contracted to administer the survey. SRL has more than 40 years of experience designing and conducting health surveys, particularly in vulnerable communities on the south and west sides of Chicago. They proposed the best plan and the most feasible budget to administer a survey.

Studies have shown that sampling through residential telephone lines was less effective in locating members of vulnerable subpopulations, particularly because of disconnected or missing telephone numbers (Northridge, Morabia, and Ganz, 1998) and the advent of widespread cell phone use. It was thus deemed important to gather data face-to-face. In addition, SRL recommended that each interview take no more than 1 hour to administer, because anything longer would result in incomplete surveys. Finally, sufficient sample size was necessary to obtain a representative sample of each community surveyed. With these survey parameters, it was determined that the final survey could contain approximately 500 items and would be administered face-to-face to roughly 300 randomly selected households per community area. In keeping with the given grant budget, six communities could be surveyed.

Targeted Community Areas

Of Chicago's 77 officially designated community areas, six were selected for study. The boundaries for these areas were defined in the 1920s and thus may or may not be consistent with how individuals within a given community area define their so-called community or neighborhood. Nevertheless, these geographic areas are often used as a basis for describing the city's health conditions, implementing services, and allocating resources (Chicago Fact Book Consortium, 1995) and were thus used to administer the Sinai Survey.

The six community areas were selected to reflect the major racial and ethnic groups of Chicago residents. North Lawndale is predominantly NH Black, and South Lawndale is predominantly Mexican. These communities were selected because they are two primary communities served by the Sinai Health System. Norwood Park is located on the northwest side and has a median household income of $53,000. Although richer than the other communities surveyed, it was selected because it was the poorest predominantly NH White community in Chicago. Roseland was selected as a predominately NH Black community on the south side, with an average median household income similar to that of Chicago. Finally, Humboldt Park and West Town were selected for two main reasons. First, these two community areas are heterogeneous—that is, in 2000, West Town was about half White and half Hispanic (predominately Puerto Rican or Mexican), and Humboldt Park was about half Black and half Hispanic (predominately Puerto Rican or Mexican). They thus represented some aspects of the racial and ethnic diversity of Chicago and reflected the changing dynamics facing many urban settings. Second, SUHI had a substantial history of working with community organizations in these communities. Humboldt Park and West Town are two areas that are notable for their strong community-based organizations and for being politically active in government. Table 3-2 presents demographic characteristics for the six Chicago communities selected for study compared to Chicago and the United States.

TABLE 3-2 Demographic Characteristics of Six Chicago Community Areas Compared to Chicago and United States, Census 2000

	Humboldt Park	North Lawndale	Norwood Park	Roseland	South Lawndale	West Town	Chicago	United States
Total population	65,836	41,768	37,669	52,723	91,071	87,435	2,896,016	281,421,906
Female (%)	52	56	53	55	42	48	52	52
Average Age (years)	25	26	43	35	25	30	32	
Non-Hispanic Black (%)	47	94	1	98	13	9	36	12
Non-Hispanic White (%)	3	1	88	1	4	39	31	69
Hispanic (%)	48	5	6	1	83	47	26	13
Mexican (%)	24	3	3	0	76	25	18	7
Puerto Rican (%)	18	0	0	0	1	16	4	1
High school graduates (%)[a]	50	60	83	77	37	70	72	80
Median household income	$28,728	$18,342	$53,402	$38,237	$32,320	$38,915	$38,625	$41,994
Unemployment Rate (%)[b]	18	26	3	17	12	7	10	6

Source: Whitman, Williams, and Shah, 2004, p. 4.
Notes:
[a] Among those 25 years and older.
[b] Percentage of resident civilians older than 16 years who did not have a job and were actively seeking work.

TABLE 3-3   Community Representatives of the Survey Design Committee and Their Affiliations

Organization	Survey committee participant
Big Brothers Big Sisters, Humboldt Park	Phil Smith, Community Coordinator and Resident of Humboldt Park
Block Club Federation, Humboldt Park	Feliz Villafane de Palacios, Director and Resident of Humboldt Park
Chicago Department of Public Health, Behavioral Health Division	Jamila-Ra, Program Manager, Chicago Department of Public Health and Co-Chair of the Cook County West District Community Health Council
Chicago Youth Centers, Roseland	Cassandra Robinson, Chicago Youth Centers and Resident of Roseland
Community Action Group, North Lawndale	Jo Ann Bradley, Executive Director and Resident of North Lawndale
Community Outreach Intervention Program, School of Public Health, University of Illinois at Chicago	Jaime Delgado, Director
Chicago Cook County Community Health Council	Anna Yuan, Executive Director
El Hogar del Nino, South Lawndale	Concepcion (Connie) Chavarria, Program Director and Resident of Pilsen (South Lawndale)
Westside Future, West Town	Angela Ellison, Executive Director

Survey Design Committee

Full participation of and ownership by the community was sought out and understood to be critical to the survey's success. Therefore, a Survey Design Committee (SDC) was convened to guide the development of the survey and lay the foundation for the project. Some members of the committee came from local community based organizations or social service agencies and/or had several years of experience working in the target communities or neighboring areas. They were community organizers, leaders, or residents (some played a dual role) and served as the *community representatives* on the SDC. Their names and affiliations are listed in Table 3-3. Other members included administrative leaders from the Sinai Health System and epidemiologists from the Sinai Urban Health Institute, who staffed the SDC.

Survey Development

The primary function of the SDC was to develop the survey instrument that would gather information relevant to improving health in the targeted communities. Over the course of 6 months, a collaborative process ensued to design the survey. Meetings were held every other week from January through March 2002, followed by 3 months of review and testing. Although no monetary incentive was received, the majority of committee members attended all six meetings. When unable to attend, they offered input via e-mail or phone. The continuity of involvement on the SDC was a reflection of each member's commitment and Sinai's philosophy of working with communities, both consistent with Community Based Participatory Research philosophy and practices (Heaney, 1993; Drevdalh, 1995; Minkler and Wallerstein 2003).

SDC meetings focused on selecting key topics and questions for the survey. There was a consensus to ask questions about common health conditions (such as hypertension, asthma, and diabetes) to assess prevalence. Questions for these topics were adapted from existing national surveys (e.g., BRFSS or NHIS). There was also general agreement on asking about well-known behavioral risk factors such as tobacco and other substance use, poor nutrition, and physical inactivity, which were also commonly asked on national health surveys.

Early on, community representatives on the SDC wanted to clarify their role and asked who would make the final decisions regarding health topics and questions if/when there were disagreements. Without hesitation, investigators responded that, "you (the community representatives) would." There was overwhelming agreement that the community leaders and residents would have the final say in shaping the survey questions. Knowing that their opinions were valued on this diverse committee, the community representatives of the SDC opted not to accept the stipends that were offered to them.

Many topics were proposed by community representatives that were not initially considered by the study investigators but proved to be most relevant to the community. Examples of such topics were: whether and how often residents reused cooking oils, grocery shopping habits, access to mental health services, how community members felt about needle exchange programs, and the use of alternative medicines. Other proposed topics led to an energetic and stimulating debate. For example, SUHI researchers suggested asking questions regarding social capital. These questions would measure feelings of trust and safety, levels of community engagement, and tolerance of diversity. However, community representatives of the SDC felt it offensive and even racist to ask these questions because this concept had been over-studied and, in the end, would not effectively inform programs. Similarly, community representatives felt questions on drug use would not be useful and could potentially even be unsafe for interviewers to ask about. They also felt that adequate information on community drug use was available from other data sources and that asking sensitive questions to individuals in their homes would not be appropriate or realistic. Thus, neither social capital nor drug use were included as topics on the survey.

While developing the instrument, the SDC decided only to administer the survey to adults ages 18 to 75 years and primary caregivers of children ages 0 to 12 years. The upper age limit for adults was set at 75 years because the SDC expressed concern about the ability of older seniors to accurately answer all of the questions and for children at 12 years because they believed that primary caregivers may not be knowledgeable about children over age 12.

Community representatives of the SDC also recognized a unique opportunity to distribute much-needed health information to the community. In fact, they believed it was the project's responsibility to do so. For example, if interviewers asked knowledge questions about diabetes management from the survey, then it was important to provide answers to these questions, especially when respondents were unsure of their responses. A packet of health information was thus left with each household after completing the interview and if respondents had immediate questions or wanted additional information for the future they could contact the Sinai Community Institute.

Once the questions were finalized, the survey instrument underwent extensive review and pretesting between April and August 2002. The adult and child modules of the instrument and all supporting materials were translated into Spanish. Modifications were made after cognitive interviews and pretesting with interviewers who were also native Spanish speakers from the community (both from Puerto Rican and Mexican heritage). The instrument was programmed for computer-assisted personal interviewing (CAPI) to ensure more efficient data collection and to minimize errors.

The final instrument contained 469 items/questions on the adult questionnaire and 144 on the child questionnaire (Sinai Urban Health Institute, 2009). Table 3-4 presents the major topic areas of the Sinai Survey, which are categorized as: health conditions, health behaviors and attitudes, healthcare access and utilization, quality of life, and other social or environmental factors. The final survey instrument, along with other study materials, was approved by the Institutional Review Boards at the University of Illinois at Chicago and the Sinai Health System.

Sample Selection

SRL was also responsible for designing the sampling frame for data collection. They constructed a three-stage probability sampling design with the goal of obtaining a representative sample of adults and children from each of the six selected community areas, as illustrated in Figure 3-1: Humboldt Park, North Lawndale, Norwood Park, Roseland, South Lawndale, and West Town. At the first stage, 15 census blocks from each community area were selected using probability proportional to size sampling (Sudman, 1976,

TABLE 3-4 Sinai's Improving Community Health Survey Topics

Health-care access and utilization	Health conditions	Health risk factors: knowledge, behaviors and attitudes	Quality of life	Other social and environmental factors
Health coverage	Arthritis	Alcohol use	Self-rated health	Acculturation
Health-seeking behavior	Asthma	Anger management skills	Health-related quality of life	Education
Prescription medications	Chronic respiratory problems	Diet/Nutrition	Perceived stress	Employment
Alternative/ Complimentary medicines	Depression	HIV/AIDS testing	Perceived Racism/Discrimination and	Food shopping habits
Prenatal care	Diabetes	Needle exchange programs	coping	Perceived violence
Cancer screening	Heart problems	Parenting skills		Phone service
Mental health services	Hypertension	Physical activity/exercise		Mode of transportation
	Obesity	SIDS knowledge		
		Tobacco Use		

Source: Sinai's Improving Community Health Survey, 2002–2003.

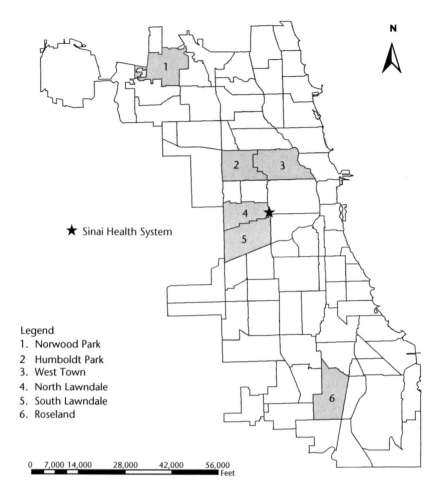

Figure 3-1 Six of Chicago's 77 Community Areas Surveyed by Sinai's Improving Community Health Survey, 2002–2003

pp. 134–138; Graf and Foote-Retzer, 2003, pg. 2). This meant that the blocks in each community area were selected in a manner proportionate to the number of adults (ages 18 years and older) living on these blocks according to the 2000 U.S. Census. Second, 37 households were selected at random from the blocks. When there were fewer than 37 housing units on a given block, equal numbers of households from the remaining blocks in the community area were randomly selected. At the third stage of selection, interviewers administered a household screener to enumerate all household members and select a random adult (18–75 years) and a child (0–12 years) respondent using the Trodahl–Carter–Bryant methodology (Trodhal and Carter, 1964). At the end of the adult interview, if there were any children in the household age 12 years or younger, the questionnaire was programmed to randomly select from among the eligible children in the household and then the adult with the most knowledge of that child's health care was interviewed. Additional details about the overall survey methodology have been published elsewhere (Graft and Foote-Retzer, 2003; Dell et al., 2005).

Survey Administration

The survey was administered face-to-face in respondents' homes from September 2002 through April 2003. All selected households received advance letters introducing the project and notifying the household of the interviewer's visit. The advance letters were jointly signed by the investigators and the respective community organization leaders for the area.

Because of the diversity of the SDC, it became clear that the project also needed a logo with a common message for all residents in the six communities. The Committee felt that the collective partnership of the SDC needed to be represented as its own entity, as opposed to individual work or community affiliations. Thus, after weeks of going back and forth, the SDC agreed to a project logo (Fig. 3-2) with hands reaching toward the sky, signifying the contributions of all in improving the health of communities. The logo was used in newsletters and project materials moving forward.

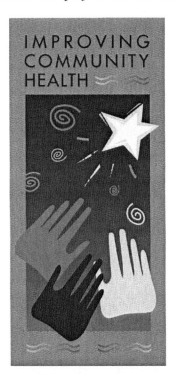

Figure 3-2 *Sinai's Improving Community Health Survey* Project Logo

Table 3-5   Total Number of Completed Surveys by
Community Area

Community Area	Adult	Child
Humboldt Park	300	160
North Lawndale	304	172
Norwood Park	190	70
Roseland	302	129
South Lawndale	300	198
West Town	303	82
Total	1699	811

Source: Sinai's Improving Community Health Survey,
2002–2003

Interviewers were recruited from local newspapers and received more than
20 hours of formal training. Roughly one-third of them were native Spanish
speakers or bilingual. They visited homes during the day, evenings, and week-
ends to contact the selected survey participant or the selected child's primary
caregivers. If no one was home to complete the survey or the adult selected
to be interviewed was unavailable, interviewers would return to complete the
survey. They left follow-up notes regarding a return visit and/or scheduled
an appointment for a later visit. Similarly, interviewers would return to interview the primary caregiver of the randomly selected child when they were
not available. In most instances, the individual who answered the door and
completed the screener was different from the adult or primary caregiver of
the child selected to be interviewed. To gain access to hard-to-reach households, interviewers contacted neighbors or key informants and made up to 12
attempts at different times of the day and days of the week before assigning
a final disposition code of "non-contact."

On average, the adult interview lasted approximately 1 hour and the child
interview lasted about 15 minutes. Respondents were given the option to
conduct the interview in either English or Spanish. Close to 20% of all interviews were completed in Spanish. Respondents received $40 for completing
the adult questionnaire and $20 for the child questionnaire. All households
received a packet of general health information, as described earlier. In the
end, data on 1,699 adults and 811 children were gathered. Table 3-5 presents
the total number of completed adult and child surveys by community area.

Response, Contact, and Cooperation Rates

Several measures were calculated to evaluate and monitor survey administration. Of the original 4,888 household addresses selected for this study, 10.5%

were non-residential; among them, 23.7% were unavailable or could not be contacted. Of the remaining 3,337 households approached and screened, 2,354 (92.2%) households were eligible. There were thus 1,953 eligible persons contacted, and among them, 1,699 adult surveys were completed, along with 811 child surveys.

The official response rate measures the overall proportion of eligible respondents who complete the survey. It was calculated by dividing the number of completed interviews by the sum of all eligible respondents, which includes refusals, non-contacted eligibles, and an estimated proportion of households whose eligibility was unknown. Based on this American Association for Public Opinion Research definition, the response rate for the Sinai Survey was 43.2% (American Association for Public Opinion Research, 2000; Johnson and Owens, 2004).

Another important measure, particularly in hard-to-reach communities that are often in transition, is the contact rate. This is the proportion of selected addresses that could be contacted, which was 76% for all six communities. The lowest contact rates were in North Lawndale (70.5%) and Humboldt Park (73.2%), two non-White communities with the lowest median household income, and the highest was in Norwood Park (85.3%), a predominately White community with the highest median household income (Table 3-2).

Once contact was established, it is important to note that the Sinai Survey had extraordinarily high cooperation rates, despite literature suggesting that it is difficult to conduct surveys in vulnerable communities and that non-White populations are not interested in participating in research (Wendler et al., 2006). The cooperation rate is the proportion of contacted adults who completed the screener and/or the survey. In this case, the cooperation rate was 76.5% for the screener and 87.0% for the survey.

These exceptionally high cooperation rates were likely the result of several factors. For one, there was strong community involvement, as described earlier, in introducing the survey to residents by sending advance letters and promoting the survey in local newspapers. In addition, the interviewers were persistent and flexible in reaching out to individual households. They visited homes during evening and weekend hours, contacted neighbors and key informants, offered the survey in English and Spanish, and made up to 12 personal attempts at different times to contact each household before the household was declared as a "non-respondent."

Despite the extra effort put forth, interviewers faced some challenges in survey administration. For instance, there was a higher-than-expected number of non-residential vacant lots, unoccupied homes, and "locked gate" housing units. Some housing projects were not receptive to our administering the survey, despite writing additional letters to their management company for their approval, and interviewers were in turn denied entry. In addition, there were two incidents of crime that were reported to officials. One interviewer was caught in crossfire shooting, and another was robbed at knifepoint. Interviewers were well-aware of and familiar with issues of safety in their assigned communities. And although they understood the dangers and received training and support on how to handle such situations, they could not avoid all risk.

"Urbanicity" is a well-documented correlate of survey non-response (Groves and Couper, 1998). The Sinai Survey response and contact rates reflect this increasing difficulty of conducting survey research in urban environments. Physical barriers to participation, restricted-access apartment buildings in particular, and respondent concerns with crime and privacy, the latter of which is reflected in strong IRB assurances and protections, made the collection of survey data in Chicago challenging but not impossible.

Data Analysis

Observations were analyzed using SAS, version 9 (SAS Institute Inc., 2002–2003) and Stata, version 8.0 to account for sampling design effects (Stata Corporation, 2003). Based on established survey design theory, two sampling weights were calculated and applied to survey observations: a probability of selection weight (at the block, household, and respondent levels) and a post-stratification weight (to assure the sample accurately reflected the age, sex, and race/ethnicity of the 2000 U.S. Census base population).

Survey Results

Although there are many important findings on the survey, a select few are described here. Topics shown include: health-care access and utilization, chronic health conditions, and health risk factors. Whenever possible, Sinai Survey data are compared with Chicago or U.S. averages from existing health surveys such as BRFSS and NHIS.

Health-Care Access and Utilization

An individual's ability to access health care is closely tied to his/her health and well-being. The lack of health insurance coverage is at the forefront on our nation's health agenda today, yet little is known about how local communities utilize services. There are several measures of health-care access and utilization on the Sinai Survey. These include topics such as access to primary care, preventive services, prescription medications, complimentary and alternative medicines, and insurance coverage. Table 3-6 presents a few selected outcomes.

Table 3-6 Selected Findings on Health-Care Access and Utilization

Health-care access and utilization	Humboldt Park (%)	North Lawndale (%)	Norwood Park (%)	Roseland (%)	South Lawndale (%)	West Town (%)	Comparison (%)
Currently insured (18–64 yrs)	61	61	93	70	46	73	73[a]
Did not obtain needed dental care in past year	33	28	9	30	25	34	...
Did not obtain needed prescription medications in past year	23	24	4	15	12	18	...
Pap Smear in last 3 years[b]	87	94	71	93	90	83	88[b]
Mammogram in the last 2 years (women >40years)	76	77	80	85	90	74	83[c]

Source: Sinai's Improving Community Health Survey, 2002–2003.

Notes: Data are weighted and age adjusted to the 2000 Standard Population, except when noted.
[a]Comparison data from Chicago BRFSS 2002.
[b]Pap Smear data are not age-adjusted. Comparison data from U.S. BRFSS 2002.
[c]Comparison data from U.S. BRFSS 2002.

The proportion of non-elderly adults (<65years) with insurance coverage ranged from 46% in South Lawndale (a mostly Mexican immigrant community) to 93% in Norwood Park (a mostly NH White community). Thus, a resident in South Lawndale was nine times more likely to be *without* insurance compared with a resident in Norwood Park ($p < 0.001$). Coverage varied for most communities (11 of the 15 pairwise community comparisons) and when compared to Chicago (73%) (Shah, Whitman, and Silva, 2006). Interestingly, among those with insurance (with the exception of Norwood Park), more than half relied on public health insurance, suggesting that employer-based coverage is not sufficient (data not shown).

One consequence of having no insurance coverage is limited utilization of routine preventive health services. Respondents living in the five non-White communities were significantly more likely to delay seeking dental care and prescriptive medications compared to Norwood Park ($p < 0 .001$). The uninsured were also up to four times more likely to have never had a mammogram and never had their blood pressure taken (Whitman, Shah, and Williams, 2004, data not shown). On the contrary, those with insurance were nearly twice as likely to have been diagnosed with chronic conditions like hypertension, diabetes, and asthma, suggesting that the uninsured are less likely to get diagnosed appropriately. Because those without insurance may have limited access to a health- care provider, their opportunity to be screened and their utilization of preventive services were lower than those with insurance.

Results also indicate that the majority of women in all six communities are receiving routine cervical and breast cancer screenings (Table 3-6). Access to Pap Smear tests is consistent with declining trends in the prevalence of and mortality from cervical cancer for most women in the United States. In fact, the overwhelming majority of women in all six communities had received a Pap Smear test in the last 3 years, with the lowest rate reported by White women in Norwood Park. Similarly, the majority of women 40 years and older reported having had a mammogram in the prior 2 years. In fact, despite low insurance coverage in South Lawndale, 90% of women had received a recent mammogram, the highest estimate reported by the Sinai Survey.

Chronic Health Conditions

In addition, for the first time, the severity of several chronic health conditions facing these Chicago communities was assessed. Most survey questions used to measure disease prevalence came from existing national health surveys and asked whether respondents had ever been diagnosed with a particular health outcome, such as: "Has your doctor or a health professional ever told you that you have diabetes?"

Table 3-7 presents five common health conditions affecting Chicago communities: hypertension, diabetes, obesity, depression, and asthma. Five non-White communities reported a disproportionately high burden of poor health on these measures. For example, about 40% of adults in Roseland and North Lawndale were living with high blood pressure compared to 23% of adults in Chicago ($p < 0.001$). In these two African American communities, despite differences in their median household income, a greater proportion of adults diagnosed with high blood pressure were younger and female, which has important implications for targeting interventions.

The prevalence of diabetes was also significantly higher in four of the six communities (all eight pairwise comparisons were significant at $p < 0.001$). When stratified by race and ethnicity, the diabetes prevalence among Puerto Ricans was particularly higher than other groups (Whitman, Silva, Shah, 2006; see Chapter 10). For example, the percentage of Puerto Ricans with diabetes was significantly higher than the percentage of Mexicans and Whites (20.8% vs. 4.1% and 3.1%, respectively; $p < 0.025$ for both). Prevalence estimates for Hispanics in Chicago are generally available from the Chicago Department of Public Health but are rarely available for Hispanic subgroups like Mexicans and Puerto Ricans. Without the Sinai Survey, the disproportionate burden of diabetes among Puerto Ricans almost certainly would have never been known.

Table 3-7 also presents other important variations in health documented by the Sinai Survey. Rates of obesity (adult and pediatric), depression, and asthma (adult and pediatric) were consistently lower in the White community of Norwood Park compared to the non-White communities. The mostly Black communities reported high rates of obesity, whereas the predominately Mexican immigrant community reported the highest rate of depression. Asthma was most notable in the mixed communities of West Town and Humboldt Park, which are undergoing urban transition. The burden of poor health, although far worse among the non-White communities in general, varied among the communities. This emphasizes the need to identify specific health problems facing each community and to tailor interventions addressing them.

Health Risk Factors

The Sinai Survey also asked many questions related to health risk factors associated with knowledge, attitudes, and behaviors. Again, these results are most relevant to shaping new interventions and directing resources to address health problems to local communities. Selected results on smoking, HIV testing, and diet/nutrition are described here.

The prevalence of smoking was disproportionately higher in the minority communities, reaching 39% in North Lawndale compared to 24% in

TABLE 3-7 Selected Findings on Chronic Health Conditions

Chronic Health Conditions	Humboldt Park (%)	North Lawndale (%)	Norwood Park (%)	Roseland (%)	South Lawndale (%)	West Town (%)	Comparison (%)
High blood pressure	35	41	26	39	17	28	23
Diabetes	16	10	4	12	6	14	7
Obesity	36	41	20	38	37	31	22
Pediatric obesity	48	46	12	56	34	42	17[a]
Depression	21	15	9	13	21	23	—
Screened depression	20	17	6	19	20	13	16[b]
Asthma	18	18	13	14	1	19	11
Pediatric asthma	17	16	9	15	6	20	12[c]
Pediatric screened asthma	11	7	6	8	6	8	—

Source: Sinai's Improving Community Health Survey, 2002–2003.

Notes: Data are weighted and age adjusted to the 2000 Standard Population. Comparison data are age-adjusted from Chicago BRFSS 2002 (Shah, Whitman, and Silva, 2006), except when noted.
[a]Pediatric obesity comparison data from U.S. NHANES 2003–2004 obesity; data for children ages 2–5 (13.9%) and 6–11 (18.9%).
[b]Screened depression comparison data is the lifetime prevalence of major depressive disorder from National Comorbidity Study, 2002.
[c]Pediatric asthma data for children age 0-12 years for physician diagnosed asthma. Comparison data from National Health Interview Survey, 1998.

Chicago ($p < 0.001$; Table 3-8). The extraordinary rate of smoking in this Black community is comparable to smoking rates from the early 1970s, before the Surgeon General's report on the dangers of smoking (Satcher, 2000). The Sinai Survey also asked about smoking habits and cessation efforts, which indicated that many current smokers had recently tried to quit or would like to quit in the near future. These data were used to obtain a grant from the Illinois Department of Public Health to address disproportionately high rates of smoking in the North Lawndale community compared to Chicago overall and other community areas surveyed. Chapter 7 presents these Sinai Survey results and details how these local data were used to design a culturally specific, community-based smoking cessation intervention.

In addition, there were several questions related to HIV testing and attitudes toward safe sex and injection drug use. The proportion of residents in North Lawndale ages 18 to 64 years who were ever tested for HIV was significantly higher than every other community ($p < 0.05$). This community also had the highest AIDS incidence rate. Yet, for South Lawndale, a neighboring community area where AIDS incidence rate is moderately high, the HIV testing rate was quite low. Results also showed that proportion recently tested for HIV (in the last 12 months) was three times higher North Lawndale, Roseland, and Humboldt Park than those recently tested nationally (Table 3-8).

In general, residents in the surveyed communities favored needle exchange programs, providing HIV information in high schools and elementary schools and distributing condoms in high schools. Attitudes were less favorable regarding pharmacies selling clean needles and condom distribution in elementary schools. These survey findings have profound implications for community-based HIV prevention strategies and for nationally designed programs often implemented at the local level (using federal funding), which do not support needle exchange programs and condom distribution in schools (Allgood et al., 2009).

Dietary habits and nutrition are important risk factors, but accurately measuring these topics proved challenging. Results based on standardized questions on consumption of daily fruits and vegetables from national surveys were inconsistent, suggesting that respondents may have interpreted questions differently (data not shown, Shah and Whitman, 2005). In some instances, responses to questions that were suggested by the SDC were more informative. For example, as many as 40% of adults in the non-White communities reported that they did not understand nutritional guidelines and that nutritious foods were too costly compared to only 10% to 13% in Norwood Park (data not shown). Although these are not common questions, the community representatives of the SDC thought it would be relevant to shaping new educational programs and advocating for access to cheaper healthy food options in the community.

TABLE 3-8 Selected Findings on Health Risk Factors

Health behaviors	Humboldt Park (%)	North Lawndale (%)	Norwood Park (%)	Roseland (%)	South Lawndale (%)	West Town (%)	Comparison (%)
Current smokers	35	39	18	33	20	32	24[a]
Ever HIV-tested	60	77	50	68	41	65	44[b]
HIV-tested in last 12 months	29	38	11	37	11	22	12[b]
Favor distributing HIV information							
In elementary schools	90	91	85	92	91	94	—
In high schools	95	97	98	97	96	100	—
Favor condom distribution							
In elementary schools	55	53	22	47	66	53	—
In high schools	90	90	74	88	88	93	—
Favor needle exchange programs	61	59	70	63	62	77	—
Favor pharmacies selling clean needles	41	37	58	41	39	56	—

Source: Sinai's Improving Community Health Survey, 2002–2003.

Notes:
Data on current smokers are weighted and age-adjusted to the 2000 Standard Population.
All other data are weighted and only include respondents aged 18–64 because the national comparisons only include this age group.
[a]Comparison data from Chicago BRFSS 2002.
[b]Comparison data from U.S. BRFSS 2002.

Other Survey Topics

The Sinai Survey results presented here are only the tip of the iceberg. Other health topics examined broader social forces influencing health, such as perceived stress, anger management, and perceived racism, as outlined in Table 3-4. The survey also included common questions on quality of life and overall demographics, such as education, occupation, income, acculturation, primary mode of transportation, and so forth. A comprehensive study of many results has been published in two Sinai Survey reports (Whitman, Williams, and Shah, 2004, Shah and Whitman, 2005) and several journal articles (Dell et al., 2005; Shah, Whitman, and Silva, 2006; Margellos-Anast, Shah, and Whitman, 2008; Whitman et al., 2007; Allgood et al., 2009).

Interpreting Results

It must be emphasized that Sinai Survey results do not reflect the health of all communities or of all racial and ethnic groups in Chicago. As described by the sampling design, the results represent the health of the six specific community areas selected. Because Chicago is uniquely "hypersegregated" (Massey and Denton, 1993), results for a given community area are associated with the predominant racial or ethnic group that resides there. For example, the insurance rates are quite low among adults in South Lawndale, who are predominantly Mexican immigrants. These findings may or may not represent the insurance status of other Mexicans living in Chicago.

Although this distinction is important, when designing community interventions, some organizations found that the health of a given community area may be similar to those in neighboring areas, particularly when the neighboring two communities shared similar demographic characteristics (e.g., age, sex, race, and income). For example, the health of adults living in South Lawndale was used to describe the health of a neighboring area, Back of the Yards, and the health of adults living in North Lawndale was assumed to be similar to that of East and West Garfield Park because of their similar demographic profiles. Thus, the Sinai Survey results have often been used by organizations located in neighboring areas of the targeted surveyed communities.

The Sinai Survey is unique because it measures important disparities in health and health care. It quantified the magnitude of several health problems and identified associated risk factors. Specifically, tabulated responses to several questions were substantially higher than national and city level comparison data, revealing health concerns that were never before known. In addition, because of the manner in which the Sinai Survey was developed, its questions are culturally sensitive to social norms, and its outcomes are most relevant and meaningful to shaping effective community interventions.

Impact of the Sinai Survey

Seven years after receiving the original Robert Wood Johnson Foundation award in 2002, no one could have predicted the substantial impact of the Sinai Survey. It has led to notable transformation in the way health data are measured, tabulated, and utilized by community organizations, foundations, public health providers, health-care facilities, and academic institutions in Chicago. The overwhelming evidence pointed to significant disparities in health based on socio-economic status, place of residence, and race and ethnicity. Although such findings may have been suspected, the Sinai Survey made it local and personal. As a result, community and public health leaders often mobilized to take action and formulated key recommendations on how to address many specific inequalities in health. This proactive response generated a "buzz" in the community that captured the attention of community leaders and media, primed funders to direct resources based on need, and led to meaningful new interventions for improved health in some of Chicago's most underserved communities.

This process of translating local data into meaningful local action, in general, followed a specific pattern of release. Once the data were collected, the health findings were analyzed and compared to national and city level estimates. Second, data were published in community reports or peer-review journals. And third, they were shared with the public by hosting a health forum or press conference to report back on results, agree on interpretation of results, and discuss next steps. The following pages describe how these steps were taken to disseminate and share the Sinai Survey results with those who needed to know and respond.

Dissemination

Dissemination activities of the data from the survey were supported by three annual grants awarded by a local foundation, The Chicago Community Trust, between 2004 and 2007. During these years, SUHI staff responded to numerous data inquiries, made many presentations locally and nationally, and published several articles and reports (Sinai Urban Health Institute, 2009).

The first published release of the Sinai Survey data was in January 2004 in a report entitled, *Sinai's Improving Community Health Survey, Report 1* (Whitman, Williams, and Shah, 2004). This report described 10 key findings from the survey and revealed extraordinary disparities in health between the six communities and compared to averages for Chicago or the United States. It was released at a press conference, organized by the Sinai Health System, and was featured in several headlines in local newspapers (Fig. 3-3) and on television and radio. Examples of a few headlines from prominent newspapers are: "Study finds wide health care gap: Minority, poor neighborhoods lag in treatment" from the *Chicago Tribune*, January 8, 2004; "Puerto Rican, black child asthma soaring: Racial, economic chasm in Chicago's health seen in study" from the *Chicago Sun Times*, January 8, 2004; and "Disparidaddes médicas entre comunidades: Un studio muestra que los niños puertorriqueños

METRO

CHICAGO SUN-TIMES
SUNDAY, JANUARY 4, 2004

EDITOR: Don Hayner | TO REACH US: (312) 321-2522 metro@suntimes.com   ☆ PAGE 7A

Wide race gap in epidemic of obese kids

City's black, Hispanic youth far more likely to be overweight: study

BY JIM RITTER
Health Reporter

Chicago's childhood obesity epidemic has a surprisingly large racial divide, a study has found.

In the mostly white Norwood Park neighborhood, 23 percent of kids ages 2 to 12 are overweight, while in predominantly black North Lawndale, 68 percent of kids are overweight. In mostly Hispanic South Lawndale, 58 percent of kids are overweight.

Researchers from Sinai Health System surveyed 1,699 households in six Chicago neighborhoods on obesity, AIDS, asthma and other health issues. They expected to find higher childhood obesity rates among blacks and Hispanics, based on findings from other studies. But they were so astonished at how wide the gap is in Chicago, they initially doubted their findings.

Childhood overweight rates were 64 percent in Roseland (which is mostly black), 62 percent in Humboldt Park (mostly black and Hispanic) and 65 percent in West Town (mostly Hispanic and white).

Compared with kids nationwide, Chicago kids are heavier, and the racial gap is wider. Nationwide, 26 percent of whites, 36 percent of blacks and 39 percent of Hispanics were overweight, in a sample of kids ages 6 to 11 conducted in 1999-2000.

The Chicago findings are based on parents' answers to questions

BY THE NUMBERS

Percentage of children 2-12 who are overweight or obese:

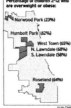

Norwood Park (23%)
Humbolt Park (62%)
West Town (65%)
N. Lawndale (68%)
S. Lawndale (58%)
Roseland (64%)

SUN-TIMES

about children's height and weight, said study director Steve Whitman. To verify their findings, researchers asked a North Lawndale school nurse to take height and weight measurements of 164 students. The findings "were fully consistent with our survey results," researchers wrote in their report, Improving Community Health Survey.

Experts have suggested several reasons low-income and minority kids are more likely to be overweight. High-fat, high-calorie food is cheaper than more-healthful fare, and corner grocery stores in many inner-city neighborhoods have poor selections of fruits and vegetables. Parents often can't afford recreation programs or fear

Itzel Tejeda, 8, has lost 22 pounds since July, thanks to more-healthful eating and exercise, including a karate class. -BRIAN JACKSON/SUN-TIMES

the parks aren't safe to play in. Poor and minority families also tend to be less informed about sound nutrition.

Parents' attitudes also may play a role. The Chicago survey found that at least 85 percent of parents in Humboldt Park, North Lawndale and Roseland believed their children are the right weight or underweight.

"We have to find a way to educate caretakers about the optimal weight for their children and their health," researchers wrote. "Otherwise, most efforts to improve the

situation will not be effective."

A determined parent can make a difference. Last July, Griselda Tejeda of Berwyn decided her 8-year-old daughter, Itzel, needed to lose weight. So Tejeda limited Itzel's portions, stopped frying food and switched to low-cal foods. She also enrolled Itzel in a karate class and is helping her learn how to ride a bike.

Itzel's weight has dropped from 102 pounds to 80. She can run around now without getting tired, and "her self esteem is great," her mom said.

Gary Diocese says 7 priests accused of abuse since '57

BY CAROLE CARLSON

Since 1957, 13 people have alleged they were sexually abused as children by seven priests serving the Diocese of Gary, Ind., Bishop Dale J. Melczek has announced.

Six of the complaints were made against three diocesan priests. Five complaints were made against two priests who served the diocese but worked for religious orders.

The diocesan response team dismissed two allegations against two priests as not credible.

The findings, released Friday, were part of two reports required of dioceses across the country in response to the priest sex abuse scandal that has rocked the Roman Catholic Church. Details of the nationwide study will be released Feb. 27.

The three diocesan priests accused have died. Allegations against two were found credible. The third wasn't investigated.

Melczek removed one of the priests from the ministry in the early 1990s, when an allegation was proved. That priest was retired at the time of the allegation and died soon after, Melczek said.

"He was not allowed to say mass publicly or give the sacraments. There was a preponderance of evidence," he said.

Allegations against the third priest weren't fully investigated because the accuser did not wish to pursue it further.

Since the accusations were made, the four-county diocese of 186,000 Catholics has spent about $60,000 for counseling services for victims, Melczek said.

Post-Tribune, with AP contributing

1 killed, 9 ejected in van accident

The driver of a van with 13 passengers from the Chicago area died Saturday after he fell asleep at the wheel and crashed on Interstate 57 in Downstate Cumberland County, Illinois State Police said.

Nine of the 13 passengers were ejected from the 1999 green Ford 350, as it overturned. It was bound for a Downstate prison.

William Scott, 49, of Chicago, was found dead at the scene after the 10:27 a.m. crash south of Mattoon. All 13 passengers were being treated at local hospitals. Their names and conditions were not being released.

The van was traveling south on I-57 when it went off the road and overturned, police said.

Ford Heights cops' woes continue as suspect escapes

BY KATE N. GROSSMAN
Staff Reporter

It's been a rough week for the Ford Heights Police Department.

First, on Dec. 26, an officer for the south suburb was charged in an armed robbery. And then Friday, a domestic battery suspect escaped from the police station garage. He remained on the loose Saturday.

An officer was leading Rodney Eugene Lewis, 28, into the station

when Lewis fled around 8 p.m. Friday, said Police Chief Cecil Cook. He would not say whether Lewis was in handcuffs or how he managed to get out of the garage.

The officer ran after Lewis, and other officers joined in the search. None could find him, said Sgt. Earl Bridges.

Lewis, of the 600 block of Carroll Parkway in Glenwood, had not been charged when he fled, Cook said. He is now wanted for domestic battery

and escape, Bridges said.

Lewis' record includes weapons and drug offenses, Bridges said.

Cook, who has been on the job six months, said Friday's was not the first escape from the garage, though it was the first under his watch.

The escape came after Michael Miller, 30, a Ford Heights police officer, was charged with six counts of armed robbery for being part of a crew that allegedly took $1,700 from victims in Chicago's

West Garfield Park neighborhood.

Prosecutors allege Miller and three others were working security Christmas night at a nightclub that was forced to close early. They were not paid, so they decided to attempt a robbery, the Cook County state's attorney's office said.

Miller was fired, and Cook said authorities are investigating whether he was involved in any other crimes.

Figure 3-3   One Example of Media Coverage from the Initial Release of Sinai's Improving Community Health Survey Results, *Chicago Sun-Times*, Jan 4, 2004.

presentan las tasas más altas de asma en toda el área de Chicago" from hola-Hoy.com, viernes 9 de enero de 2004. Although the Sinai Survey report was the culmination of the original Robert Wood Johnson Foundation award, it was just the beginning of how the Sinai Survey changed the way resources for health interventions are allocated in the city of Chicago.

Following the release of initial findings, there were many requests for additional data analyses, and SUHI became a clearing house for community-level survey data in Chicago. Inquiries came from community organizations, health-care providers, researchers, and even the Chicago Department of Public Health in pursuit of grants or in planning new health initiatives. In some instances, the entire dataset was shared. Professors from the University of Illinois at the Chicago School of Public Health used the dataset to teach community health research, and doctoral students requested use of the dataset for their dissertations. Extensive analyses of the data ensued on such diverse issues as barriers to accessing healthy food or use of needle exchange programs in communities. Along with these analyses, students and researchers offered recommendations for improved programs to the health department, policymakers, and foundations. In other instances, academic researchers used the survey data to work collaboratively with communities in developing culturally appropriate health initiatives facing vulnerable communities. Box 3-1 portrays an example of how one researcher from the University of

---

BOX 3-1 Theory Into Practice: Research Helps Latino Community Help Itself

The partnership between the School of Public Health and Chicago's Humboldt Park community illustrates what is possible when academic theory meets real life. The result is an innovative research approach that helps create culturally sensitive, mutually beneficial programs.

In 2004, a Sinai Health Systems report brought to light health disparities in Chicago and the need for preventive community-based health interventions. Armed with these findings and grants from the Centers for Disease Control and Prevention, UIC's School of Public Health partnered with Humboldt Park community representatives to explore how they deploy resources to solve problems like psychological distress, poor educational and economic resources, prevalence of asthma and diabetes, HIV/AIDS and housing shortages.

Researcher Michele Kelley is the driving force behind the collaborative relationship between UIC and the Humboldt Park community, located

(continued)

BOX 3-1 (*continued*)

on Chicago's West Side. "Sinai's report was extremely valuable to us," said Kelley. "We are trying to build on the momentum of that report and fill in some of the gaps, especially on adolescent health."

The neighborhood is interested in improving its ability to heal itself. By engaging with the community, Kelley helps its members identify, think through and answer their own health questions.

"We can't assume we will go into a community and create change," said Kelley. "The community has locally relevant insight and knowledge, and it's my job to try to understand it so that I don't inadvertently get in the way of the learning process we're sharing with each other. Our collaboration advances public health science, and we are learning how to be more effective in reducing and eliminating ethnic disparities in health."

Kelley currently is working on plans for the community's first-ever survey on adolescent health. The survey will identify critical health issues for youth as well as factors that may hold them back from becoming healthy adults.

Working with teens from Café Teatro Batey Urbano, a youth-driven alternative cultural arts and community action organization, Kelley will show them how to conduct their own research and analyze results. Youth in the community have first-hand knowledge about their peers and can provide advice on the survey while helping Kelley determine strategies to engage the interest of families to increase the response rate.

Ultimately the group will convene a youth summit to discuss their findings and develop a health action plan. Kelley foresees the group tapping into Batey Urbano's new radio station as a way to disseminate health information to local teens. By working with the community to conduct their own research, she is one step closer to accomplishing her goal.

José López, a leader in the community and executive director of the Puerto Rican Cultural Center, has watched the partnership with the School of Public Health encourage community growth.

"The university does not come into the community and impose precepts and concepts but works with us to find ways to deal with health issues," said López. "It not only has created consciousness, but has brought the concept of participatory research to us. It's a process of continuous dialogue."

Source: Reprinted from University of Illinois at Chicago School of Public Health Newsroom. Theory into practice: Research helps Latino community help itself. Online. Available: http://www.uic.edu/sph/news/news_122.html. Accessed: December 17, 2009.

Illinois did exactly this. She partnered with community groups in Humboldt Park and began to make sustainable change in social norms toward improved health.

There were also requests for information on the Sinai Survey data collection procedures. For example, the survey instrument and methodology report were shared with several organizations beyond Chicago. These included the Winnebago County Department of Public Health in Illinois, the Los Angeles County Department of Public Health, the Philadelphia Health Management Corporation, and the Morehouse School of Medicine, to name a few. The Sinai Survey became a model for gathering community level data and examining health disparities locally. Between 2004 and 2007, there were over 200 data inquires, including 30 signed data-sharing agreements and 12 doctoral students who completed their dissertations with Sinai Survey data. A detailed list of these are available in donor reports online (Shah and Whitman, 2005; Shah and Whitman, 2006; Sinai Urban Health Institute, 2009), and this process of sharing the Sinai Survey continues today.

Furthermore, nearly 200 presentations were made between 2002 and 2008 at professional conferences, academic centers, community organizations, foundations, and government agencies locally and nationally. Presentations were made at the National HIV Prevention Conference, Community-Campus Partnerships, the American Public Health Association, the International Society for Urban Health, and so forth. Invitations to present at grand rounds and luncheon discussions were common, and it was rare that a meeting on health disparities in Chicago did not mention the Sinai Survey results. In fact, the findings were featured at and the impetus for a city-wide summit on health disparities in December 2004, sponsored by the Institute of Medicine of the National Academy of Sciences, the Institute of Medicine of Chicago and others. Data findings were shared at numerous research institutions and prestigious academic health centers outside of Chicago, including the Cleveland Clinic in April 2004, because of the implications to address disparities in other urban settings. Additionally, in September 2007, the Sinai Survey served as a model for the Delaware State Department of Health in guiding their efforts to conduct community health surveys and identify the health needs of some of their most vulnerable populations.

There are also several reports and publications describing the Sinai Survey data. To date, there are two Sinai Survey Reports, the first (as mentioned earlier) was released in January 2004 (Whitman, Williams, and Shah, 2004), and the second, which built upon the first, highlighted 10 new findings and was released in September 2005 (Shah and Whitman, 2005). It included descriptions of topics such as arthritis, hypertension, cancer screening, and physical activity. There are also six journal publications (Dell et al., 2005; Shah, Whitman, and Silva, 2006; Whitman, Silva, and Shah, 2006;

Whitman et al., 2007; Margellos-Anast, Shah, and Whitman, 2008; Allgood et al., 2009). All published materials are currently available online (Sinai Urban Health Institute, 2009).

Reactions

Reactions to the Sinai Survey dissemination activities were widespread and far-reaching. At the community level, several organizations responded by coming together and prioritizing health concerns. For example, the Puerto Rican Cultural Center in Humboldt Park immediately convened a Health Summit in March 2005 and invited community residents, social services providers, and policymakers to learn about the data. They organized as part of the Greater Humboldt Park Community of Wellness and focused on issues of most relevance to their community, ranging from depression to diabetes. They decided what was most pressing based on the data and this empowered them to drive some of the health initiatives described in Section 3.

The Healthy Schools Campaign, a not-for-profit organization that advocates for a healthy school environment, also benefited from the Sinai Survey data. They used pediatric asthma and obesity findings to support their successful application for a $1 million grant from the National Institutes of Health. In addition, many parents of school children did not believe that asthma and obesity were issues facing their children. With the Sinai Survey data, the Healthy Schools Campaign was able to demonstrate the severity of asthma and obesity by using community-based participatory practices and thus engaged many parents in seeking and implementing effective solutions. This work was instrumental to examining the school meal program and physical education classes through a social justice lens. As a result of their initial success in two Latino Schools, they created the Parents United for Healthy Schools/Padres Unidos para Escuelas Saludables Coalition and have expanded to more than 40 schools in other racial and ethnic minority communities of Chicago. Other community groups, such as Centro Sin Fronteras, the Resurrection Project, and the Little Village Development Corporation (now known as En Lace), to name a few, likewise sought data to obtain funds for new initiatives in the communities they served.

Reactions by the donor community were also significant. The Sinai Survey results related to arthritis, activity limitations, and obesity were shared with the Arthritis Foundation of Chicago. Because the prevalence of arthritis in North Lawndale was higher than in other communities, the Foundation adopted this community and brought one of its free physical activity programs for adults with arthritis to this neighborhood. In addition, when invited to share findings about pediatric obesity at a Consortium to Lower Obesity in Chicago Children (CLOCC) quarterly meeting, the executive director of the Otho A. Sprague Foundation was so appalled by the disproportionate burden of obesity in some communities that he immediately sought local community groups eager to address obesity, leading to the Humboldt Park obesity initiative (described in Chapter 8 of this book). Finally, as noted previously, local foundations reported that many of the proposals they received referenced results from the Sinai Survey to demonstrate community health needs, target interventions, and evaluate progress.

Sinai Survey results received considerable media attention as well. Numerous stories and articles appeared on local news stations and in local newspapers following the release of the initial report, *Sinai's Improving Community Health Survey Report 1* (Whitman, Williams, and Shah, 2004) in January 2004 (Fig. 3-3). In fact, substantial media attention materialized after almost every published article or community event. These stories helped galvanize communities and researchers to identify solutions, respond collectively, and demand that resources be distributed to these communities in need. The media helped make the data even more visible and brought it to the attention of policymakers, community leaders, and others with influence to take action.

There were also examples of how the Sinai Survey data were used to improve public health policy. For example, advocates used the data to urge the state legislature to establish mechanisms for BMI surveillance among children in public schools and to develop the Illinois Childhood Obesity Prevention Consensus Agenda, which resulted in the passage of four public acts (CLOCC, 2009). Sinai Survey data were also used by CLOCC and the Chicago Department of Public Health to form the City of Chicago's Inter-Departmental Task Force on Childhood Obesity, which is comprised of eight city departments focusing on policy and program development to prevent childhood obesity (Becker, Longjohn, and Christoffel, 2008). In addition, following release of the smoking data publication, a press conference was held on "World No Tobacco Day" in 2005 by the Chicago Chapter of the American Lung Association. This event helped activists who were working to make public spaces smoke-free in the city. Smoke-free legislation passed in Chicago in 2007 and a year later in the State of Illinois.

Overall, the Sinai Survey results brought to light that in Chicago, where one lives, how much money one has, and the color of one's skin determines how healthy one is. Dissemination of such disparities in health first led to outrage, as highlighted by the media. Ultimately, this information motivated community stakeholders, researchers, and political leaders to organize and respond with targeted, community-driven solutions. The most effective community responses resulted when evidence of disparities from the Sinai Survey were linked to solutions or recommendations for improved health. The results then resonated with communities, engaged stakeholders (such as politicians and funders), and enabled them all to design new interventions and implement change to combat disparities as detailed in later chapters.

Lessons Learned

The successes and challenges faced in translating data into meaningful programs have provided many lessons to those affiliated with the survey. The experience of preparing a community to respond to findings from the Sinai Survey varied depending on its readiness. New initiatives emerged in some communities because of their ability to engage with political leaders and to be organized and advocate collectively with one voice. For example, in Humboldt Park, the Community of Wellness, the Puerto Rican Cultural Center and other stakeholders formed a persuasive example of such an organization and were thus critical to driving change in their communities (see Chapter 12).

Several presentations were made in all of the surveyed communities. Yet, for some, few new interventions (to our knowledge) were developed or resources obtained. The exact reasons for this are unclear but may result from a lack of key local partners or the infrastructure for community groups to organize with a focus on a specific health priority. Although individual leaders, such as community organization executive directors and/or hospital administrators, expressed interest in the Sinai Survey findings, there was a lack of any collective reaction to the dissemination activities. In evaluating this effort, it appeared that competing priorities may have limited substantial health initiatives in these communities.

Although data are essential, without organizing the community and the political will to support it, the ability to make change is challenging. For example, because of the strong community organizations and the support of local politicians, greater funding and resources came to Humboldt Park. Successful interventions ranged from a newly formed academic–community collaborative with federal funding to support a major diabetes initiative to an individual commitment to leading a walking club and aerobic sessions at the local park fieldhouse (see Chapter 10). These actions, big or small, were stimulated by Sinai Survey results and vivified by the community's pre-existing infrastructure and organization.

Conclusions

The Sinai Survey has begun to achieve its goal of utilizing data as a catalyst for change by gathering evidence to redirect resources to communities most in need. The survey and its development has been an important example of how meaningful data can be effectively gathered with

community involvement and support. Findings revealed substantial variations in health outcomes that were never before known. It also stimulated
many groups to design new interventions and bring more than $15 million
in resources to underserved communities in Chicago. Dissemination of
and reaction to the Sinai Survey results were extraordinary and critical
to translating data into action. The net effect has been improved health
of communities at multiple levels, as illustrated in Section 3 of this book.
It is hoped that the Sinai Survey and this story will continue to serve as
a national inspiration for other community hospitals, community groups,
and public health practitioners for driving change toward greater health
equity in the future.

Acknowledgments

There are many individuals and community organizations that ought to be
acknowledged for the development of the Sinai Survey and its success. To
begin, we thank The Robert Wood Johnson Foundation and The Chicago
Community Trust for their shared vision and generous financial support
of this work. The authors acknowledge all those who designed the survey, the communities who welcomed us (and even those who criticized
us), and the valiant people who have struggled for many years to improve
their health, thus inspiring us to want to help them do that. Specifically,
we are indebted to the community representatives of the Survey Design
Committee and their affiliated community organizations (as listed in Table
3-3) for the many hours they spent with us and their invaluable input. In
addition, we recognize the in-kind support from members of the Sinai
Health System who served on the Survey Design Committee: Linda Miller,
Ed Rafalski, Maurice Schwartz, Jesse Green, and Xochitl Salvador. We
especially thank Cynthia Williams, co-principal investigator on *Sinai's
Improving Community Health Survey* project, without whom the Survey
Design Committee could not have been established and maintained.
Authors are grateful to the Survey Research Laboratory at the University
of Illinois. In particular, we thank Timothy Johnson and Ingrid Graf, along
with the dedication and persistence with which the interviewers and field
staff implemented the survey. Authors also thank the committed staff of
the Sinai Urban Health Institute whose collaborative spirit made this project a success: Jade L. Dell, Jocelyn Hirschman, Helen Margellos-Anast,
and Abigail Silva. Finally, and most importantly, authors acknowledge all
of the community respondents, who completed the survey and made the
Sinai Survey possible.

References

Allgood, Kristi, Abigail Silva, Ami M. Shah, and Steve Whitman. 2009. HIV testing practices and attitudes on prevention efforts in six Community Areas of Chicago. *Journal of Community Health* 34:514–522.

Becker, Adam, Matthew Longjohn, and Kathy Christoffel. 2008. Taking on childhood obesity in a big city: Consortium to Lower Obesity in Chicago Children (CLOCC). *Progress in Pediatric Cardiology* 25(2):199–206.

CLOCC (Consortium to Lower Obesity in Chicago Children). 2009. *Illinois Childhood Obesity Prevention Consensus Agenda*. Online. Available: http://www.clocc.net/coc/policy/consensus.html. Accessed December 7, 2009.

Benbow, Nanette, Yu Wang, and Steve Whitman. 1998. The big cities health inventory, 1997. *Journal of Community Health* 23(6):471–489.

Chicago Fact Book Consortium. 1995. *Local Community Fact Book: Chicago Metropolitan Area, 1990*. Chicago, IL: Academy Chicago Publishers.

Dell, Jade L., Steve Whitman, Ami M. Shah, Abigail Silva, and David Ansell. 2005. Smoking in 6 diverse Chicago communities—a population study. *American Journal of Public Health* 95(6):1036–1042.

Drevdahl, Denise J. 1995. Coming to voice: The power of emancipatory community interventions. *Advanced Nursing Science* 18:13–24.

Graf, Ingrid and Karen Foote-Retzer. 2003. *Improving Community Health, Final Methodological Report* (SRL Project #912). Survey Research Laboratory, College of Urban Planning and Public Affairs, University of Illinois at Chicago: June.

Groves, Robert M. and Mick P. Couper. 1989. *Nonresponse in household interview surveys*. New York: John Wiley & Sons.

Heaney, Thomas W. 1993. If you can't beat'em, join'em: The professionalization of participatory research. In: *Voices of change: Participatory research in the United States and Canada*, ed. Peter Park, Mary Brydon-Miller, Budd Hall, and Ted Jackson. Westport, CT: Bergin and Garvey, pp. 41–46.

Johnson, Timothy P. and Linda Owens. 2004. Survey response rate reporting in the professional literature. In: American Statistical Association. 2003 Proceedings of the Section on Survey Research Methods. Alexandria, VA: American Statistical Association, pp. 127–133.

Margellos, Helen, Abigail Silva, and Steve Whitman. 2004. Comparison of health status indicators in Chicago: Are Black-White disparities worsening? *American Journal of Public Health* 94(1):116–121.

Margellos-Anast, Helen, Ami M. Shah, and Steve Whitman. 2008. Prevalence of obesity among children in six Chicago communities: Findings from a health survey. *Public Health Reports* 123:117–125.

Massey, Douglas S. and Nancy A. Denton. 1993. *American Apartheid: Segregation and the Making of the Underclass*. Cambridge, MA: Harvard University Press.

McGinnis, J. McGinnis and William H. Foege. 1993. Actual causes of death in the United States. *Journal of American Medical Association* 270:2207–2212.

Minkler, Meredith and Nina Wallerstein, eds. 2003. *Community-based Participatory Research for Health*. San Francisco: Jossey Bass.

Northridge, M. E., A. Morabia, M. L. Ganz, M. T. Bassett, D. Gemson, H. Andrews, et al. 1998. Contribution of smoking to excess mortality in Harlem. *American Journal of Epidemiology* 147:250–258.

SAS Institute Inc. 2002-2003. SAS statistical software, version 9.1.3 for Windows@. Cary, NC: SAS Institute.

Satcher, David. 2000. *Reducing tobacco use: A report of the Surgeon General.* U.S. Dept. Health and Human Services. Online. Available: http://www.cdc.gov/tobacco/data_statistics/sgr/2000/. Accessed April 7, 2010.

Silva Abigail, Steve Whitman, Helen Margellos, and David Ansell. 2001. Evaluating Chicago's success in reaching the Healthy People 2000 goal of reducing health disparities. *Public Health Reports* 116(5):484–494.

Shah, Ami M., Steve Whitman, and Abigail Silva. 2006. Variations in the health conditions of 6 Chicago Community Areas: A case for local-level data. *American Journal of Public Health* 96(8):1485–1491.

Shah, Ami M. and Steve Whitman. 2005. *Progress report to the Chicago Community Trust.* Grant ID#C2003-00844, May 2005. Chicago, IL: Sinai Health System.

Shah, Ami M. and Steve Whitman. 2006. *Progress report to the Chicago Community Trust.* Grant ID#C2005-01173, October 2006. Chicago, IL: Sinai Health System.

Silva, Abigail, Steve Whitman, Helen Margellos, and David Ansell. 2001. Evaluating Chicago's success in reaching the Healthy People 2000 goal of reducing health disparities. *Public Health Reports* 116(5):484–494.

Sinai Urban Health Institute. 2009. *Research/evaluation project: Sinai's Improving Community Health Survey.* Online. Available: http://www.suhichicago.org/research-evaluation-detail,suhi_project;0838b6603278f8ebf520f4cd8a72edfb.html. Accessed December 16, 2009.

Sudman, Seymour. 1976. *Applied Sampling.* New York, NY: Academic Press.

Standard Definitions: Final dispositions of case codes and outcome rates for surveys. 2004. Ann Arbor, MI: American Association for Public Opinion Research.

Stata Corporation. 2003. STATA statistical software, version 8.0 for Windows@. College Station, TX: Stata Corp.

Trodhal, Verling C. and Roy E. Carter. 1964. Random selection of respondents within households in phone surveys. *Journal of Marketing Research* 1:71–76.

Wennberg, John and Alan Gittelsohn. 1973. Small area variations in health care delivery: A population-based health information system can guide planning and regulatory decision making. *Science* 14; 182(4117):1102–1108.

Whitman, Steve, Cynthia Williams, and Ami M. Shah. 2004. *Sinai Health System's community health survey: Report 1.* Chicago, IL: Sinai Health System.

Whitman Steve, Ami M. Shah, Abigail Silva, and David Ansell. 2007. Mammography screening in six diverse communities in Chicago-A population study. *Cancer Detection and Prevention* 31:166–172.

Whitman Steve, Abigail Silva, and Ami M. Shah. 2006. Disproportionate impact of diabetes in a Puerto Rican community of Chicago. *Journal of Community Health* 31(6):521–531.

4

THE JEWISH COMMUNITY HEALTH SURVEY OF CHICAGO: METHODOLOGY AND KEY FINDINGS

Maureen R. Benjamins

Introduction

Motivated by the findings of the *Sinai Improving Community Health Survey* described in the Chapter 3 (Shah and Whitman, 2010), Jewish leaders within Chicago envisioned a similar survey for their own community. Just as that survey revealed substantial differences among groups, these leaders recognized that certain health issues may also be more (or less) prevalent within the Jewish community. They understood that collecting this type of detailed health information could lead to more successful interventions and policy changes and that the findings would allow the agencies serving this population to more accurately tailor their services. Thus inspired, they began to mobilize an effort to collect similar data in two of the most densely populated Jewish neighborhoods in the city. This is how Chicago became one of the first (if not the first) cities to implement a population-based health survey specifically for a Jewish community.

Lack of Existing Health Data for Jewish Individuals

Valuable information about the Jewish population in America comes from the National Jewish Population Survey (NJPS), from regional Jewish data surveys such as the Metropolitan Chicago Jewish Population Study (MCJPS), and from a variety of other community-level data sets. However, these studies are not designed to measure components of individual health and well-being, such as physical and mental health status and access to health care. In addition, obtaining information about the Jewish population from more general health data sources is also difficult because most do not include information on religious affiliation. Moreover, Jewish populations are generally widely dispersed and are often minorities even in the most concentrated of communities. Thus, small sample sizes render national, state, and even city health surveys insufficient for deriving accurate estimates for these communities (Fielding and Frieden, 2004).

Importance of Collecting Health Data for Jewish Individuals

Collecting health data is important for ethnic minority groups such as Jews because they may have significantly different health profiles than other individuals. This is because both the cultural norms shared by those with a Jewish background and the religious beliefs held by many Jews may influence health-related behaviors and outcomes (Jacobs and Giarelli, 2001). Orthodox Jews, in particular, live according to a distinct set of rules that often impact health-related behaviors, such as dietary choices. In addition, Jewish children often attend private day schools, which differ from public schools in the foods they offer, the health-related information provided in their curricula, and the presence of physical education and extracurricular activities. Therefore, health risk factors and outcomes for both adults and children could be expected to differ from the general population. This is supported by diverse findings from previous research, such as studies that show that Jews have higher rates of depression (Kennedy et al., 1996; Levav et al., 1997) and breast cancer (Egan et al., 1996) but lower rates of other health problems, such as alcoholism (Levav et al., 1997) and cervical and penile cancer (for review, *see* Koenig, McCullough, and Larson, 2001).

Partnerships and Funding

The leadership of this initiative came from the Jewish Federation of Metropolitan Chicago. The Jewish Federation is the largest not-for-profit social welfare institution in Illinois and the hub of Chicago's Jewish community. In addition to being the first to initiate an adapted use of the Sinai survey, the Jewish Federation accomplished the essential feat of getting the data collection effort funded. Specifically, the survey was enabled by generous grants provided through two local sources, the Polk Bros. Foundation and the Jewish Federation's Fund for Innovation in Health (supported by the Michael Reese

Health Trust). Additional funding for the second phase of the project (data analysis) came from the Fund for Innovation in Health, the Irvin and Ruth Swartzberg Foundation, and the Fel-Pro Mecklenberger Supporting Fund.

Once funding was secured, an additional partner was added to the group. As with the *Sinai Improving Community Health Survey* (described in Chapter 3; Shah and Whitman, 2010), the logistics of data collection were handled by the University of Illinois at Chicago's Survey Research Laboratory. Specifically, this organization was responsible for the survey design, sampling, and interviews. Work done by the Sinai Urban Health Institute during the data collection phase was performed as "in-kind" contributions. More details about each step of the data collection process are provided below.

Methodology

Questionnaire Development

The development of the survey questionnaire began with a series of meetings held with the stakeholders, community leaders, and agency professionals. This community group was first introduced to the *Sinai Improving Community Health Survey* (Sinai Survey) instrument and then charged with determining if any questions were irrelevant and which (if any) additional topics should be covered. In the end, approximately 50 additional questions were included to focus on health and religious issues important to the Jewish population. For example, topics such as genetic disorders, disability, and participation in Jewish religious activities were covered. To make room, questions deemed less relevant to the Jewish population or less of a priority were removed from the original survey. Removed questions included those on Hispanic ethnicity, STD testing, needle exchange programs, presence of a working telephone in the home, and selected discrimination measures, for example. As with the original Sinai Survey, the questions used were taken verbatim from national and state surveys whenever possible so that comparison data would be available. In total, the Jewish survey included 475 adult and 100 child questions.

Sampling

The group of community leaders and agency professionals was also in charge of selecting the target area to be surveyed. They chose a community made up of two contiguous neighborhoods: West Rogers Park and Peterson Park. This community on the north side of Chicago was selected because of the high concentration of Jewish individuals residing there and a presumed need for additional services and resources.

A three-stage sampling design was employed to get a representative sample from the designated community. In the first stage, 45 census blocks were randomly selected from the two geographic areas. After the blocks were selected, interviewers recorded each housing unit on each block. This resulted in 1,719 households. In the second stage, all of the households from each of the census blocks were included. The blocks were assembled into seven groups, to be selected at random over time as needed to reach the target sample size. In the third stage, one eligible respondent was selected at random from each household.

The inclusion criteria for adults specified that they must identify themselves as Jewish, be at least 18 years of age, and live in the designated study area. Once the adult interview ended, respondents were asked if there were any children 12 years of age or younger in the household. If so, one of the children was randomly selected and the adult with the most knowledge about that child's health was interviewed. Note that this may not be the same as the original adult respondent.

Survey Administration

The data for this study were collected between August 2003 and January 2004 by researchers from UIC's Survey Research Laboratory. Interviews were done face-to-face using computer-assisted technology. In all, 201 Jewish adults and 57 caregivers of Jewish children were interviewed in their homes. The adult interviews took 1 hour, on average, and the child interview generally took 15 minutes. As a token of appreciation, respondents were given $20 for an adult interview and $10 for a child interview.

Response Rates

Interviews were attempted at 1,124 households. Of these, 286 were nonresidential, unable to be contacted, or refused to participate. An additional 529 were ineligible. Three measures summarizing the rates of responses and refusals are described here. The response rate measures the proportion of eligible respondents who completed an interview. To calculate this, the number of eligible people who completed the interview is divided by the sum of all of those in the numerator, plus refusals, noncontact of eligibles, and a proportion of households whose eligibility status is unknown (AAPOR, 2000). The response rate for this survey using this conservative calculation was 50.9%.

Another helpful measure is the refusal rate. This measures the proportion of eligible respondents who either refused to complete the interview or who broke off the interview. The refusal rate for the current survey was 16.6%. Finally, the cooperation rate is used to determine how many of the eligible individuals completed an interview. Here, 75.2% cooperated. This cooperation rate is much higher than other national surveys. For example, the response rate for the 2000 National Jewish Population Survey was 28% and the cooperation rate was 40% (United Jewish Communities Report, 2004).

The high cooperation rate for this survey may at least partially result from the efforts undertaken to make the community aware of the importance of the survey. For example, before respondents were approached by the interviewers, they first received a letter explaining the survey and the importance of this type of data for the community. These letters, which were printed on letterhead from the Jewish Community Council of West Rogers Park, were signed by leaders of the community, including the chief rabbinical judge of the Chicago Rabbinical Council (Fig. 4-1). In addition, the interviewers underwent rigorous training, both in general interviewing skills, as well as in relevant aspects of the Jewish culture. Care was taken to avoid conflicts, such as asking for interviews on the Sabbath or during Rosh Hashanah.

Weighting

The adult frequencies are weighted to make the sampled population resemble the demographic characteristics of the population surveyed. In other words, the weight accounts for various differences between the sample and the population, as well as differences in the selection probabilities. The weight is equal to the inverse of the probability of selection. The child data is not weighted because the sample was too small.

Results

The demographic and social make-up of this Jewish community is discussed first. Whenever possible, results will be compared to other populations. Specifically, comparable data from the National Jewish Population Survey (NJPS), the Chicago Behavior Risk Factor Surveillance System (BRFSS), the U.S. Census, and other national surveys are provided (when available). Following this, a brief overview of the primary health-related findings from this survey are provided, including health-care access and utilization, disease prevalence, mental health status, and health behaviors. Again, comparison data is given when available. Several specific areas of concern are highlighted (Table 4-1). In addition, information about three vulnerable populations within this community is given. All findings in this section reflect the adult sample unless otherwise noted.

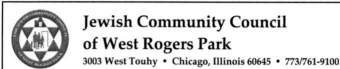

**Jewish Community Council
of West Rogers Park**

3003 West Touhy • Chicago, Illinois 60645 • 773/761-9100

Summer/Fall, 2003

Dear Friend,

<u>**We are asking for your help.**</u> The Jewish Federation of Metropolitan Chicago and Sinai Urban Health Institute are working with the Survey Research Laboratory of the University of Illinois at Chicago to conduct a health survey of Jewish households in West Rogers Park and Peterson Park for the Jewish community.

In this survey, eligible community members ages 18 and older will have the chance to share their experiences on health-related topics such as access to healthcare, diet, exercise, and many other issues. The results of the survey will be used to identify gaps in health and human services, and to advocate for improved health programs and greater resources for your community.

An interviewer from the Survey Research Laboratory will soon make a visit to your home and ask for your participation. All of the interviewers will go through a training program to ensure that they are sensitive to the religious and modesty concerns of the community. Your participation in this health survey is completely voluntary. We have taken every step possible to ensure that the information that you provide is <u>**confidential.**</u> Your responses will be analyzed with others from your community; no individual will be identified in reports or data files.

There are two parts to the survey: the first part asks about the health of an *adult* in the household and takes about one hour to complete, and the second part, which takes 15 minutes, asks about the health of a *child* in the household. Some questions may appear intrusive, but they are necessary to ensure that the Jewish community receives all of the supportive services that it needs.

Because your contribution and time are important, if you are eligible and selected to participate you will be paid $20 for completing the adult portion of the survey; if an eligible household contains a child aged 12 or younger, you would receive an additional $10 for completing that questionnaire.

If you want additional information about the survey, we encourage you to ask the interviewer questions when he or she visits your household. Also, feel free to call Ingrid Graf, the project coordinator at UIC at (312) 431-0492. Thank you in advance for your participation in this endeavor.

Sincerely,

Alice Segal	Rabbi Gedalia Schwartz	Rabbi Shmuel Fuerst
Jewish Community Council	Chicago Rabbinical Council	Dayan, Agudath Israel
of West Rogers Park		

Senator Ira Silverstein Alderman Bernard Stone

Figure 4-1 Letter From Local Politicians and Religious Leaders to Encourage Participation in the Jewish Community Health Survey

Sample Characteristics

Demographic Characteristics

The sociodemographic characteristics of the community are shown in Table 4-2 and are briefly summarized here. The gender distribution shows that the population represented by the current survey included slightly more females than males (52% vs. 48%). These numbers are similar to U.S. Census estimates, whereas in the national Jewish population there were even more

TABLE 4-1   Selected Health Topic Results for the *Jewish Community Health Survey*

Topic 1: Health Status. The majority of adults rated their own health as good or better, although approximately half had at least one of the most common chronic conditions. The most prevalent chronic condition was high blood pressure, which was reported by more than one-fourth of adults.

Topic 2: Health Behaviors. Levels of physical activity were slightly higher than city and national estimates but still below recommended amounts. Relative to other groups, levels of smoking, drinking, and marijuana use were low.

Topic 3: Health-Care Access and Utilization. Most adults had health insurance and a usual place to go for health care; they also received routine check-ups and recommended preventive services. However, almost one-fourth of the sample reported being unable to obtain certain needed medical services.

Topic 4: Overweight and Obese Adults. Over half of Jewish adults were overweight, including 25% who were obese.

Topic 5: Overweight and Obese Children. Like adults, the majority of children 2 to 12 years old were overweight (54%). This includes 26% of all children who qualified as obese.

Topic 6: Depression. More than one-fifth of individuals reported having been diagnosed with depression at some point in their life. In addition, 17% were screened as currently depressed using the CES-D scale of depressive symptoms.

Topic 7: Disability. Almost one-fourth of the adults in this community lived with someone with some type of a disability. Furthermore, nearly half of the disabled individuals reported special care needs such as therapists or mobility devices.

Topic 8: Experiences with Violence. One-quarter of adults had witnessed domestic violence and nearly one-third reported that a member of their household had been a victim of physical, verbal, or sexual violence.

Topic 9: Genetic Testing. Within these Jewish neighborhoods, 58% of adults had never been screened for genetic disorders. Of these, many reported not being aware of the tests or did not consider them necessary.

females. Of the individuals in this sample, 20% were born outside of the United States. The majority of these were born in the former Soviet Union or Israel. This percent of immigrants is almost double the overall U.S. estimate. The age distributions (not displayed) show that this Jewish community tends to be older than the general U.S. adult population. It is important to note that approximately 20% of Jewish adults living here were older than 65 years of age. This is greater than the overall national estimates (17%) but slightly lower than national Jewish estimates (24%). The mean age of the adult population in this Jewish community was 49.3 years.

Socio-Economic Status

Individuals in this community are highly educated. Notably, two-thirds had a college degree or higher, and nearly one-third had a graduate degree (Table 4-2). This exceeds the levels of education seen in the national NJPS

TABLE 4-2   Comparison of Selected Demographic and Socioeconomic Characteristics

	WRP (%)	MCJPS (%)	NJPS (%)	Chicago[a] (%)	United States[a] (%)
Gender					
Female	52	52	56	51	51
Male	48	48	44	49	49
Nativity					
U.S.-born	80	87	85	78	89
Foreign-born	20	13	15	22	11
Marital status					
Married	73	57	57	40	54
Divorced/ separated	7	9	10	12	12
Widowed	7	11	8	7	7
Never married	13	23	25	41	27
Education					
Some college or less	35	31	45	74	75
College degree	38	41	30	16	16
Graduate degree	27	29	25	10	9
Annual Household Income					
Less than $25,000	14[b]	14	22	33	29
$25,000– $74,999	38[b]	44	44	47	48
More than $75,000	47[b]	43	34	20	23
Employment Status					
Employed	60	64	61	61	65

Sources: Jewish Community Health Survey, 2003; Metropolitan Chicago Jewish Population Study (MCJPS), 2000–2001; National Jewish Population Survey (NJPS), 2000–2001; U.S. Census, 2000 (for Chicago and U.S. data).

Note: Percentages may not add to 100 because of rounding.
[a]Age ranges vary slightly. Specifically, education is asked of adults ≥25 and employment status for those ≥16. All others reflect adults ≥18.
[b]Income categories differ for the current survey. They are as follows: Less than $30,000, $30,000–$69,999, and More than $70,000.

(slightly) and in the United States and Chicago (greatly). For example, the percentage of individuals in this community with a graduate degree is three times higher than the national average. Like education, individuals in the current survey also had relatively high incomes. For example, nearly half of the sample reported a household income of more than $70,000 per year. This is substantially higher than levels in the national Jewish estimates, Chicago, and the U.S. However, it is important to consider differences in average family size. As discussed below, families in this Chicago Jewish community tend to be larger, and thus, the "per capita" income levels would be lower. In other words, the financial situation of this population may not be as favorable as the income data suggests. Finally, 60% of the individuals in this sample were currently employed. This estimate is very similar to that of the NJPS and Chicago (both at 61%) and just slightly below national levels.

Family Structure

In this population, nearly three-quarters of the individuals were married (Table 4-2). Compared to national Jewish estimates and the U.S. population, Jews in the current survey were much more likely to be married and approximately half as likely to be single/never married. Only 10% of individuals in this community lived alone (data not shown). This estimate is much lower than those for the national Jewish population or the U.S. population and may speak to the importance placed on family within this culture. At the other end of the spectrum, the survey found that more than one-third of individuals lived in a household with five or more total occupants. This is not surprising as individuals in the current survey also tended to have more children.

Religious Characteristics

Adults living in this Jewish community showed high levels of religious involvement, even compared to Jewish individuals nationally (Table 4-3). For example, more than 80% percent of individuals in the current study belonged to a synagogue compared to 46% in the NJPS. Of the synagogue members, the majority of individuals (89%) belonged to Orthodox traditions. This is in sharp contrast to national estimates, which show more balanced memberships in Orthodox, Conservative, and Reform affiliations. Other measures of Jewish connections include keeping a Kosher home and marrying within the faith. In the current sample, the majority reported keeping a Kosher home (79%) and nearly all of the married individuals had Jewish spouses. Markers of other issues specific to Jewish communities showed that more than one-fourth of the respondents reported that they had received services from Jewish-affiliated agencies in the past year. In addition, one-fourth of the sample reported that their income was insufficient to meet their religious obligations. These religious obligations could include belonging to a synagogue, keeping Kosher, belonging to a Jewish Community Center (JCC), or going to Israel.

TABLE 4-3 Religious Characteristics Among Jewish Adults in West Rogers Park/Peterson Park, Chicago, and the United States

	WRP(%)	MCJPS(%)	NJPS(%)
Synagogue affiliation			
Orthodox or Traditional	72	5	11
Conservative	5	13	15
Reform	3	19	17
Reconstructionist	0	2	1
Other	1	3	2
Not affiliated	19	58	54
Keeps a Kosher home	79	20	21
Jewish spouse (if married)	96	82	69
Received Jewish services in past year	28	—	—
Income insufficient for religious obligations	25	35	—

Sources: Jewish Community Health Survey, 2003; Metropolitan Chicago Jewish Population Study (MCJPS), 2000–2001; National Jewish Population Survey (NJPS), 2000–2001.

Health Care Access and Utilization

Access to health-care services, as well as the appropriate use of these services, is strongly linked to many health outcomes. Although issues such as a lack of health insurance and an inability to afford the rising costs of health care are plaguing the United States as a whole (DeNavas-Walt, Proctor, and Lee, 2005; Lasser, Himmelstein, Woolhandler, 2006), little is known about the health care needs of the Jewish population in general. Even less is known about the needs of Jews at the local level.

Access to Care

The findings showed that almost all adults in this Jewish sample reported having health insurance, regardless of age (Table 4-4). Notably, almost all adults younger than 65 years of age in this Jewish sample had private insurance compared to only 70% of adults nationwide. Of older adults, about half had private insurance (in addition to Medicare), which is slightly below the national average. The percent of individuals who reported not getting the services that they needed provides additional insight into how well individuals can access health care. In this sample, nearly one-quarter of respondents reported not getting some type of health care when they needed it (this includes medical care, prescription medications, mental health care, dental care, and eye care). Respondents were asked about this issue in another way as well. Specifically, they were asked, "Do you feel that your family income is sufficient or insufficient to meet your current health needs, irrespective of

TABLE 4-4   Health-Care Access and Utilization Within a Jewish Community in Chicago and the U.S. General Population

	Jewish Community (%)	United States (%)
Health insurance		
Any insurance		
18–64 years of age	95	81
65 years and older	99	99
Private insurance		
18–64 years of age	91	70
65 years and older	48	61
Did not get health care when needed	23	—
Income insufficient for health-care needs	28	—
Usual source of care	90	84
Gets routine check-ups	70	65
Visited doctor in the past year	89	68
Visited hospital in the past year	32	—

Sources: Jewish Community Health Survey, 2003; U.S. Data from Current Population Survey, 2003; National Health Interview Survey, 2001; Medical Expenditure Panel Survey, 2002.

health insurance?" In response, 28% reported that their income was insufficient to meet their health care needs.

Health-Care Utilization

Numerous questions were asked regarding the individuals' use of various health-care services (Table 4-4). To begin, nearly all adults reported having a "particular clinic, doctor's office, or health care facility" that they usually frequented when sick or seeking advice about health. Also referred to as having a "usual source of care," this is an important issue to examine because it is correlates with better health outcomes, greater use of preventive services, and reduced medical costs, among other things (De Maesneer et al., 2003; DeVoe et al., 2003; Starfield and Shi, 2004). Fortunately, almost all adults in this Jewish community reported having a usual source of care. This estimate was slightly higher than levels seen for all adults in the United States. Likely facilitated by this, the majority of adults reported getting regular check-ups with their physician and visiting a physician in the past year. In addition, nearly one-third visited a hospital in the past 12 months.

As seen in Table 4-5, individuals in the Jewish Community Health Survey reported high levels of preventive service utilization for almost all types of services. For example, most individuals (88%) had their blood pressure screened in the previous year. This is likely to be similar to rates of

TABLE 4-5   Preventive Health-Care Utilization Rates for a Jewish Community in Chicago, the Overall City of Chicago, and the United States

	Jewish Community (%)	Chicago (%)	United States (%)
Blood pressure test (all, in past year)	88	—	95[a]
Colonoscopy or sigmoidos-copy (≥50 years, ever)	52	46	37
Blood stool test (all, ever)	51	41	45
Mammogram (females, ≥40 years, in past 2 years)	80	80	70
Pap smear (females, ≥18 years, in past 3 years)	89	88	83
PSA (males, ≥50 years, ever)	36	—	57

Sources: Jewish Community Health Survey, 2003; Chicago data is for Cook County from the Behavioral Risk Factor Surveillance System, 2002 and 2003; U.S. data is from the Behavioral Risk Factor Surveillance System, 1999, 2000, 2002; National Health Interview Survey, 1998, 2000, 2003.

Note: [a]In past 2 years.

screening in national samples, which here are measured within the previous 2 years. Approximately half of the current sample reported ever having a colonoscopy (or sigmoidoscopy) and a blood stool test. These numbers are both slightly higher than local and national averages.

For female services, large percentages of women in the appropriate age ranges reported regular mammograms and Pap smears (80% and 89%, respectively). The fact that these numbers are both higher than national averages (Smith, Cokkinides, and Eyre, 2007) is surprising given the cultural barriers faced by Orthodox women based on guidelines concerning modesty issues and interactions between adults of opposite genders. Perhaps targeted messages regarding the higher likelihood of Jewish women to have the gene mutations linked to breast and ovarian cancer (USPSTF, 2009) and to have been diagnosed with breast cancer (Egan et al., 1996) have motivated women in this group to be more proactive about screening, despite their discomfort with the process. Men in this sample, on the other hand, have shown lower-than-average rates of screening for prostate-specific antigen (PSA) tests. Although more than half of the men in the national sample reported having this test in the past year, only 36% of the men in the current sample did.

The use of complementary and alternative medicine (CAM) has grown significantly throughout the past decade within the general U.S. population. High levels of CAM use are also seen in the current sample, where almost half of adults have visited at least one type of alternative care provider. This level is similar to those seen in the most recent national study, which found that approximately 37% of adults have used some form of CAM (not including prayer) at some point in their lives (Barnes et al., 2004). Certain types of CAM treatments are used more frequently by those in this community. For example, although only 20% of adults in the United States have ever been to a chiropractor, more than one-third of those living here have done so. Similarly, nationwide only 4% of adults have used acupuncture compared to 14% of those in the current sample (Barnes et al., 2004).

Physical Health Outcomes

Self-Rated Health

The first measure of overall health status was determined with a question that asked respondents, "In the last 12 months, would you say your health in general has been excellent, very good, good, fair, or poor?" This measure, often called self-rated health, is a commonly used indicator of health status because it is strongly predictive of mortality risk, even after accounting for other risk factors such as age, low education and income, high blood pressure, obesity, and other measures of health status (Idler and Benyamini, 1997). In other words, individuals who report that their health is poor are more likely to die in a given period compared to individuals who say their health is good, even if these two individuals have the same number of health problems. Using this global measure of health status, it was found that the vast majority of adults in this Jewish community considered themselves to be in "good" health or better. Just more than one-quarter were at the highest end of the scale ("excellent"), whereas only 5% said they had "poor" health.

Disease Prevalence

Another important indicator of health and well-being—particularly for adults—is the prevalence of chronic conditions. Respondents were asked if they had ever been diagnosed with each of the six most common conditions (Table 4-6). (Few health questions were asked of Jews nationwide or in Chicago. Therefore, most of the comparison data for this area will come from national health surveys.) When adjusted for age, the first finding shows that over one-fourth of the Jewish sample reported a diagnosis of hypertension. This is slightly higher than the percentages seen in the national sample. Hypertension, also known as high blood pressure, is important to study because it is one of the leading causes of cardiovascular morbidity and mortality in the United States. It also increases an individual's risk of other health problems such as stroke and kidney failure. Fortunately, once detected, many simple changes (such as eating a healthy diet, exercising

TABLE 4-6   Prevalence of Chronic Conditions in the Jewish
Community Health Survey and the United States

	WRP (%)	United States (%)
Hypertension	28	21
Diabetes	7	7
Cancer	7	7
Heart problems	13	11
Arthritis	25	21
Asthma	10	11
Any of these	51	—

Sources: Jewish Community Health Survey, 2003 (age-adjusted);
National Health Interview Survey, 2002.

regularly, not smoking or drinking, and/or taking medication) can reduce
the risks related to this condition (NHLBI, 2005). Unfortunately, the Centers
for Disease Control and Prevention (CDC) estimate that nearly one-third of
all cases of high blood pressure are undetected. This means that the rates
seen here are likely to greatly underestimate the number of individuals with
unhealthy blood pressure levels (for all groups).

Levels of other chronic conditions, including diabetes, cancer, and asthma,
were similar to national estimates. For all of these, less than 10% of the
adult population had been diagnosed with the condition. Larger percentages
of individuals reported having arthritis and heart problems. Again, both of
these rates are comparable to national estimates. Overall, just more than half
of the adults reported having at least one of these six conditions.

The prevalence of other chronic conditions was also assessed. Particular
attention was paid to diseases that are often more prevalent in Jewish populations. However, the majority of these diseases, and others, were reported
by so few respondents that reliable estimates could not be produced. For
example, less than 5% of the sample reported being diagnosed with Crohn's
Disease, colitis, Hepatitis B or C, tuberculosis, or bipolar disorder.

Although levels of many of the most common chronic conditions were
comparable to national estimates (and affected fairly small percentages of
individuals), it is important to pay attention to these rates for several reasons.
For one, rates of conditions like diabetes were low but may be growing rapidly. As discussed later in this chapter, levels of obesity in this population
are high (even among young children), and it is well-established that being
overweight is a major risk factor for diabetes (as well as other chronic conditions, such as high blood pressure and heart problems). Thus, the prevalence
of these conditions is likely to increase in this population in the coming
years. In addition, having chronic condition rates equal to those seen for the
country as a whole is not necessarily an impressive accomplishment. For

many measures of health, the United States routinely ranks at the bottom of all industrialized countries. For example, the average life expectancy at birth for the United States is only the 48th highest in the world (World Fact Book, 2005). Finally, the community should not be satisfied with the current levels of chronic conditions because these conditions significantly affect an individual's quality of life, yet a large percentage result from preventable causes. Thus, continually lowering the prevalence of these conditions is a reasonable, and worthy, goal for all communities.

Obesity

More than half of both adults and children in this community were overweight or obese. Specifically, 33% of adults were overweight and an additional 24% were obese. For children, 28% were overweight and an additional 26% were obese. More information on the data related to childhood obesity is presented in Chapter 9, along with a description of the intervention developed to address this important health risk (Benjamins, 2010). Of the overweight and obese adults, 87% rated themselves as slightly or very overweight. The remaining 13% said they were about the right weight or underweight. This is important to know because those overweight or obese individuals who perceive themselves as the right weight (or underweight) would not be aware of the need to lose weight. Half of all adults (most of whom were overweight or obese) said they were currently trying to lose weight, whereas an additional 37% were working to maintain their weight. Nearly one-fourth of the adult respondents were both exercising and eating healthier to lose weight. Unfortunately, less than half of overweight or obese adults reported that their doctor had advised them to lose weight. In fact, only 22% of all adults had received this advice.

Mental Health Outcomes

Mental health is as essential to overall health and well-being as physical health. Moreover, mental illnesses, such as depression, are risk factors for many chronic conditions and can have a negative influence on the course and management of these conditions (Chapman, Perry, and Strine, 2005). Therefore, depression is expected to be the second leading source of the global burden of disease by 2020 (Murray and Lopez, 1996). As shown in Table 4-7, over half of the sample reported emotional health problems (defined by the respondent). Unfortunately, these problems had a large impact on individual's lives, such as restricting overall productivity and even limiting an individual's ability to work. More specific information on one of the most common mental health conditions—depression—is provided below.

TABLE 4-7   Mental Health Problems in the Jewish Community Health Survey

	Percent
Emotional Health	
Ever had emotional health problems	53
Days in past month when emotional health was not good	
1–7 days	22
8 or more days	14
Accomplished less because of emotional problems	
Some of the time	20
All or most of the time	7
Did not work because of emotional problems	
Some of the time	16
All or most of the time	3
Depression	
Ever diagnosed with depression	21
Screened depressed (CESD)	17
Depressed in the past month	32

Source: Jewish Community Health Survey, 2003.

Three different measures of depression were examined within this Jewish population. For the first measure, respondents were asked if they had ever been told by a physician that they were depressed. In contrast to this measure of clinical diagnosis, the second measure used a set of questions to screen for probable depression. These questions, called the Center for Epidemiological Studies Depression (CES-D) scale, included a set of 10 statements, such as "I felt depressed" or "I felt everything was an effort" (Radloff, 1977). Individuals with four or more positive responses to these statements were considered likely to be depressed. Finally, individuals were asked if they were depressed in the past month.

In this sample, more than one-fifth of individuals reported having been diagnosed with depression at some point in life. This is slightly higher than recent national estimates, which have found that lifetime depression is reported by 16% of adults (Kessler et al., 2003). In addition, nearly as many adults screened positive for current depression (using the CES-D scale). Although recent national comparisons for this measure are not available, older data shows that this estimate is similar to the general public's rate of depression.

Finally, approximately one-third of adults in this sample reported that they had been depressed in the past month. Again, no good comparison data could be found, but this number is substantially higher than national estimates of depression within the past *year* (Kessler et al., 2003). In other words, Jewish adults in this community are much more likely to consider themselves as having been depressed compared to other adults in the United States. Moreover, overweight and obese individuals were two to three times more likely to screen positive for depression compared to those who were normal or underweight.

Physical and Mental Disability

Respondents were not asked directly if they were disabled (because of practical and ethical reasons), but they were asked about the presence of disability within their household. From this question, it was estimated that nearly one-fourth of individuals (23%) in this community lived with an individual with a disability. This is significantly higher than the rate reported for all Jewish households in Chicago (15%). It is more difficult to compare this with American households overall because the Census uses a broader measure of disability (and finds a 29% rate with this measure). The absolute, and relative, magnitude of disability in this community warrants further attention.

Individuals who responded that they lived with an individual with a disability (note that this could be the respondent as well) were then asked what type of disability the individual had been diagnosed with. Approximately half of this group reported a learning disability. An additional 20% reported a general physical disability. More specific responses were also given, such as blindness, deafness, and emotional problems. Not unexpectedly, a substantial proportion (45%) of the individuals with a disability had special care needs. These needs were diverse, reflecting the wide range of disabilities reported. Many involved either some type of health-care provider or a mobility device. In addition, other service providers, such as tutors and caregivers, were needed by many of the disabled individuals.

Certain characteristics were more commonly seen in adults living with someone with a disability compared to those living in households without a disabled individual. Perhaps most importantly, individuals living with someone with a disability were more likely to report certain health problems themselves. For example, the percentage of individuals who screened positive for depression was nearly twice as high in this group than in the general population. Levels of poor subjective health were also higher for adults in this group. Not surprisingly, individuals living in a household with a disabled individual were more likely to face financial difficulties as well. More specifically, more than half of these individuals reported that they had insufficient funds to meet their needs. Likely for this reason, almost half of this group (44%) had used Jewish services in the past year.

Health Behaviors

Because of the increasing awareness of the role that health behaviors play in maintaining wellness, numerous questions were asked to gauge the level of behavioral risk factors in this population. This section summarizes eating habits, physical activity, smoking, drinking, and drug use.

Eating Habits

The majority of respondents (66%) said that diet and nutrition were very important to them. A similar percentage (62%) reported being satisfied with their current eating habits. However, when this question is examined by weight status, large differences are found. Specifically, normal or under-weight individuals were much more likely to be satisfied with their eating habits (80%) than overweight individuals (62%) or obese individuals (34%). Overall, access to food did not seem to be a problem for most individuals. For example, the vast majority of individuals had a grocery store within 15 minutes of their home. Furthermore, almost two-thirds of individuals were very satisfied with the food selection available to them. Finally, 84% said that their income was sufficient to buy the food they wanted.

Several unhealthy eating behaviors were reported for both adults and children within this community. For example, more than one-fourth (29%) of all adults reported eating fast food once a week or more (Table 4-8). Unfortunately, nearly one-third of children (32%) also reported eating out at least once a week, and this percentage was higher for overweight or obese children (38%) than for normal weight children (28%). In addition,

TABLE 4-8   Comparisons of Selected Health Behaviors in the Jewish Community Health Survey

	WRP (%)	Chicago (%)	United States (%)
Eating habits			
Eats fast food regularly (≥1 time/ week)	29	—	—
Physical activity			
Moderate activities (≥3 times/ week)	50	43	47
Vigorous activities (≥3 times/ week)	27	22	25
Cigarette use			
Current smoker	4	23	22
Former smoker	30	23	25
Alcohol use			
Current drinker (≥1 drink in last month)	48	60	59
Drug use			
Smoked marijuana in past month	4	7	6

Source: Jewish Community Health Survey, 2003; Behavioral Risk Factor Surveillance System, 2002, 2003; National Survey on Drug Use and Health, 1998, 2001.

approximately two-thirds of all children failed to eat the recommended daily five servings of fruits or vegetables. This number would be even higher if fruit juices were not included in the question. Other issues, such as a deficiency in dairy intake for girls, were also seen.

Physical Activity

Respondents were asked about levels of both moderate and vigorous physical activity. Examples that were given to define moderate activities included brisk walking, bicycling, vacuuming, gardening, or anything else that caused small increases in breathing or heart rate. Examples of vigorous activities included running, swimming laps, aerobics, heavy yard work, or anything else that caused large increases in breathing or heart rate. For each level, respondents were asked how many times per week they engaged in the activities for at least 20 minutes at a time.

It is generally recommended that adults engage in moderate physical activities for at least 30 minutes on 5 or more days of the week (CDC, 2005). In addition, Healthy People 2010, a collection of health goals for the United States, recommends that individuals engage in vigorous physical activity 3 days or more per week for 20 minutes or more at a time (USDHHS, 2000). Meeting either (or both) of these goals has been shown to provide individuals with extensive health benefits. Unfortunately, in this community, levels of both moderate and vigorous activity fell below recommended amounts of exercise. Approximately one-half of individuals participated in moderate activities and one-fourth in vigorous activities three times or more a week (Table 4-8). These levels are both slightly higher than Chicago averages but similar to those for the United States.

Some differences in activity levels exist when looking at demographic and socio-economic characteristics (not shown). For example, women were significantly more likely to report regular moderate exercise but were slightly less likely to report participating in vigorous activities. Although no differences are seen for education, individuals with lower incomes were less likely to report moderate exercise compared to those who earn more. Finally, foreign-born individuals have much lower levels of physical activity for both moderate and vigorous intensities. Many of these trends are similar to those seen in other populations (USDHHS, 2000).

Smoking

On a more positive note, questions regarding cigarette use found that only 4% of the sample reported being a current smoker (Table 4-8). This is well below the rates of smoking noted in the general population. Interestingly, the percentage of individuals who had smoked in the past was slightly higher for the Jewish sample. Note that a social desirability bias may result in individuals underreporting their actual smoking levels. This may be particularly true in a predominantly Orthodox community where rules (and norms) prohibiting smoking exist (such as explicitly prohibiting smoking on the Sabbath). Although these findings are thus likely to underestimate the actual level of smoking in this community, the bias toward underreporting is thought to occur (to some extent) in all populations. Thus, actual levels of smoking in this sample are likely to be higher than reported but still lower than other populations.

Drinking Alcohol

It was also found that approximately half of the adults in this Jewish sample consumed alcoholic beverages in the past month. This level is lower than both the Chicago and U.S. population estimates. Further analyses showed that the vast majority of these "drinkers" had one drink or less per week, on average. A series of questions was also asked to assess the prevalence of drinking problems. These questions concerned topics such as feeling guilty about drinking, drinking in the morning, drinking and driving, and being advised by a doctor to stop drinking. For each of these questions, no more than 3% of the sample reported a problem.

Drug Use

Finally, only 4% of the adults reported smoking marijuana in the past month. This rate is slightly lower than Chicago or U.S. rates. No additional questions on drug use were included here.

Other Health-Related Issues

Domestic Violence

The issue of domestic violence has been attracting an increasing amount of attention within the Jewish community. The population estimates provided by the current study complement the more qualitative data obtained from a previous needs assessment done in Chicago (Altfeld, 2004) and, to our knowledge, provide the first prevalence estimates of domestic violence within any Jewish community in Chicago. Specifically, the survey revealed that one-fourth of individuals in this community had witnessed domestic violence (data not shown). This is very similar to *suspected* prevalence rates reported in the Needs Assessment on Domestic Abuse in the Chicago Jewish community, which used key informant interviews and surveys of community members and leaders to estimate that the rate of abuse in Jewish households was 23% to 25% (Altfeld, 2004). Unfortunately, this type of information is often underreported (within all populations), so these rates most likely underestimate the actual prevalence of this type of violence. The sensitive nature of domestic violence information is highlighted by the fact that less than half of the individuals in the current sample (39%) who witnessed this type of violence actually reported it. Individuals were also asked if they, or members of their household, had ever been a victim of physical, verbal, or sexual violence. Nearly one-third of the sample responded affirmatively. This is lower than estimates from a national survey of women in the United States (Plichta and Falik, 2001).

Genetic Testing

Individuals of Jewish descent, particularly Ashkenazi Jews (82% of this sample), have a higher risk for carrying mutations for certain genetic diseases. The American College of Obstetrics and Gynecology recommends that Ashkenazi Jews be offered carrier screening for four specific disorders: Tay-Sachs disease, Canavan disease, cystic fibrosis, and familial dysautonomia. Rates of these disorders can be as much as 20 to 100 times higher in this population (Chicago Center for Jewish Genetic Disorders, 2005). It is particularly important to examine rates of screening within the Jewish population of Chicago because existing data show low rates of testing for at least one "Jewish" genetic disorder. More specifically, rates of testing for Tay-Sachs disease in the Chicago area were significantly lower than rates seen for other cities with large Jewish populations (JUF website, 2005).

The current survey revealed that within this Jewish community in Chicago, 42% of all adults had been screened for some type of genetic disorders (data not shown). Rates were highest among those of child-bearing age, those who were currently married, and those who had children. In addition, individuals with college degrees, higher incomes, and current employment were more likely to report having been screened. Finally, Orthodox Jews and members of synagogues were more likely to report being screened for genetic disorders, compared to those belonging to other denominations and those who did not belong to a synagogue.

Of the individuals who reported having been screened, only a small percentage (13%) found that they were carriers for a genetic disorder. Tay-Sachs was the most commonly reported condition; however, the adults reporting this made up less than 5% of the total population. Individuals were asked several questions to better understand the motivations and barriers to being tested. About half of those who had been screened said that they had done so after being told by their doctor or rabbi about Dor Yeshorim, a program based in New York to facilitate the confidential screening of Jewish individuals for relevant conditions. Approximately one-fourth said that they had been tested because of family concerns. A smaller percentage reported that a family history of genetic disorders prompted their screening. The reported barriers fell into three main groups: those who did not feel like it was neces-sary, those who never considered testing, and those who did not know such tests existed.

These findings suggest that interventions aimed at educating and encourag-ing doctors and rabbis within these communities to provide information and referrals may be an effective means of increasing screening rates. Additional efforts to raise community awareness may also be valuable because many reasons given for not being screened involved a lack of knowledge about the tests and their importance. Educational campaigns offered through syna-gogues, women's organizations, community centers, campus Hillels, and mass media should all be expanded. Finally, although not frequently reported as a barrier here, cost is often a major impediment to screening. Programs that offer free or reduced cost screenings are crucial for increasing rates.

Vulnerable Groups

Finally, because some individuals shoulder a disproportionate amount of the burden posed by the health problems discussed above, the health status of potentially vulnerable groups is examined here. In particular, adults with large families, single parents, older adults, and Russian-speaking immi-grants were all expected to have special needs. For example, families with four or more children were more likely to have insufficient funds for impor-tant needs such as health care, food, or education. More disturbingly, nearly half of all single parents lived below the poverty line (based on approxima-tions using the 2003 federal poverty guidelines) (USDHHS, 2005). In addi-tion, more than half lived in a household with someone with a disability. Perhaps for these reasons, single parents had more depressive symptoms and were more likely to report being depressed in the past month compared to other adults.

Adults older than 65 years of age were relatively advantaged financially, yet they still faced a disproportionate amount of health problems. These problems included elevated rates of high blood pressure (63%), arthri-tis (65%), and activity limitations (37%). Finally, there was a substantial Russian-speaking immigrant population in this Jewish community. Although this group made up only 5% of the sample, they represent an estimated 1,150 adults in the community and warrant special attention because of the disad-vantages they face. For example, nearly half of the individuals in this group reported having insufficient funds to meet their health-care and food needs. Health concerns were also common. For example, levels of heart disease were more than twice as high as levels seen in the total sample (and in national estimates), and these individuals were also much more likely to have weight problems.

Overall Survey Impact

Dissemination and Reactions

A variety of dissemination strategies were used to share these findings with community members, health service providers, and other relevant groups and individuals. To begin, these findings were shared with the community through the publication and distribution of an in-depth report. Specifically, it summarized the methodology and main results of the survey in layman's terms for all interested individuals and agencies (Benjamins et al., 2006a). Since its publication, this report has been made available (free of charge) to any interested group or individual. It can also be downloaded from the SUHI website (www.SUHIchicago.org).

To coincide with the publication of this report, a "release event" was held to present the findings and to allow community members a chance to ask questions and make comments and suggestions (Fig. 4-2). This event was held at the local Jewish Community Center. All respondents to the survey were invited back, and information about the presentation was distributed through numerous avenues (including synagogue newsletters) to reach the maximum number of individuals. Approximately 40 individuals attended this session, which included opening remarks from a vice president of the Jewish Federation and the CEO of Mount Sinai Hospital. Healthy refreshments were served and the project dietitian provided healthy recipe cards and other health promotion materials. Despite the relatively low attendance, the project staff felt that this important part of the research process helped to strengthen the relationship between the research team and the community, as well as to begin generating conversations about health among individuals and organizations.

Following this, a multipage article about the event and the survey findings was published in a community newspaper, the Chicago Jewish News. For other researchers and those in the academic world, a summary article was published in the *Journal of Community Health* (Benjamins et al., 2006b). In addition, for those who provide services within the Jewish community, an article was published in the *Journal of Jewish Communal Service* (Benjamins et al., 2007). This article had the distinction of being the first article focused on health ever published in this journal.

Finally, the findings were presented to community stakeholders, including lay leaders, community agency professionals, rabbis, and school administrators, through a series of meetings held with all interested groups. Each meeting began with a presentation by the project director of the study background, methodology, and results. The second half of each meeting was organized like an informal focus group, facilitated by

Figure 4-2   Advertisement for Community Meeting to Discuss Findings of the Jewish Community Health Survey

a member of the project steering committee from the Jewish Federation. To begin, time for questions about the findings was allowed. Then, everyone present was asked to comment on the following questions: *(1)* What are the most pressing health concerns?; *(2)* How should these issues be addressed?; and *(3)* Who should be involved? Through these sessions, health problems were prioritized, potential intervention ideas were developed, and future partners were identified.

Interventions and Other Uses of the Data

The first intervention developed based on findings from this survey was the Jewish Day School Wellness Initiative. This four-year project, which uses a culturally-appropriate model of school wellness to reduce levels of childhood obesity within Jewish schools in Chicago, is described in detail in Chapter 9 (Benjamins, 2010). Other interventions have also been developed based on findings from the current survey.

In particular, data regarding the prevalence of domestic violence factored into the recent creation of a pilot program targeting synagogues as a vehicle to promote safe and healthy relationships. Through this model certification program, synagogue clergy, professionals, and lay leadership participate in a series of core trainings and institutional policy review to improve their capacity to both prevent abuse, as well as to respond to congregants experiencing abuse in a way that is appropriate, effective, spiritual, and healing. Another intervention informed by the survey data promotes health and well-being among older adults in the targeted survey community. Specifically, a well-known model of promoting aging in place was adapted and implemented in an Orthodox community with a large proportion of residents who are 60 years and older. This adapted Naturally Occurring Retirement Community (NORC) model is now known as LaBriut ("To Your Health") and is in its third year. It brings a range of wellness programs (e.g., chronic disease self-management classes, fall prevention classes, nutrition and exercise programs, health screenings, shopping shuttle) to more than 250 seniors annually.

Conclusions

This chapter summarizes findings from the groundbreaking *Jewish Community Health Survey*. Overall, the findings indicate that the individuals in this community were as healthy (or healthier) than the average residents of Chicago or the United States; however, many serious health concerns still exist for both adults and children. Perhaps the most striking health problems involve weight. In fact, it was discovered that more than half of all adults and children were overweight. In addition, elevated rates of hypertension, disability, and depression were apparent. The current survey was also instrumental in collecting local data on other health-related behaviors and experiences. For example, it was discovered that more than half of adults had not been screened for genetic disorders. A more distressing finding is that a large proportion of individuals had witnessed or experienced some type of violence. In addition to these health concerns, many of the respondents were found to have financial limitations, unmet health-care needs, and other issues that could prevent them from achieving optimal levels of physical and emotional health. Moreover, certain groups of individuals shouldered a disproportionate amount of these financial and health-related burdens. In particular, members of large families, single parents, and older adults were found to have special needs and remain important targets for the provision of social services.

This type of in-depth health information for a Jewish community is rare and has not been available before in Chicago or in most other cities. The findings have greatly increased the awareness of health issues within this community and have provided an impetus for change. The findings are also being used to guide health promotion and disease prevention activities at the individual, organization, and community level. Through these means, this health survey continues to be a valuable asset for the Jewish community of West Rogers Park/Peterson Park. Finally, it is hoped that this effort will spur similar surveys in Jewish communities around the country.

Acknowledgments

The catalyst of this initiative was Joel Carp of the Jewish Federation of Metropolitan Chicago. His leadership enabled the project to gather both community support and sufficient funding. His colleague, Dana Rhodes, and the director of the Sinai Urban Health Institute, Steven Whitman, were also valuable members of the survey steering committee and consistently provided guidance and support for the project. The generous grants from the Polk Bros. Foundation, the Jewish Federation's Fund for Innovation in Health (supported by the Michael Reese Health Trust), the Irvin and Ruth Swartzberg Foundation, and the Fel-Pro Mecklenberger Supporting Fund must be recognized again. Furthermore, the author would like to thank the University of Illinois at Chicago's Survey Research Laboratory, which so competently handled the logistics of data collection. Thanks are also due to members of the Sinai Urban Health Institute, especially Kristi Allgood, who provided numerous "in-kind" contributions. Finally, and most importantly, much appreciation is due to the community respondents who completed the survey and made this unique effort possible.

References

Altfeld, Susan. 2004. *Domestic abuse in the Chicago Jewish community: Needs and priorities.* Report prepared for Jewish Women International.

American Association for Public Opinion Research (AAPOR). 2000. *Standard Definitions: Final Dispositions of Case Codes and Outcome Rates for Surveys.* Ann Arbor, MI: AAPOR.

Barnes, Patricia M., Eve Powell-Griner, Kim McFann, and Richard L. Nahin. 2004. *Complementary and alternative medicine use among adults: United States, 2002.* CDC Advance Data Report #343.

Benjamins, Maureen R. 2010. Fighting childhood obesity in a Jewish community. In *Urban health: Combating disparities with local data,* ed. Steven Whitman, Ami M. Shah, and Maureen R. Benjamins. New York: Oxford University Press.

Benjamins, Maureen, Dana M. Rhodes, Joel M. Carp, and Steven Whitman. 2006a. *Report on the findings of the Jewish Community Health Survey: West Rogers Park & Peterson Park.* Chicago, IL: Jewish Federation of Metropolitan Chicago.

Benjamins, Maureen, Dana M. Rhodes, Joel M. Carp, and Steven Whitman. 2006b. A local community health survey: Findings from a population-based survey of the largest Jewish community in Chicago. *Journal of Community Health* 31(6):479–495.

Benjamins, Maureen R., Dana M. Rhodes, Joel M. Carp, and Steven Whitman. 2007. Conducting a health survey: Rationale, results, and advice for other Jewish communities. *Journal of Jewish Communal Service* 82:83–95.

Centers for Disease Control and Prevention (CDC) website. *Physical Activity for Everyone: Recommendations.* Online. Available: http://www.cdc.gov/nccdphp/dnpa/physical/recommendations/index.htm. Accessed October 4, 2005.

Chapman, D. P., G. S. Perry, and T. W. Strine. 2005. The vital link between chronic disease and depressive disorders. *Preventing Chronic Disease.* January, 2005. Online. Available: http://www.cdc.gov/pcd/issues/2005/jan/04_0066.htm. Accessed December 1, 2009.

Chicago Center for Jewish Genetic Disorders website. 2005. *About Jewish Genetic Disorders.* Online. Available: http://www.jewishgeneticscenter.org/what/. Accessed October 4, 2005.

De Maesneer, Jan M., Lutgarde De Prins, Christiane Gosset, and Jozef Heyerick. 2003. Provider continuity in family medicine: Does it make a difference for total health care costs? *Annals of Family Medicine* 1(3):144–148.

DeNavas-Walt, Carmen, Bernadette D. Proctor, and Cheryl Hill Lee. 2006. U.S. Census Bureau, Current Population Reports, P60-231, *Income, Poverty, and Health Insurance Coverage in the United States: 2005,* U.S. Government Printing Office, Washington, DC.

DeVoe, Jennifer E., George E. Fryer, Robert Phillips, and Larry Green. 2003. Receipt of preventive care among adults: Insurance status and usual source of care. *American Journal of Public Health* 93(5):786–791.

Egan, Kathleen M., Polly A. Newcomb, Mathew P. Longnecker, Amy Trentham-Dietz, J. A. Baron, D. Trichopoulos, et al. 1996. Jewish religion and risk of breast cancer. *Lancet* 347:1645–1646.

Fielding, Jonathan E. and Thomas R. Frieden. 2004. Local knowledge to enable local action. *American Journal of Preventive Medicine* 27(2):183–184.

Idler, Ellen L. and Yael Benyamini. 1997. Self-rated health and mortality: A review of twenty-seven community studies. *Journal of Health and Social Behavior* 38:21–37.

Jacobs, Linda A. and Ellen Giarelli. 2001. Jewish culture, health belief systems, and genetic risk for cancer. *Nursing Forum* 36:5–13.

Jewish United Fund (JUF) website. 2008. JUF/JF Directory of Services: Chicago Center for Jewish Genetic Disorders. Online. Available: http://www.juf.org/services_resources/directory.asp?id=0035. Accessed September 7, 2005.

Kennedy, Gary J., Howard R. Kelman, Cynthia Thomas, and Jiming Chen. 1996. The relation of religious preference and practice to depressive symptoms among 1,855 older adults. *Journals of Gerontology* 51B:P301–P308.

Kessler, Ronald C., Patricia Berglund, Olga Demler, et al. 2003. The epidemiology of major depressive disorders: Results from the National Comorbidity Survey Replication (NCS-R). *Journal of the American Medical Association* 289(23):3095–3105.

Koenig, Harold G., Michael E. McCullough, and David B. Larson. 2001. *The Handbook of Religion and Health.* Oxford: Oxford University Press.

Lasser, Karen E., David U. Himmelstein, and Steffie Woolhandler. 2006. Access to care, health status, and health disparities in the United States and Canada: Results of a cross-national population-based survey. *American Journal of Public Health* 96(7):1300–1307.

Levav, Itzhak, Robert Kohn, Jacqueline M. Golding, Myrna Weissman. 1997. Vulnerability of Jews to affective disorders. *American Journal of Psychology* 154:941–947.

Murray, Christopher J. L. and Alan D. Lopez, editors. 1996. *Summary: The Global Burden of Disease.* Boston (MA): Harvard School of Public Health.

National Heart, Lung, and Blood Institute (NHLBI) website. 2005. *Your Guide to Lowering High Blood Pressure.* Online. Available: http://www.nhlbi.nih.gov/hbp/index.html. Accessed September 22, 2005.

Plichta, Stacy B. and Marilyn Falik. 2001. Prevalence of violence and its implications for women's health. *Women's Health Issues* 11(3):244–258.

Radloff, Lenore S. 1977. The CES-D scale: A self-report depression scale for research in the general population. *Applied Psychological Measurement* 1(3):385–401.

Shah, Ami M. and Steven Whitman. 2010. Sinai Health System's Improving Community Health Survey: Methodology and Key Findings. In *Urban Health: Combating Disparities with Local Data*, ed. Steven Whitman, Ami Shah, and Maureen R. Benjamins. New York: Oxford University Press.

Smith, Robert A., Vilma Cokkinides, and Harmon J. Eyre. 2007. Cancer screening in the United States, 2007: A review of current guidelines, practices, and prospects. *CA: A Cancer Journal for Clinicians* 57(2):90–104.

Starfield, Barbara and Leiyu Shi. 2004. The medical home, access to care, and insurance: A review of the evidence. *Pediatrics* 113(5):1493–1498.

United Jewish Communities Report. 2004. *National Jewish Population Survey 2000–01: Strength, Challenge and Diversity in the American Jewish Population.* A United Jewish Communities Report, in Cooperation with the Mandell L. Berman Institute and the North American Jewish Data Bank. January, 2004.

U.S. Department of Health and Human Services (U. S. DHHS). 2000. *Healthy People 2010: Understanding and Improving Health*, 2nd ed. Washington, DC: U.S. Government Printing Office, November 2000.

U.S. Department of Health and Human Services (U. S. DHHS). 2005. The HHS federal poverty guidelines. Online. Available: http://aspe.hhs.gov/poverty/03poverty.htm. Accessed November 10, 2005.

U.S. Preventive Services Task Force (USPSTF). 2009. Genetic risk assessment and BRCA mutation testing for breast and ovarian cancer susceptibility. Online.

Available: http://www.ahrq.gov/clinic/uspstf05/brcagen/brcagenrs.htm.   Accessed April 20, 2009.

World Fact Book. 2005. *Rank Order: Life Expectancy at Birth.* CIA Publications. Online. Available: http://www.cia.gov/cia/publications/factbook/rankorder/2102rank. html. Accessed September 23, 2005.

5

THE CHICAGO ASIAN COMMUNITY SURVEYS: METHODOLOGY AND KEY FINDINGS

Matthew J. Magee, Lucy Guo, Ami M. Shah, and Hong Liu

Introduction

Despite Chicago's diverse population, existing data that describe racial and ethnic minority health are lacking, particularly among the Asian population (Walter, 2004). Data are limited because they are typically aggregated for all Asians[1] and are rarely available at the state, city, or community level. The availability of health data for specific racial and ethnic groups enables policymakers, researchers, and service providers to develop appropriate agendas that most effectively improve health outcomes, monitor progress in reducing disparities, and plan targeted interventions.

Inspired by the *Sinai's Improving Community Health Survey* (Sinai Survey), the Asian Health Coalition of Illinois (AHCI) and its community partners began implementing a similar local assessment of health in three Asian populations in Chicago. They conducted health surveys in the Chinese, Cambodian, and Vietnamese communities; together these are called the Chicago Asian Community Health Surveys (Asian Surveys). In this chapter, the background, methods, and key findings are discussed briefly to highlight the processes, achievements, and impact of the Asian Survey project. The intent is that this description will motivate and guide other institutions, agencies, or communities interested in conducting a similar community health survey.

Background and Rationale

The Chicago Asian population grew from 102,938 in 1990 to 125,974 in 2000 (Misra et al., 2005). The Asian community is one of the fastest growing racial and ethnic groups in the city, yet little is known about its health status (Tao, Han, and Shah, 2006). Consequently, developing strategic plans and implementing health programs is challenging for community-based organizations (CBOs) serving the Chicago Asian population. How does one monitor success in improving access to health care or the health status of communities? How do funders know that their goals have been met without such health data?

To our knowledge, few agencies have surveyed the health needs of the Chicago Asian community in the past. Surveys that had previously been conducted used convenient sampling techniques that may not have achieved a sufficient sample size to estimate population level characteristics. Although previous efforts are notable, the results are unpublished and it is unclear whether these data were useful to quantify important health problems, shape health programming, and direct resources to these communities.

In the United States, Asians have historically been stereotyped as the "model minority" (Peterson, 1966). Yet, limited health data that do exist in Chicago for this population suggest otherwise. Data indicate that the Asian community is in fact in great need of additional public health programming, and many health outcomes show a slower rate of improvement for this population compared to Chicago at large. For example, from 1997 to 2005, the infant mortality rate in Chicago increased among Asians whereas it stabilized or decreased for Whites, Blacks, and Hispanics. Overall, the Chicago Department of Public Health reported an increase in Asian age-adjusted all-cause mortality rates between 1990 and 2000, from 416 to 466 per 100,000 (Misra et al., 2005). During the same time period, all-cause mortality rates decreased in Chicago as a whole. Such data indicated several important health disparities and prompted local community leaders to take action to help explain these startling poor health trends.

Three principal factors motivated the Asian Surveys. First, these health surveys would further explore the important health disparities that already exist and identify other areas of health need. Second, providing information about specific Asian ethnicities would augment each community's ability to plan effective programs and interventions. Third, data from these health surveys would inform policymakers and funders of how resources for the Asian community should be best distributed. The success of the Sinai Survey served as a model project for the Chicago Asian community to adapt for its own use, with the hope of generating awareness of the need for Asian specific health resources.

Partnerships

To meet the Chicago Asian communities' need for accurate and scientific local health data, AHCI and its partners gathered new health data about the Chinese, Cambodian, and Vietnamese populations in Chicago. In collaboration with the Sinai Urban Health Institute, AHCI received funding from the Illinois Department of Public Health, the United Way of Metropolitan Chicago, and the Retirement Research Foundation to implement this project. Specifically, the Asian Surveys aimed to: *(1)* document the general health status of Asian immigrants and Asian American residents in Chicago; *(2)* compare the results to other racial and ethnic groups with local data from the Sinai Survey (Whitman, Williams, and Shah, 2004) and other comparable local, state, and national health statistics; and *(3)* use the findings to motivate community organizations, guide targeted interventions, and bring greater resources to the community to increase efforts for improved health overall. To achieve these ends, AHCI partnered with three well-established and dynamic CBOs to implement the project: Chinese American Service League, Cambodian Association of Illinois, and Chinese Mutual Aid Association. These organizations were pivotal to guiding survey development, ensuring cultural sensitively, and promoting community acceptance of the survey. They were also essential to data collection and interpretation of the survey results.

Methodology

Sample Selection

Because of the diversity of the Asian population living in Chicago, AHCI needed to select specific Asian subgroups to be surveyed. These groups were selected based on where Asians were most populated and where there was greatest community interest. AHCI first examined existing health and socio-economic data, which are often displayed by Chicago's 77 officially designated community areas. Areas with the greatest proportion of Asian adults and the overall number of Asians living in one of the community areas were identified based on data from the U.S. 2000 Census. Second, AHCI considered its community partners, their proximity to the location of AHCI, and their level of support and interest in local data. Based on these factors, three community areas were selected for the Asian Survey project.

Armour Square, home of Chicago's largest Chinese community and commonly known as Chinatown, was the first community area selected. It was selected for two reasons. First, based on the U.S. 2000 Census, 61% of its residents reported their race or ethnicity to be Asian (Bocskay et al.,

2007). The high concentration of Asians living within a given geographic area best facilitated use of the door-to-door study design that was modeled after the Sinai Survey. In addition, a strong community partner, the Chinese American Service League, is located in this area. They understood the value of health data for the Chinese population it serves and agreed to partner in this endeavor with AHCI. They supported the project with community relations and data collection.

Another community area selected was Albany Park. According to the 2000 U.S. Census, it has the second largest number of Asians overall in Chicago, consisting of Indians, Filipinos, Vietnamese, Koreans, and Cambodians. However, because of the smaller individual population sizes, there are no published Census data about these Asian subgroups. They are instead aggregated into a category of "other." Researchers decided to work with the Cambodian population in this community because of AHCI's longstanding relationship with the Cambodian Association of Illinois, located in this community area. This partner agency has served the Cambodian community since 1976. Unlike the relatively dense residential layout of the Chinese population in the Chinatown neighborhood (in Armour Square), the Cambodian population is geographically dispersed within a diverse community area.

Third, Uptown, located on Chicago's north side, was also chosen to be part of the Asian survey project. Uptown is a diverse community area and historically a home to recent Asian and African immigrants. Based on the 2000 U.S. Census, nearly 13% of Uptown residents are Asian and 7% of the Chicago Asian population resides here (Misra et al., 2005, Bocskay et al., 2007). Uptown was identified as a neighborhood of high need by several local foundations, which carefully assess the social service needs of communities. In 2000, 34% of the Uptown population was foreign-born and 25% lived in poverty. In addition, AHCI and its community partner, the Chinese Mutual Aid Association, are both located in Uptown. Because Vietnamese individuals represent 27% of all Asians residing in Uptown, the largest Asian subgroup, this ethnicity was chosen to be surveyed. Just as with the Cambodian population in Albany Park, the Vietnamese population in Uptown is less concentrated.

To summarize, the three Asian ethnicities (in distinct Chicago communities) targeted were the Chinese population in Armour Square, the Cambodian population in Albany Park, and the Vietnamese population in Uptown (Fig. 5-1). Although the community areas represented the geographic boundaries for the Asian Surveys, the project focused on gathering health information from the three Asian subgroups residing within them. The community areas are referenced by the specific Asian ethnicities (i.e., Chinese, Cambodian, and Vietnamese) in the remainder of this chapter.

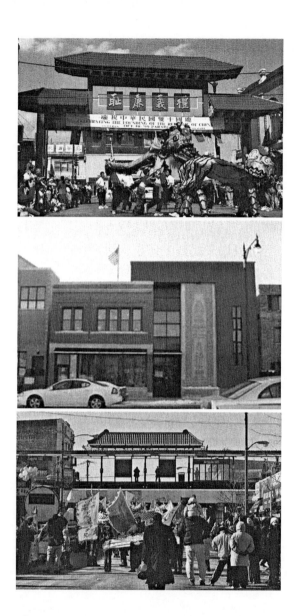

Figure 5-1 Chinese, Cambodian, and Vietnamese Communities in Chicago (Top) Chicago's Chinatown is on the near south side in the Armour Square community area. It is home to number of banks, Chinese restaurants, gift shops, grocery stores, Chinese medicine stores, and so forth. It is a community hub for Chinese people in Chicagoland, a business center for Chinese in the Midwest, as well as a popular destination for tourists and locals alike. (Middle) The Cambodian Association of Illinois is comprehensive social service organization founded in 1976. It was founded by a group of Cambodian refugee volunteers having fled the tyranny, brutality, and torture of the Khmer Rouge genocide in which 2 million people perished. It is the only nonprofit organization in the

Questionnaire Development

The Asian Surveys sought to create a comprehensive questionnaire that would cover a wide variety of health topics while maintaining the ability to compare results to analogous state and national data. Additionally, from the project's inception, AHCI and its partners committed to ensuring that the communities being interviewed would have input into the questionnaire design. Because the local leaders and partner CBO staff know their communities' health needs best, they were recruited to review the survey instrument by participating in the study's Project Advisory Board.

Chinese Health Survey

AHCI initially designed the Chinese Survey based on existing health survey instruments. They first used the Sinai Survey to assess those health topics they wanted to keep (Whitman, Williams, and Shah, 2004). The Sinai Survey was modeled after several national health surveys, including the Centers for Disease Control and Prevention's Behavioral Risk Factor Surveillance System (BRFSS), the National Health and Nutrition Examination Survey (NHANES), and the National Health Interview Survey (NHIS). Most health measures for the Asian Surveys were taken directly from the previously mentioned national surveys. Some questions were taken from other established measures. For example, measures of mental health were taken from the previously validated Center for Epidemiologic Studies-Depression Scale (CES-D). Nutrition questions were derived from NHANES and modified by the Project Advisory Board to offer response choices that were more appropriate for the Chinese community's diet. When appropriate, questions were adapted from New York City Community Health Survey (NYC Department of Health and Mental Hygiene, 2005), which had also been administered with a Chinese population. The survey only included culturally specific questions that the Project Advisory Board determined as important to the Chinese community's health.

The survey instrument was translated and back-translated from English to Chinese, and both versions were modified several times. Both the Chinese and

---

Chicago metropolitan area that provides bilingual programming to address the interrelated social and economic needs of the Cambodian-American population. (Bottom) The elevated train stop on Argyle St. in Uptown, Chicago is on the north side of Chicago. Chicago's Uptown neighborhood is home to many ethnic Chinese Southeast Asian (Vietnamese, Laotian, Cambodian, etc.) residents and businesses.

Sources: Illinois Bureau of Tourism: http://www.enjoyillinois.com/illinoismediacenter/images/pics/HighRes/Chicago/chinatown_festival.jpg; Michael Golamco www.michaelgolamco.com; Uncommon Photographers, Argyle El Stop Online http://www.uncommonphotographers.net/?m=20090203

TABLE 5-1   Topics Included in the Chicago Asian Community Surveys, 2006–2008

Health conditions	Health behaviors and attitudes	Health-care access	Other social or environmental factors
Tuberculosis	Diet/Nutrition	Primary care	Education
Hepatitis	Smoking	Health coverage	Employment
Diabetes	Alcohol	Cancer screening	Income
Hypertension	HIV/STDs	Vaccination	English proficiency
Cholesterol	Obesity	Medication/	Sense of
Other diseases	Accident prevention	Supplements	community[a]
	Mental health		
	Self-rated health		

[a]Only on Cambodian and Vietnamese Asian Surveys.

English versions were pilot-tested in Mandarin and Cantonese among 20 community residents in Armour Square with the help from the community partner. The final set of questions for the initial Chinese community survey contained 159 items and covered a range of health topics detailed in Table 5-1.

Cambodian and Vietnamese Health Surveys

The development of the survey instruments for the Cambodian and Vietnamese populations followed a similar process. First, staff from their respective community organizations met with project staff to review the instrument utilized in Chinatown. The survey for the Cambodian and Vietnamese was identical; additionally, whenever possible the same questions utilized in the Chinese survey were included in the Cambodian and Vietnamese survey instruments. Some questions were removed and others added according to the suggestions of community partners and based on response rates of questions in the Chinese survey.

The principal changes in the Cambodian and Vietnamese survey instruments were to the nutrition and diet section. Rather than documenting the participants' nutritional intake, the questions asked about the nutritional value of certain foods (e.g., "Do you think mangos are high or low in added sugar?"). Questions asked about foods that were common to the Asian diet, such as rice noodles, tofu, and soy milk. Additionally, because the physical activity section had a low response rate in the Chinese survey, it was omitted for the Cambodian and Vietnamese instrument. Finally, a section was added to include the Sense of Community Index in an effort to capture participants' perception of safety and comfort in their community (Chavis and Wandersman, 1990).

A Project Advisory Board for the Cambodian and Vietnamese surveys functioned identically to the Chinatown Board. Members met over a period of

5 weeks and reviewed the project's sampling design, survey instrument, and management plans. Questions on the survey instrument were modified according to the Board's suggestions. The survey instruments were translated into Khmer and Vietnamese and back-translated into English. Additionally, each question was reviewed independently to ensure the meaning was accurately translated. Interviewers pilot-tested the survey instrument informally with approximately 10 community volunteers at each study partner site. Interviewers also practiced the instrument with volunteers from the community organizations and afterward shared any difficulties with the Board. The practice sessions gave interviewers the opportunity to administer the survey questions adhering to protocol guidelines. Moreover, this phase of survey development offered the interviewers and overall project an opportunity to make final changes to specific questions and phrases that were problematic during the practice interviews. The final set of questions for the Cambodian and Vietnamese surveys contained 203 items and included topics listed in Table 5-1.

All three final Asian survey instruments, along with the study protocol and interviewer training materials, were approved by the Sinai Health System Institutional Review Board in Chicago, Illinois.

Survey Administration

The first step of data collection was to choose a scientific sampling method that was feasible for each community. Study staff explored a variety of potential sampling methods. Telephone and Internet surveys were two feasible study designs; however, AHCI felt that many Asian community residents, particularly those with heavier health burdens, would be more receptive to face-to-face interviews. The details of how the Chinese, Cambodian, and Vietnamese individuals were identified and selected to participate in the survey are described below.

Chinese Survey Instrument

As previously mentioned, because the Chinese survey was conducted in the Chinatown neighborhood of Armour Square (where the community was densely populated with Chinese residents), it was possible to conduct random door-to-door sampling. In collaboration with The University of Illinois at Chicago's Survey Research Laboratory (SRL), AHCI implemented a three-stage probability sampling design to gather the most accurate health profile of the Asian population within this community. In the first stage, four census tracts in Armour Square were chosen for having the highest percentage of Asian adults living in the area according to the 2000 U.S. Census. Sampling in these tracts increased the probability that a randomly selected individual was Asian, and most likely Chinese. Next, 30 census blocks were randomly selected among the four census tracts. Utilizing U.S. Postal Service data,

SRL compiled a list of addresses for every household and apartment building on these blocks and assigned identification numbers to each household. Every household on these randomly selected blocks were then approached to participate in the survey as the second stage of the sample. In the third stage, one member from each household was selected using a random selection tool derived from the Troldahl–Carter–Bryant selection matrix (Troldahl and Carter, 1964) for participation in the study. Random selection of household respondents reduced selection bias and enabled a diverse sample of participants by sex and age. The selection matrix insured that household members were selected at random, independent of who answered the door or who was most likely at home during interviewer hours. Household members were eligible if they self-identified as Asian, were at least 18 years of age, provided written informed consent, and lived in the community for at least the past 6 months.

AHCI hired and trained eight interviewers for the Chinese Survey, five of whom were residents of Chinatown. All of the interviewers spoke English and either Cantonese or Mandarin. All interviewers received training on how to follow study protocols, speak about and introduce the project, administer the survey, and gather feedback about the questionnaire's translation, when necessary. The Sinai Urban Health Institute and SRL both assisted with the trainings to provide comments from their experiences in other communities.

Data collection for the Chinese health survey took place in two phases; data was first collected from November 2006 to January 2007 and resumed again from June 2007 to March 2008 because of funding constraints. Interviewers visited a total of 904 households and 572 (63%) of units were eligible (i.e., current residencies). Interviewers subsequently made contact with 447 eligible household members, of which 385 agreed to participate and complete the survey. The participation rate, defined as the number of interviews divided by the number of eligible respondents, was 86.1%. Similarly, the overall response rate, defined as the number of interviews divided by the eligible sample, was 67.2% (American Association of Public Opinion Research, 2006).

The questionnaire took about 45 minutes to complete. Interviewers conducted surveys in the participants' preferred language. Upon completion of the survey, participants received $20 as compensation for their time. Interviewers completed 19 blocks and collected 385 surveys in approximately 7 months of data collection.

Cambodian and Vietnamese Health Survey Instruments

Compared to the Chinese population, the Cambodian and Vietnamese populations were far less densely populated in their respective community areas. The relative dispersion prohibited AHCI from using the door-to-door approach employed for the Chinese Survey. In attempt to maximize resources, survey the largest number of Cambodians and Vietnamese individuals, and maintain scientific sampling, AHCI elected to pilot the use of a relatively new but scientifically established technique known as Respondent-Driven Sampling (RDS) (Heckathorn, 1997).

RDS has emerged as an important scientific sampling method for reaching populations that are traditionally hard to recruit. Similar to snowball sampling, after completing an interview RDS asks participants to invite their peers to join the study. However, RDS collects more information than snowball sampling to ensure random and representative sampling. Typically, three "seeds" are chosen to initiate the survey and then are given recruitment coupons to distribute to their peers. After the seeds are chosen, the only participants eligible for the study are those with a coupon. Each coupon is given a serial number and the relationship between participants and their recruits is recorded.

To begin sample recruitment, RDS seeds (individual respondents) were chosen from a phonebook based on common Cambodian and Vietnamese surnames. Relative to the overall size, two seeds from the Cambodian population and four seeds for the Vietnamese were selected. Each seed was given three coupons printed on color-coded paper. The coupons contained study contact information, eligibility criteria, and a serial number that was linked to the seeds' name in a database. The seeds were asked to distribute the coupons to their peers and instructed that for each coupon brought in by a new eligible participant, the seed would receive $5. Upon completing the survey, each new survey participant received the same instructions.

Eligible participants were 18 years of age or older; self-identified as Cambodian or Vietnamese; spoke English, Khmer, Vietnamese, or Cantonese; provided proof of residency in the designated community areas of Albany Park or Uptown based on zip code; and presented a valid study coupon. Interviewers obtained written informed consent from all new eligible participants. Each returned coupon number was recorded in a database, and according to RDS procedures, all new participants were asked to estimate their social network size and to describe the type of relationship between themselves and the referring participant. After completing the survey, participants were compensated $20 for their time. Recruitment and interviewing went on until the project goals were achieved. By 13 weeks, 150 interviews with Cambodian participants were completed, and in 22 weeks, 250 interviews with Vietnamese participants were completed.

Survey Analyses

To make the data from the surveys more representative of the Asian population from each community area selected, when possible survey design specific weighting techniques were followed. The Chinese Survey data were weighted to the probability of selection and were age-adjusted to the 2000 U.S. standard population. Data from the Cambodian and Vietnamese surveys were weighted to social network size using RDS Analyses Tool (RDSAT) version 5.6 (Volz et al., 2007). These survey data were weighted to respondents' social network sizes to obtain a population based representative sample within each specified geographic area. All data presented in this chapter are weighted and age-adjusted the standard population, unless otherwise noted. Age-adjusted 95% confidence interval estimates were calculated (Keyfitz, 1966).

Results

Sample Characteristics

The demographic characteristics of the three Asian study populations varied (Table 5-2). The Chinese Survey respondents consisted of a large elderly population, more than 37% of the sample was 65 years or older, and more than 15% were 80 years or older. Cambodian survey respondents were younger and more likely to be female. Roughly half of study participants had a

TABLE 5-2   Socio-Demographic Characteristics of Chicago Asian Community Survey Participants

Characteristic Sample Size (n)	Chinese 368%	Cambodian 150%	Vietnamese 250%	U.S. Asian —%
Female	55.8	64.0	58.6	51.7
Age				
18–44 years	28.5	48.7	28.9	57.7
45–64 years	34.3	32.8	45.5	30.5
65+ years	37.2	16.7	25.6	11.7
Education				
High school or more	45.8	45.2	49.3	85.4
Annual household income				
<$30,000 USD	68.9	59.9	80.7	—
Unemployed	18.0	37.8	59.1	3.4
Foreign-born	93.4	80.2	100.0	67.2
10+ years in United States[a]	58.2	55.8	62.7	75.4
Spoken English proficiency[b]				
Less than "very well"	90.3	81.7	97.3	36.1

Sources: Chicago Asian Community Survey Project, 2006–2008; U.S. Asian data come from 2005 to 2007 American Community Survey 3-year estimates for Asians alone.

Notes: All estimates in this table are weighted for the probability of selection.
[a]Among participants who are foreign-born.
[b]Participants who reported their first language was not English were asked to rate their English speaking ability.

high school education or more—notably less than the U.S. national average of 85% for Asians (American Community Survey, 2005–2007 estimate). The substantial majorities in all three communities reported an annual household income less than $30,000 and Vietnamese residents reported a lower income compared to the other respondents. They were also more likely to be unemployed. The vast majority of all three Asian populations were foreign-born, and among them, the majority had lived in the United States for more than 10 years. Compared to U.S. Asians, the study sample were more likely to be recent immigrants and less likely to report English proficiency.

Key Health Outcomes

Results demonstrate specific health-related needs for Chicago's Chinese, Cambodian, and Vietnamese communities. An overview of major health outcomes is presented in this section, with an emphasis on the topics that AHCI and its partners have identified as areas of significant health concern.

Obesity and Diabetes

Although the overall prevalence of obesity is low among Asians, national surveys indicate substantial variation in obesity between different Asian ethnicities (Barnes, Adams, and Powell-Griner, 2008). Survey respondents were asked to report their weight and height and were considered obese if their body mass index (BMI), calculated as weight in kilograms divided by height in meters squared (kg/m^2), based on standard CDC calculations for the U.S. population, was 30 or greater.

Age-adjusted obesity proportions ranged from 2% among Vietnamese respondents to 11% among Cambodian respondents (Table 5-3). These obesity rates are approximately half that of the overall proportions for Chicago (22%) and the United States (26%, not age-adjusted) (CDC, 2008). The Cambodian obesity prevalence was significantly higher than the Chinese and Vietnamese proportions ($p < 0.05$), but similar to the national Asian estimate (9%). Such variation is consistent with national surveys, indicating the need for disaggregating data for different Asian nationalities.

In addition, studies have shown that the increased risk for cardiovascular disease, diabetes, and mortality may be more pronounced at lower BMI values for some Asian populations (Bell, Adair, Popkin, 2002; McNeely and Boyko, 2004; Shai et al., 2006; Wen et al., 2008), suggesting the need to lower the BMI cut-off points to 25 kg/m^2 for obesity (Deurenberg-Yap and Deurenberg, 2003, World Health Organization Expert Consultation, 2004; Razak et al., 2007; World Health Organization, 2009). In fact, when considering this lower cut-off point (BMI > 25), 40% of Cambodians, 33% of

TABLE 5-3   Prevalence of Diabetes and Obesity Among Chinese, Cambodian, and Vietnamese Residents Compared to U.S. Asians

Condition	Chinese % (95% CI)	Cambodian % (95% CI)	Vietnamese % (95% CI)	U.S. Asians % (95% CI)
Obese (BMI ≥30 kg/ m²)	3.9 (1.9, 5.9)	11.4 (6.0, 16.8)	1.9 (0.2, 3.6)	8.9 (7.0, 10.8)
Diagnosed with diabetes	7.1 (4.3, 9.8)	12.0 (6.5, 17.5)	12.9 (8.5, 17.3)	8.9 (6.9, 10.9)

Sources: Data are from the Chicago Asian Community Survey, 2006–2008; U.S. Asian data come from National Health Interview Survey, 2007.

Notes: All estimates in this table are weighted and age-adjusted to the 2000 U.S. Census standard population. The 95% confidence interval estimates were calculated according to Keyfitz, 1966.

Chinese, and 20% of Vietnamese residents were considered be at increased risk of poor health.

In recent years, the prevalence of diabetes among Asians has increased more than other racial and ethnic groups, despite lower BMIs. Studies have shown growing rates of diabetes among Asians, with even slight increases in weight gain (McBeen, Gilbertson, and Collins, 2004; McNeely and Boyko, 2004, Shai et al., 2006). However, limited research exists to determine the obesity and diabetes prevalence among U.S. Asian subgroups and its associated social, cultural, and behavior risk factors. Far less is known about Asians or Asian subgroups in an urban center like Chicago.

The survey asked several questions about diabetes and its associated risk factors with the intention of providing these data to CBOs for improved health programming in this area. Consistent with most national surveys, diabetes was measured by asking whether respondents were ever diagnosed with the condition. Table 5-3 presents the prevalence estimates for each Asian community surveyed compared to the United States.

Age-adjusted estimates of diabetes in the Cambodian and Vietnamese communities were higher than the averages for the United States (8%, BRFSS, 2001, not age-adjusted) overall and U.S. Asians (9%, NHIS 2007, age-adjusted), despite very low rates of obesity. Of particular note, 13% of Vietnamese respondents reported that they had ever been diagnosed with diabetes, but only 2% of respondents were considered obese. The proportion of obese respondents was lower among the Vietnamese compared to the Cambodian and Chinese respondents. For all three Asian Surveys, the diabetes prevalence was higher among women than men (data not shown). The gender difference found in the Asian Surveys was consistent with other research demonstrating a more pronounced increased risk of diabetes among women associated with BMI and weight gain (Shai et al., 2006).

Finally, participants who lived in the United States for more than 10 years had a higher prevalence of obesity and diabetes compared with those who were here for less than 10 years, again consistent with studies from national data (Sanghavi-Goel et al., 2004; Oza-Frank, Stephenson, and Narayan, 2009).

In response to these data trends, the Asian Survey data now offer prevalence estimates for obesity and diabetes for a Cambodian, Chinese, and Vietnamese communities in Chicago. It also draws attention to how obesity rates should be interpreted for some Asian subgroups and what these rates could mean to individuals who may be at increased risk of cardiovascular disease and diabetes. Survey findings also detail other risk factor information about diet- and nutrition-related to Asian specific foods that would be meaningful to shaping community-based interventions that address diabetes and other health problems in these Chicago Asian communities.

Cardiovascular Disease Risk Factors: Hypertension, Cholesterol, and Smoking

Cardiovascular disease is the leading cause of death in the United States. In addition to diabetes, the survey collected information on three of the most important risk factors for cardiovascular disease: hypertension, high cholesterol, and smoking. To assess hypertension, respondents were asked, "Have you ever been told by a doctor, nurse, or other health professional that you have high blood pressure or hypertension?" Respondents were also asked about smoking. Based on the standard definition, "current smokers" were defined by the proportion of respondents who have smoked at least 100 cigarettes in their lifetime and smoke now. These cardiovascular disease questions matched the questions on the CDC's BRFSS in an effort to ensure the data was comparable to Chicago and U.S. figures.

The prevalence of hypertension ranged from 22% among Chinese respondents to 28% among Vietnamese respondents (Table 5-4). All three communities reported proportions of hypertension that were higher than the U.S. Asian estimate of 20% (NHIS, 2007). As expected, an increase in hypertension prevalence was also seen with older age: 24% of participants aged 50 to 65 years and 75% of participants 82 years and older reported hypertension. Interestingly, women were significantly more likely than men to report high blood pressure (35% vs. 18%, not age-adjusted, univariate analysis). This proportion is also double the national estimate for Asian women (15%, BRFSS, 2005, not age-adjusted).

Although proportions reporting high blood pressure were higher than the U.S. average for Asians, the proportions reporting high cholesterol were lower. The prevalences of high cholesterol were 17%, 25%, and 26% for

TABLE 5-4   Prevalence of Cardiovascular Disease Risk Factors Among Participants

Condition	Chinese % (95% CI)	Cambodian % (95% CI)	Vietnamese % (95% CI)	U.S. Asians % (95% CI)
Hypertension	22.1 (18.3, 25.9)	25.7 (18.1, 33.2)	28.4 (22.5, 34.3)	19.5 (17.0, 22.0)
High cholesterol	16.5 (13.3, 19.7)	25.4 (18.4, 32.4)	25.6 (20.9, 30.3)	35.0 (33.3, 36.7)
Current smoker	13.3 (9.7, 16.9)	12.7 (7.4, 18.0)	7.6 (4.4, 10.8)	9.2 (7.4, 11.0)

Sources: Chicago Asian Community Survey, 2006–2008; U.S. Asian data from National Health Interview Survey, 2007 (for hypertension and current smoker) and Behavioral Risk Factor Surveillance System Survey, 2005 (for high cholesterol).

Notes: All estimates in this table are weighted and age adjusted to the 2000 US Census standard population. The 95% confidence interval estimates were calculated according to Keyfitz, 1966.

Chinatown, Cambodian, and Vietnamese, respectively (Table 5-4). The proportion of residents with high cholesterol from all three Asian communities was significantly lower than the national average for Asians (35%).

Based on the 2007 National Health Interview Survey, the proportion of Asian adults that smoke is half that of all adults in the United States (20%, CDC, 2008, not age-adjusted). From the Asian Surveys, smoking prevalence ranged from 8% among Vietnamese respondents to 13% among Chinese respondents, compared to 9% for U.S. Asians (NHIS, 2007, age-adjusted). Although estimates of current smoking in the Asian community appear low, substantial disparities were found by gender. National Asian data indicate that men are far more likely to smoke than women (16% vs. 4%, CDC, 2008). From the Asian Survey, 31% of Chinese and 26% of Cambodian men were also more likely to smoke compared to only 2% of Chinese women and 8% of Cambodian women. The smoking proportions found among Asian men in these two Asian communities are higher than those reported by other racial and ethnic groups nationally (except 37% of NH American Indian/Alaska Native, CDC, 2008).

Health Insurance Coverage

In the United States, insurance coverage ensures appropriate use of healthcare services and, consequently, better health outcomes. Nationally, nonelderly Asians are more likely to be uninsured compared to non-Hispanic Whites. Where limited research on Asian subgroups exists, data indicate some variation in insurance coverage by Asian subgroup (Kaiser Family Foundation, 2008). The Asian surveys sought to determine the level of

TABLE 5-5   Percentage of Chicago Asian Community Survey Participants with Insurance Coverage by Community and Various Subgroups

Insured group	Chinese % (95% CI)	Cambodian % (95% CI)	Vietnamese % (95% CI)	U.S. Asians %
18–64 years	51.1 (44.4, 57.7)	68.9 (59.8, 76.9)	69.9 (63.0, 76.2)	83
65 years and older	92.0 (86.1, 95.9)	90.0 (76.5, 97.7)	95.3 (86.9, 99.0)	98
Male	47.2 (39.4, 55.2)	66.7 (52.5, 78.9)	71.8 (62.1, 80.3)	—
Female	57.1 (50.0, 63.0)	80.2 (70.8, 87.6)	80.3 (72.9, 86.4)	—

Sources: Chicago Asian Community Survey, 2006–2008; U.S. Asian data come from March Current Population Survey, 2004–2006, three year pooled data.

Notes: Estimates in this table are *not* weighted by the sampling probabilities or age-adjusted to a standard population. All 95% CI were calculated using Fischer's Exact Methods.

Reference: Kaiser Family Foundation and APIAHF "Race, Ethnicity and Health Care" Fact Sheet, April 2008.

health insurance in the three communities to better explain how Chinese, Cambodians, and Vietnamese residents access and utilize health-care services in Chicago.

Table 5-5 presents the prevalence estimates of health insurance for the three Asian communities. Less than three-fourths of participants ages 18 to 64 years in all three communities reported some health insurance coverage. The proportion of non-elderly adults who were uninsured was particularly low among the Chinese population (51%). This was likely influenced by the lower percent of respondents in this population with public insurance and the higher proportion that were self-employed compared to Cambodian and Vietnamese respondents (data not shown). Overall, men had lower insurance coverage than women for all three Asian populations. In addition, given the availability of public insurance for seniors, the proportion of respondents age 65 years and older who had insurance coverage was lower than expected in the three surveyed communities.

The Asian Surveys also measured whether residents received culturally and linguistically appropriate services, which is an important factor that likely contributes to racial and ethnic disparities in access to health care. For example, respondents were asked in what language they preferred to communicate with their doctor. The vast majority of the Vietnamese population (89%) preferred to communicate in a language other than English (Vietnamese), followed by 70% of Chinese (Mandarin or Cantonese) and 65% of Cambodians (Khmer). This is consistent with other survey findings indicating that more than 80% of respondents spoke English "less than very well." Few had access to translator services and to compensate in the Chinese community, survey data found that half of respondents reported that they "usually/always" brought a family member or friend to translate for them. These findings have important overall implications to interventions aimed at improving health and, specifically, to informing local health-care delivery systems serving these Asian populations.

Utilization of Cancer Screening and Tests for Various Infectious Diseases

One measure of how well individuals utilize health services is whether they access routine health screenings. The survey thus assessed whether Chinese, Cambodian, and Vietnamese residents had utilized routine cancer screenings and screening tests for infectious diseases.

Survey results identified limited utilization of routine cancer screening as a major health problem. For one, data were examined to determine whether women age 40 years and older had received a mammogram within the last 2 years. Fewer than half of women from the Chinese and Cambodian surveys reported that they had a mammogram in the last 2 years (Table 5-6). These rates were about the same as that of U.S. Asians (54%) but substantially lower than the overall U.S. rate (83%).

Screening for cervical cancer was also an important indicator of health. Table 5-6 presents age-adjusted prevalence of women age 18 years and older who had a Pap smear in the previous 3 years. Similar to mammography

TABLE 5-6   Prevalence of Diagnostic and Preventative Screenings Among Chinese, Cambodian, and Vietnamese Participants

	Chinese % (95% CI)	Cambodian % (95% CI)	Vietnamese % (95% CI)	U.S. Asian %
Had a mammogram in last 2 years[a]	45.7 (43.8, 54.0)	43.0 (34.3, 50.0)	59.0 (53.2, 64.6)	54.0 (47.1, 60.9)
Had a Pap Smear in last 3 years	43.1 (37.9, 48.2)	48.4 (27.9, 67.8)	69.8 (47.8, 85.3)	63.9 (58.6, 69.2)
Ever had a colonoscopy[b]	23.3 (19.1, 28.1)	31.0 (13.4, 52.4)	28.7 (15.8, 44.2)	34.2 (28.1, 40.3)
Ever had an HIV test	13.4 (11.1, 15.7)	24.8 (12.2, 41.6)	26.1 (13.7, 39.6)	30.9 (27.8, 34.0)
Ever been tested for Tuberculosis	59.0 (54.0, 63.9)	69.5 (54.1, 86.7)	87.7 (77.8, 95.5)	—
Ever been tested for Hepatitis B[†]	17.9 (14.3, 22.1)	13.3 (8.6, 19.5)	29.2 (23.8, 35.1)	—

Sources: Chicago Asian Community Survey Project, 2006–2008; U.S. Asian data come from Agency for Healthcare Research and Quality, National Healthcare Disparities Report, 2007.

Notes: Estimates are weighted and age adjusted to the 2000 U.S. population unless otherwise noted (†). 95% confidence intervals were calculated according to Keyfitz, 1966.
[a]Among women ≥ 40 years.
[b]Among adults ≥ 50 years.

utilization, less than half of Chinese and Cambodian women had a routine cervical cancer screening. Cervical cancer screening in all three communities was low compared to the national average of 83% (BRFSS, 2002) and U.S. Asians (64%). Consistent with national data for colon cancer screening, respondents ages 50 years and older were asked if they had ever had a colonoscopy or sigmoidoscopy. Twenty-three percent of Chinese, 31% of Cambodian, and 29% of Vietnamese adults reported a lifetime history of a colonoscopy, compared to 34% of U.S. Asians and 62% of the overall U.S. population (BRFSS 2008, not age-adjusted). For all three Asian populations, women were slightly more likely to report having had a colonoscopy than men.

Finally, participants were asked if they had been tested for three infectious diseases: HIV, tuberculosis, and hepatitis B virus (HBV). Only one-fourth of Cambodian and Vietnamese respondents reported ever receiving an HIV test; this number was even lower among Chinese residents. This is in contrast to one-third of U.S. Asians (NHIS, 2007) who reported having received an HIV test. The majority of respondents received a screening for tuberculosis, but a lower percentage had been screened for HBV. Given the well-documented increased risk of HBV for Asians, the low utilization of HBV screening, particularly among Cambodian and Chinese residents, is most concerning and highlights important work for community-based organizations serving these communities.

Mental Health and Quality of Life

Despite increased efforts to better evaluate minority health concerns, issues of mental health and depression among Asians in the United States are poorly understood (Ma, 2000; Collins et al., 2002). Cause-specific mortality data has shown that suicide rates are far greater among Asians than Whites, especially among Chinese women (Liu and Yu, 1985; Yu, Chang et al., 1985). Data suggest that Asians are less likely to seek help for their mental health problems compared to Whites (Li et al., 1999; Takeuchi et al., 2007). There are significant barriers to meeting their mental health needs, and one study suggests that immigration factors such as age at immigration and time in the United States are associated with mental health disorders (Takeuchi et al., 2007). More research is needed to inform culturally appropriate interventions to address those issues.

The mental health section of the survey included a shortened version (10 items) of the Center of Epidemiologic Studies Depression Scale (CES-D) (Radloff, 1977). The CES-D is a validated scale that covers a range of different types of depressive symptoms. An individual who responds positively

TABLE 5-7   Mental Health Burden and Self-Rated Health among Chinese, Cambodians, and Vietnamese

Characteristic	Chinese % (95% CI)	Cambodian % (95% CI)	Vietnamese % (95% CI)
CES-D 10 (score ≥4)[†]	15.1 (11.2, 19.0)	17.3 (10.6, 24.0)	13.6 (9.0, 18.2)
Responded positive to at least one depressive symptom[†]	83.9 (79.8, 87.5)	88.0 (81.7, 92.7)	63.2 (56.9, 69.2)
Self-rated health (fair/poor)	36.9 (31.1, 42.7)	46.9 (36.7, 57.1)	46.2 (38.5, 53.9)

Sources: Chicago Asian Community Survey, 2006–2008.

Notes: Estimates are weighted and age-adjusted to the 2000 U.S. population unless otherwise noted (†). 95% CI were calculated using Fisher's Exact Method for the depressive symptoms. Self-rated health 95% confidence intervals were calculated according to Keyfitz, 1966.

for at least four questions of the shortened version is considered to be experiencing depressive symptoms, and it suggests that they have a high mental health burden (Whitman, Williams, and Shah, 2004). Nationally, 20% of Black and White adults scored above the threshold for depression (16 or higher on the 20-point CES-D scale) (Jones-Webb and Snowden, 1993).

The majority of participants reported at least one depressive symptom in all three communities (Table 5-7). High mental health burden was observed among 15% Chinese, 17% Cambodian, and 14% Vietnamese respondents. Recent immigrants (those who have lived in the United States for less than 5 years) and those with lower household income (less than $30,000) reported higher mental health burden. Overall, CES-D scores suggest a low burden of mental health; participants in all three surveys reported an average of two depressive symptoms.

Using one last question to assess quality of life, respondents were asked to assess their own health as "excellent," "very good," "good," "fair," or "poor." Studies have shown that one's perception of their own health is predictive of subsequent mortality (Idler and Benyamini, 1997; Benyamini and Idler, 1999; McGee et al., 1999). From the Asian Surveys, 37% of Chinese, 47% of Cambodian, and 46% of Vietnamese respondents reported that their health was "fair" or "poor" (Table 5-7). These proportions were all significantly higher than national estimates for U.S. Asians (11%, NHIS, 2007, age-adjusted). In general, survey findings offer insight into mental health status and quality of life of some Asian communities in Chicago. The data suggest that many are not enjoying life to its fullest and may be experiencing some underlying burden of disease that is not captured by health outcomes measuring disease prevalence only.

Dissemination

AHCI and its partners committed to using data collected from the Asian surveys in a wide variety of public contexts. The key results described here are only a small fraction of the data available and are intended to provide a sample of the type of information now available for Chinese, Cambodian, and Vietnamese communities in Chicago. To translate these data into meaningful programs, several steps were taken to publish and disseminate the Asian Survey findings. Since completing these Asian Surveys, findings have been presented at national conferences, meetings of Chicago community-based organizations, and in public health journals.

Preliminary results from the first few months of the project were presented to the 2007 American Public Health Association (APHA) meeting (Guo et al., 2007, Magee et al., 2007; Shah et al., 2007) and to the 2007 National HIV Conference hosted by the CDC (Magee et al., 2007). In 2008, preliminary findings from the final surveys were presented to the annual APHA meeting (Shah et al., 2008; Cheung et al., 2008) and the International Conference on Urban Health (Guo et al., 2008). Additionally, AHCI and its partners have presented community specific survey results to each of its community-based organization partners, Northwestern University Medical School, University of Illinois at Chicago School of Public Health, and DePaul University.

In addition, as this chapter is being written, a summary report highlighting key findings is being prepared for dissemination to Asian communities in Chicago (The Asian Health Coalition of Illinois, 2010). The report aims to serve as a resource for CBOs writing grants and shaping their community efforts to prevent disease and improve health in the Chinese, Cambodian, and Vietnamese communities of Chicago. The hope is that it will also inspire other Asian subgroups to implement similar health surveys in their neighborhoods.

Bringing appropriate resources to the Asian communities surveyed was also an important goal of the project. Demonstrating the community's specific health needs through scientific surveys was an important first step toward raising local public health funds. Publishing the survey findings in scientific journals is an important means to reach this goal of the project. To date, one article has been published in the *International Journal of Health and Aging Management* (Simon et al., 2008) and another accepted for publication in The Journal of Urban Health (Shah et al., Forthcoming). Future publications will focus on specific health topics—namely, diabetes, cancer screening, and access to care.

Challenges and Lessons Learned

The process of developing and carrying out the Asian Surveys demonstrated many valuable lessons to the stakeholders involved. Although the project was overwhelmingly successful from the perspective of the community members and CBO staff, this success required overcoming challenges. Those that might be useful to consider for others embarking on such local health surveys are described here.

First, the project was directly funded by three distinct types of agencies. AHCI was responsible for seeking grants to fund all aspects of the survey project and did so by submitting grants to the state government, a local nonprofit service organization, and a national nonprofit research organization. Each supporting agency had different grant requirements, and AHCI had to balance the agencies' funding priorities, reporting mechanisms, and schedu les. As a result, the project demanded significant administrative efforts from AHCI, and project staff was required to fill various roles. Additionally, because the project was funded by three agencies over a period of 2 years, the Asian Survey project did not have funding for an interval of four months in 2007 and had to suspend data collection. Future health surveys administered would benefit if the funding stream came from one principal donor (similar to the Sinai Survey, Chapter 4).

Second, attempting to employ rigorous scientific research methodologies was challenging for CBOs that focused on providing direct services. The three CBOs that partnered in this project had strong organizational histories of serving their communities and were committed to the Asian Survey project. Although they provided invaluable input to the survey design and administration, their staff often had competing priorities and other existing programs running concurrently to the Asian Surveys. Without sufficient resources to support additional staff and/or time away from their existing work, the CBO staff was pulled in several directions. Employing scientific methods to capture a representative survey sample required agencies to develop research infrastructure. For future surveys, it will be important to sufficiently fund and support CBOs to partner in such endeavors.

Finally, AHCI's extraordinary effort to capture the health status of the Cambodian and Vietnamese communities in Chicago is notable. They are commended for their innovative approach to adapting RDS methodology because these populations were so disperse and spread out. The novelty of the RDS approach was conducive, for the most part, to meeting the objectives of the Asian Surveys, although it had never been used before in this context. Validation of RDS was not one of the objectives of the survey project, and determining appropriate sample size estimates and analytic techniques for the RDS methods remains a limitation. Nevertheless, the Cambodian and Vietnamese surveys represent the first documented effort to adapt RDS in a community setting beyond its traditional sampling purposes. More research is needed to understand the feasibility of using RDS methodology for other community health surveys.

Conclusions

The Chicago Asian communities are ethnically and culturally diverse, continue to increase in population, and contribute significantly to the city's prosperity. The monitoring of health status and development of adequate health programming are fundamental public health processes essential to creating sustainable and healthy communities for Asians in Chicago. The Asian Survey project sought to assess and accurately document the general health status of three specific Asian subgroups. AHCI and its partners successfully implemented the Asian Surveys with strong community input and participation.

The Asian Surveys identified several areas of health concern for the Chinese, Cambodian, and Vietnamese populations. The prevalence of diabetes was found to be high, especially among Asians who have lived in the United States for more than 10 years. Another concern highlighted in this chapter was the prevalence of risk factors for cardiovascular disease (e.g., hypertension, smoking, and cholesterol) found in the three Asian communities. The cardiovascular disease risk factors were particularly concerning among men surveyed. Despite the prevalence of health risk factors, the reported practice of receiving preventative health screenings was low for the Chinese, Cambodian, and Vietnamese communities. Next, access to care was discussed as a widespread concern for the Asian communities. Finally, survey results suggest that the burden of mental health issues and depression is an area of concern for the surveyed populations.

The Asian Surveys stimulated much discussion and interest from other communities that wanted to conduct research in similar populations. More research is needed to understand the feasibility of using RDS methodology for community research.

The results of the project have already made important contributions to documenting the health needs of Chicago's Chinese, Cambodian, and Vietnamese communities and will continue to be used to leverage support for developing an appropriate program and policy response. The use of local level data to bring awareness, garner financial support, and implement programs targeted at specific health concerns constitutes an empowering and sustainable process for communities. Most importantly, the process of collecting and disseminating data has the potential to improve the health of individuals at the local community level.

Acknowledgments

Many persons and organizations were instrumental to the planning, implementation, and documentation of the Asian health surveys. The authors would first like to thank the staff of Asian Health Coalition of Illinois for their contributions—namely, William Cheung and Sandhya Krishnan, Project Coordinators. Implementing the surveys in each respective community would not have been possible without the executive directors and staff at the Chinese American Service league, Cambodian Association of Illinois, and Chinese Mutual Aid Association. In addition, the tireless work of the project interviewers who were critical to the survey's success, particularly Tola Chuon and Sarouen Soeun from the Cambodian Association of Illinois and Huy Tran from the Chinese Mutual Aid Association. Additional support was also provided by Survey Research Laboratory of the University of Illinois at Chicago, most notably Karen Retzer, Ingrid Graf, and Timothy Johnson. Finally, the staff of Sinai Urban Health Institute played a critical role assisting with all data management and entry, notably Sheena Freeman.

Notes

1. The authors recognize the importance of including and defining Asian, Asian American, and Asian and Pacific Islander American correctly; moreover, they know that individuals conceptualize and characterize their race and ethnicity differently. The Chicago Asian Community Surveys focused on Chinese, Cambodian, and Vietnamese populations, and this chapter uses the term Asian to describe these three races. However, the authors intend this term to be inclusive of persons who consider their race to be Asian, Asian American, Asian and Pacific Islander American, or a combination of these and other races. The term Asian is used for brevity and to avoid repeating acronyms.
2. In addition, as this chapter is being written, a summary report highlighting key findings is being prepared for dissemination to Asian communities in Chicago.
3. To date, one article has been published in the International Journal of Health and Aging Management (Simon et al., 2008), and additional articles are under review.

References

American Association for Public Opinion Research. 2006. *Standard Definitions: Final Dispositions of Case Codes and Outcome Rates for Surveys*, 4th ed. Lenexa, KS.
The Asian Health Coalition of Illinois. *Chicago Asian Community Surveys: A Comprehensive Report*. Chicago, Illinois: Asian Health Coalition of Illinois, 2010.

Barnes, Patricia M., Patricia F. Adams, and Eve Powell-Griner. 2008. Health characteristics of the Asian adult population: United States, 2004–2006. *Advance Data from Vital and Health Statistics* 394 (January 22).

Bell, A. Colin, Linda S. Adair, and Barry M. Popkin. 2002. Ethnic differences in the association between body mass index and hypertention. *American Journal of Epidemiology* 155:346–353.

Benyamini, Yael and Ellen L. Idler. 1999. Community studies reporting association between self-rated health and mortality: Additional studies, 1995 to 1998. *Research on Aging* 21; 3 (May):392–401.

Bocskay Kirsti A., Dana M. Harper-Jemison, Kevin P. Gibbs, Kingsley Weaver, and Sandra D. Thomas. 2007. *Community Area Health Inventory, Part One: Demographic and Health Profiles*. Health Status Index Series Vol. XVI, No. V. Chicago, IL: Chicago Department of Public Health Office of Epidemiology.

Centers for Disease Control and Prevention. 2008. State-specific prevalence of obesity among adults in the United States, 2007. *Morbidity and Mortality Weekly Report* 57(28):765–768.

Centers for Disease Control and Prevention. 2008. Cigarette smoking among adults— United States, 2007. *Morbidity and Mortality Weekly Report* 57(45):1221–1226.

Chavis, David M. and Abraham Wandersman. 1990. Sense of community in the urban environment: A catalyst for participation and community development. *American Journal of Community Psychology* 18(1):55–81.

Cheung, William, Matthew Magee, Ami Shah, Lucy Guo, Hong Liu, and Steve Whitman. 2008. Respondent Driven Sampling (RDS) in Asian American health research: Preliminary recruitment analysis from a community health survey in Chicago's Cambodian and Vietnamese neighborhoods. Presented at the 136th Annual Meeting of the American Public Health Association, San Diego, October 25–29.

Collin, Karen Scott, Dora L. Hughes, Michelle M. Doty, Brett L. Ives, Jennifer N. Edwards, and Katie Tenney. 2002. Diverse communities, common concerns: Assessing health care quality for minority Americans. The Commonwealth Fund. March, 2002. Online. Available: http://www.commonwealthfund.org/~/media/Files/Publications/Fund%20 Report/2002/Mar/Diverse%20Communities%20%20Common%20Concerns%20 %20Assessing%20Health%20Care%20Quality%20for%20Minority%20Americans/ collins_diversecommun_523%20pdf.pdf. Accessed December 15, 2009.

Deurenberg-Yap, Mabel and Paul Deurenberg. 2003. Is a re-evaluation of WHO body mass index cut-off values needed? The case of Asians in Singapore. *Nutrition Reviews* 61(1):80–88.

Guo, Lucy, Ami M. Shah, William Cheung, Matthew J. Magee, and Hong Liu. 2008. Are Asian and Pacific Islander Women in Chicago receiving appropriate cancer screening? Results from 3 community health surveys. Presented at the 7th International Conference on Urban Health, Vancouver, October 29–31.

Guo, Lucy, Mathew Magee, Ami M. Shah, Steve Whitman, Hong Liu, and Sandhya Krishnan. 2007. Measuring stigmatized mental health issues in an Asian community: Preliminary results from Chicago's Chinatown community survey. Presented at the 135th Annual Meeting of the American Public Health Association, Washington DC, November 3–7.

Heckathorn, Douglas. 1997. Respondent-driven sampling: A new approach to the study of hidden populations. *Social Problems* 44(2):174–199.

Idler, Ellen L. and Yael Benyamini. 1997. Self-rated health and mortality: A review of twenty-seven community studies. *Journal of Health and Social Behavior* 38:21–37.

Jones-Webb, Rhonda J. and Lonnie R. Snowden. 1993. Symptoms of depression among Blacks and Whites. *American Journal of Public Health* 83(2):240–244.

Kaiser Family Foundation, 2008. Race, ethnicity and health care. Fact Sheet (Publication #7745). April. Online. Available: http://www.kff.org/minorityhealth/upload/7745.pdf. Accessed December 10, 2009.

Keyfitz, Nathan. 1966. Sampling variance of standardized mortality rates. *Human Biology* 38:309–317.

Li, Pui-Ling, Stuart Logan, Lydia Yee, and Sarah Ng. 1999. Barriers to meeting the mental health needs of the Chinese community. *Journal of Public Health Medicine* 21:74–80.

Liu, William T. and Elena Yu. 1985. Asian/Pacific American elderly: Mortality differentials, health status, and use of health services. *Journal of Applied Gerontology* 4:35–64.

Ma, Grace X. 2000. Barriers to the use of health services by Chinese Americans. *Journal of Allied Health* 29:64–70.

Magee, Matthew J., Kristi L. Allgood, Ami M. Shah, Sandhya Krishnan, Dahlia Christiansen, and Hong Liu. 2007. Lifetime history of HIV testing is lower among South Chinatown residents in Chicago than other community neighborhoods. Presented at the National HIV Prevention Conference, Atlanta, December 2–5.

Magee, Matthew J., Ami M. Shah, Sandhya Krishnan, Steve Whitman, and Hong Liu. 2007. Key health indicators from Chicago's Chinatown: Preliminary analysis of health disparities from an ongoing community health survey. Presented at the 135th Annual Meeting of the American Public Health Association, Washington DC, November 3–7.

McBean, A. Marshall, Shuling Li, David T. Gilbertson, and Allan J. Collins. 2004. Differences in diabetes prevalence, incidence, and mortality among the elderly of four racial/ethnic groups: Whites, Blacks, Hispanics and Asians. *Diabetes Care* 27:2317–2324.

McGee, Daniel L., Youlian Liao, Guichan Cao, and Richard S. Cooper. 1999. Self-reported health status and mortality in a multiethnic U.S. cohort. *American Journal of Epidemiology* 149:41–46.

McNeely, Marguerite J. and Edward J. Boyko. 2004. Type 2 diabetes prevalence in Asian Americans: Results of a national health survey. *Diabetes Care* 27(1):66–69.

Misra, Shyam, Kirsti. Bocskay, Antigone Kouvelis, and Sandra Thomas. 2005. *Demographic and Health Profile of the Chicago Asian Community 2000.* Chicago, IL: Chicago Department of Public Health Epidemiology Program.

New York City Department of Health and Human Hygiene. 2005. New York City Community Health Survey. Community health survey questionnaire. Online. Available: http://www.nyc.gov/html/doh/downloads/pdf/episrv/neighborhood-2005.pdf. Accessed November 10, 2009.

Oza-Frank, Reena, Rob Stephenson, and Venkat Narayan. 2009. Diabetes prevalence by length of residence among U.S. immigrants. *Journal of Immigrant Health* Online: 18 August 2009: DOI: 10.1007/s10903-009-9283-2).

Petersen, William. 1966. Success Story, Japanese-American Style. *The New York Times Magazine.* Section 6: January 9, pp. 20–43.

Razak, Fahad, Sonia S. Anand, Harry Shannon, Vladamir Vuksan, Bonnie Davis, Ruby Jacobs, et al. 2007. Defining obesity cut points in a multiethnic population. *Circulation* 115(16):2111–2118.

Radloff, Lenore S. 1977. The CES-D scale: A self-report depression scale for research in the general population. *Applied Psychological Measurement* 1:385–401.

Sanghavi-Goel, Mita, Ellen P. McCarthy, Russell S. Phillips, and Christina C. Wee. 2004. Obesity among U.S. immigrant subgroups by duration of residence. *Journal of American Medical Association* 292:2860–2867.

Shah, Ami M., Matthew J. Magee, Sandhya Krishnan, Steve Whitman and Hong Liu. 2007. Presented at the 135th Annual Meeting of the American Public Health Association, Washington DC, November 3–7.

Shah, Ami M., Matthew J. Magee, Lucy Guo, William Y. Cheung, Sheena Freeman, Hong Liu, et al. 2008. Measuring progress toward the HP2010 goals: Cancer screening in two Chicago Asian populations. Presented at the 136th Annual Meeting of the American Public Health Association, San Diego, October 25–29.

Shah, Ami M. and Steven Whitman. 2010. Sinai Health System's Improving Community Health Survey: Methodology and key findings. In: *Urban health: Combating Disparities with Local Data.* eds. Whitman, Steve, Ami M. Shah, and Maureen R. Benjamins. New York, NY: Oxford University Press.

Shah AM, Lucy Guo, Matthew Magee, William Cheung, Melissa Simon, Amanda LaBreche and Hong Liu. "Comparing Selected Measures of Health Outcomes and Health-Seeking Behaviors in Chinese, Cambodian and Vietnamese Communities of Chicago: Results from Local Health Surveys." *Journal of Urban Health.* doi:10.1007/s11524-010-9469-x.

Shai, Iris, Rui Jiang, JoAnn E. Manson, Meir J. Stampfer, Walter C. Willett, Graham A. Colditz, et al. 2006. Ethnicity, obesity, and risk of type 2 diabetes in women: A 20-year follow-up study. *Diabetes Care* 29(7):1585–1590.

Simon, Melissa A., Mathew J. Magee, Ami M. Shah, Lucy Guo, Williams Cheung, Hong Liu, et al. 2008. Building a Chinese community health survey in Chicago: The value of involving the community to more accurately portray health. *International Journal of Health and Aging Management* 2(December):40–53.

Tao, Laurent S., Jini Han, Ami M. Shah. 2006. Measuring state-level Asian American and Pacific Islander health disparities: The case of Illinois. *Asian American Pacific Islander Nexus* 4(1):81–96.

Takeuchi, David T., Nolan Zane, Seunghye Hong, David H. Chae, Fang Gong, Gilbert C. Gee, et al. 2007. Immigration-related factors and mental disorders among Asian Americans. *American Journal of Public Health* 97:84–90.

Troldahl Verling C. and Roy E. Carter. 1964. Random selection of respondents within households in phone surveys. *Journal of Marketing Research* 1:71–76.

Volz, Eric, Cyprian Wijnert, Ismail Degani, and Douglas D. Heckathorn. 2007. Respondent Driven Sampling Analyses Tool (RDSAT) Version 5.6. Itasca, NY: Cornell University.

Walter, Ashley, ed. *Strategy in Action: Eliminating Health Disparity in Illinois.* Illinois Public Health Futures Institute, 2004.

Wen, Chi Pang, Ting Yuan David Cheng, Shan Pou Tsai, Hui Ting Chan, Hui Ling Hsu, Chih Cheng Hsu, et al. 2008. Are Asians at greater mortality risks for being overweight than Caucasians? Redefining obesity for Asians. *Public Health Nutrition* 12(4):497–506.

Whitman, Steven, Cynthia Williams, and Ami M. Shah. 2004. Sinai Health System's Improving Community Health Survey: Report 1. Chicago, IL: Sinai Health System.

World Health Organization. 2009. Global database on body mass index: BMI classification. Online. Available: http://apps.who.int/bmi/index.jsp?introPage=intro_3.html. Accessed December 3, 2009.

World Health Organization Expert Consultation. 2004. Appropriate body-mass index for Asian populations and its implications for policy and intervention strategies. *Lancet* 363(9403):157–163.

Yu, Elena, Ching-Fu Chang, William Liu, and Stephan Kan. 1985. Asian-white mortality differentials: are there excess deaths? In *Report of the Secretary's Task Force on Black Minority Health*, ed. Margaret M. Heckler. Washington, DC: Department of Health and Human Services, pp. 209–254.

6

COMPARING THE HEALTH STATUS OF TEN CHICAGO COMMUNITIES

Ami M. Shah

Introduction

Over the course of 6 years, survey data—the first of its kind—were gathered from 10 local communities in Chicago (Shah and Whitman, 2010; Benjamins, 2010; Magee et al., 2010). Each survey captured the health status of diverse racial and ethnic populations living in different geographic areas of the city. The data helped highlight health concerns and risk factors associated with distinct communities and explain how a given population experienced health. The community health surveys responded to the need for local level data in urban centers (Simon et al., 2001), offering pertinent information on how to shape community-based interventions and bring greater resources to poor and underserved neighborhoods.

In addition to understanding the health of individual communities, comparing the health of different communities within a given city proved to be an important strategy for uncovering and examining disparities. Such intra-urban study offers insight into a population's health in relative terms (Galea and Schulz, 2006). It reflects the manner in which health is experienced and resources are optimally allocated, which in turn affects overall health outcomes.

This chapter has three goals. First, it briefly compares and contrasts the methods and approaches employed to conduct ten community health surveys in Chicago. Second, it examines five key results for the diverse communities surveyed. Third, the chapter illustrates the value of the community

survey data and comments on its implications for broader policies and programs in striving toward equitable health for all racial and ethnic groups
within an urban setting.

Background

The city of Chicago is divided into community areas (CAs). In the 1920s,
sociologists from the University of Chicago defined 75 CAs roughly corresponding to generally recognized neighborhoods existing at that time. Since
then, there have been two revisions. The O'Hare airport area was annexed
by the city and one community area was divided into two. Today there are
77 officially designated Chicago CAs (The Chicago Fact Book Consortium,
1995). CAs often serve as loci for describing health in Chicago, implementing community-based interventions, and allocating public health resources.

The boundaries of the CAs are aligned with Census tracks and some surveillance health data. For example, data from vital records and communicable disease registries can be geocoded to the CA level and have shown
substantial variation in health outcomes between some CAs (Whitman et al.,
2004). However, disease prevalence and risk factor data are not available at
the community area level. Such information would describe health behaviors
and other more recently defined social determinants of health. It would offer
suggestions about the causes of poor health and insight into where and how
to develop effective community-based interventions. Although such information would be valuable, it is rarely available.

In response to the need for such local data, a comprehensive health survey
was first conducted in six diverse Chicago communities. The communities
were selected for study based on the homogeneity of their racial and ethnic
demographics, their geographic location, and the community's demand for
local health data. This survey, called the *Sinai's Improving Community Health
Survey* (Sinai Survey), was one of the largest population-based, door-to-door
community health surveys in Chicago. The original survey, funded by The
Robert Wood Johnson Foundation, was administered in 2002 to 2003 in six
Chicago community areas. As detailed in Chapter 3 (Shah and Whitman, 2010),
the Sinai Survey was implemented by the Sinai Urban Health Institute (SUHI)
and its many community partners. More specifically, the Sinai Survey captured
the health of a White community on the north side (Norwood Park), two predominantly Black communities (North Lawndale and Roseland) on the west
and south sides, and a predominantly Mexican community (South Lawndale).
Also included are two racially/ethnically mixed communities (Humboldt Park
and West Town), which house the largest concentration of Puerto Ricans in
Chicago. Figure 6-1 presents a map of these geographic areas.

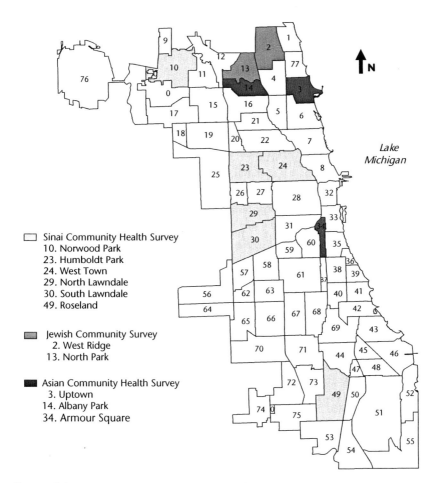

Figure 6-1   Chicago's 77 Community Areas: Chicago Communities with Local Area Health Survey Data

As preliminary findings from the Sinai Survey were disseminated, the value of local health information became apparent to other communities. To begin, the Jewish Federation of Metropolitan Chicago was inspired by the impact of the Sinai Survey to pursue a similar health assessment for its community in 2003. The Federation, which is the largest not-for-profit social welfare institution in Illinois and the hub of Chicago's Jewish community, convened Jewish community leaders and members to design a *Jewish Community Health Survey* (Jewish Survey), as detailed in Chapter 4 (Benjamins, 2010). They identified the geographic area with the largest concentration of Jewish individuals to be surveyed, selecting several neighborhoods that crossed two Chicago community areas: North Park and West Ridge (Fig. 6-1).

Similarly, the Asian Health Coalition of Illinois witnessed the usefulness of local data and took the initiative to gather data about three Asian communities (Chapter 6). First, they worked with community partners to target Chicago's Chinatown, which is part of the Armour Square CA, comprised of the largest concentration of Asians in Chicago. Thereafter, another survey was designed to be administered to the Cambodian population in Albany Park and the Vietnamese population in Uptown. These Asian communities were smaller in overall population size and were less concentrated within a given geographic area. To obtain a random sample of these populations, unique recruitment methods were employed in partnership with community-based organizations. From 2006 to 2008, a local health survey was administered by the *Chicago Asian Community Surveys* (Asian Survey) project in these three Asian communities, capturing the health of the Chinese, Vietnamese, and Cambodian populations residing in Armour Square, Uptown, and Albany Park, respectively (Magee et al., 2010).

In the end, surveys were completed in 10 Chicago communities (Fig. 6-1). Although the designated Chicago CA boundaries may not always be consistent with the distinct racial and ethnic group's community, or neighborhood, they are important to geocoding existing health data. For these purposes, they simply provide a context to understand the surveyed population. Table 6-1 outlines the designated Chicago CAs and the unique racial and ethnic group represented by each survey.

TABLE 6-1   Racial and Ethnic Groups Represented Within the Selected Chicago Community Areas

Survey	Chicago Community Area Surveyed (*Colloquial Names*)	Predominant Racial/ Ethnic Group
Sinai's Improving Community Health Survey, 2002–2003	Humboldt Park	50% Black, 25% Puerto Rican, 25% Mexican
	West Town	50% White, 25% Puerto Rican, 25% Mexican
	South Lawndale (*Little Village*)	Mexican
	North Lawndale	Black
	Roseland	Black
	Norwood Park	White
Jewish Community Health Survey, 2003	North Park/West Ridge (*West Rogers Park/Peterson Park*)	White, Jewish
Chicago Asian Community Health Surveys, 2006–2008	Armour Square (*Chinatown*)	Chinese
	Albany Park	Cambodian
	Uptown	Vietnamese

Methods

From 2002 to 2008, four major surveys were designed and implemented to gather health data about 10 communities: the Sinai Survey, Jewish Survey, Chicago Asian Chinese Survey, and the Chicago Asian Cambodian/Vietnamese Surveys. Roughly two-thirds of the survey instruments had questions with identical wording, comparable to national health surveys (e.g., Behavioral Risk Factor Surveillance System [BRFSS] Survey, National Health Interview Survey [NHIS]). The remaining questions were culturally appropriate and sensitive to the unique histories and health concerns of the specific community. All of the health surveys were comprehensive and asked questions about disease prevalence and various risk factors, although some included more questions than others. For example, the Sinai and Jewish Surveys included about 500 questions, comprised of an adult and child module, and took a little over 1 hour to complete. They were conducted using computer-assisted programming (CAPI). The three Asian surveys included between 160 and 200 questions, comprised of an adult module only, and took about 45 minutes to complete. They were administered by hand (i.e., paper surveys) and face-to-face by trained interviewers. They were offered in several different languages, each appropriate to the community surveyed. Although the Cambodian and Vietnamese Surveys were administered in different languages, they had identical questions and employed the same methodology. Table 6-2 compares and contrasts the different methods employed.

The sampling scheme shaped how the survey would be administered. It also determined what geographic and racial and ethnic population the sample selected would represent. For the Sinai Survey, individuals were selected to participate based on age (18–75 years) and place of residence. Although the survey instrument included questions on race and ethnicity, these data were not used as criteria for survey participant eligibility. The Sinai Survey data are thus representative of the population defined by the geographic boundaries of each Chicago CA.

The Jewish and Asian surveys had slightly different sampling schema. Inclusion criteria were based not only on age (18 years and older) and place of residence but also on self-identification to a specific religious group and/or nationality (e.g., place of origin). For these surveys, the data are representative of a population that self-identified as Jewish, Cambodian, or Vietnamese living within a defined geographic area or neighborhood.

In addition, the size of the population was considered when determining how best to locate individuals to be surveyed. For example, in conducting the Sinai, Jewish, and Chinatown Surveys, there were enough individuals to be surveyed with a common racial and ethnic or religious background who lived within a relatively small geographic area. These areas or

TABLE 6-2 Comparison of Chicago Community Health Survey Methods: Survey Instrument, Sampling Frame, Data Collection, Administration and Analysis

	Sinai's Improving Community Health Survey, 2002–2003	Jewish Community Health Survey, 2003	Chinese Asian Survey, 2006–2008	Cambodian and Vietnamese Asian Surveys, 2006–2008
Survey instrument	Adult module included 469 questions, child module included 100 questions	Adult module included 475 questions, child module included 100 questions	Adult module only, 159 questions	Adult module only, 203 questions
Sampling frame	Three-stage probability sampling design from six Chicago community areas (Humboldt Park, Norwood Park, North Lawndale, Roseland, South Lawndale and West Town)	Three-stage probability sampling design from designated blocks with high concentrations of Jewish families in two Chicago community areas (West Rogers Park and Peterson Park)	Three stage probability sampling design from four tracts with highest concentration of Asians (>50%) in the Armour Square community area; From these combined tracts, selected random blocks and all households were approached	Respondent-Driven Sampling; Two "seeds" (individuals selected to initiate the survey) identified for Cambodian population and four "seeds" for Vietnamese population using common surnames from the telephone book
Final data represent	Population living in the designated community area surveyed	A Jewish population living in the designated block area between West Rogers Park and Peterson Park	An Asian population living in the designated block area, which comprises Chinatown, assumed to be predominantly Chinese	A Cambodian and Vietnamese population living in the designated community area of Albany Park and Uptown, respectively

Eligibility	18–75 years of age; Resided in one of the six selected community areas	18 years and older; Self-identified as Jewish	18 years and older; Self-identified as Chinese or Asian, and lived in the Armour Square community for at least the last six months	18 years and older; Self-identified as Cambodian or Vietnamese; Proof of residency in Albany Park or Uptown based on zip code, respectively; Presented with a valid study coupon from a referring participant (starting with the seeds)
Survey administration	Interviewed in English or Spanish; Participants received on average $50 along with a packet of health information	Interviewed in English only; Participants received $20	Interviewed in English, Mandarin, and Cantonese; 96% of interviews conducted in Mandarin or Cantonese; Participants received $20	Interviewed in English, Khmer, Vietnamese, or Cantonese; Participants received $20, plus $5 for each of the three coupons that resulted in another survey participant (maximum $35)

(Continued)

TABLE 6-2 (Continued)

	Sinai's Improving Community Health Survey, 2002–2003	Jewish Community Health Survey, 2003	Chinese Asian Survey, 2006–2008	Cambodian and Vietnamese Asian Surveys, 2006–2008
Data collection	Face-to-face interviews; Gathered data using CAPI between September 2002 and April 2003; Completed 1,699 interviews with adults and 811 interviews with caregivers of children; Response rate = 43%	Face-to-face interviews; Gathered data using CAPI between August 2003 and January 2004; Completed 201 interviews with Jewish adults and 57 caregivers of Jewish children; Response rate = 51%	Face-to-face interviews; Data gathered by hand (paper-surveys) between November 2006 and January 2007; and June 2007 and March 2008; Completed 385 interviews with Asian adults; Response rate = 67%	Collected face-to-face by hand (paper-surveys) between September 2007 and March 2008; Completed 150 interviews with Cambodian adults within 13 waves over 12 weeks; 250 interviews with Vietnamese adults within 35 waves over 21 weeks
Data analysis	Employed probability of selection and post-stratification weights based on sex, age, and race of 2000 U.S. Census	Employed probability of selection weights	Employed probability of selection weights	Employed weights based on social network size

neighborhoods were well-defined (either by Chicago CA boundaries or by a community organization). From the designated geographic area, randomly selected blocks, households, and individuals were then selected. This, however, was not the case for the Cambodian and Vietnamese surveys. These populations were relatively small and not as concentrated in one geographic area. Thus, a unique sampling technique, respondent-driven sampling, was employed to obtain (what is as close as possible to) a representative sample of these minority populations. The final data gathered from these surveys are representative of the Cambodian and Vietnamese populations within the zip codes defined as part of the inclusion criteria. Additional details about each survey methodology employed are available in earlier chapters of this book (Shah and Whitman, 2010, Benjamins, 2010, Magee et al., 2010).

Statistical software was used to adjust for effects of the complex sampling design for the Sinai Survey, the Chinatown Survey, and the Jewish Surveys (SAS Institute Inc., 2004; Stata Corporation, 2003). All estimates were weighted for the probability of selection. The Sinai Survey also included a post-stratification weight to ensure that the sample resembled the distribution of age, sex, and race from each CA's population according to the 2000 U.S. Census. Post-stratification weights were not employed for the Jewish and Asian surveys because no reliable comparable data for such groups were available. Data from the Cambodian and Vietnamese surveys were analyzed using Respondent Driven Sampling Analyses Tool (RDSAT) version 5.6 (Volz et al., 2007). These survey data were weighted to respondents' social network sizes to obtain a population based representative sample within each specified geographic area.

All data presented are age-adjusted to the 2000 U.S. Standard Population.[1] Ninety-five percent confidence intervals (CIs) were estimated for all response items using statistical software, when possible, and by hand according to Keyfitz estimation (Keyfitz, 1966) when not possible. Two proportions were deemed statistically different from one another if their CIs did not overlap.

Comparison and Interpretation of Survey Results

Demographic Characteristics

Table 6-3 presents the demographic characteristics of the 10 communities surveyed. For all the data tables that follow, the 10 communities are presented in a specific order based first on completion of the survey (i.e., Sinai Survey, Jewish Survey, and Asian Surveys) and second by their racial and ethnic composition. A brief description of each follows.

First, there are two racially and ethnically diverse communities of Humboldt Park and West Town (Table 6-1). They increasingly face urban

TABLE 6-3 Demographic Characteristics of Ten Chicago Communities Survey, 2002–2008

Community Area	Humboldt Park	West Town	South Lawndale	North Lawndale	Roseland	Norwood Park	West Ridge and North Park	Armour Square	Albany Park	Uptown
Total Population	65,836	87,435	91,071	41,768	52,723	37,669	270,500[a]	7318[b]	10199[b]	8206[b]
Sample Size	300	303	300	304	302	190	201	368	150	250
Race/Ethnicity (%)										
NH White	3	40	10	1	0	88	100	—	—	—
NH Black	47	9	6	94	98	0	—	—	—	—
Hispanic-Mexican	25	25	77	1	0	2	—	—	—	—
Hispanic-Puerto Rican	18	17	1	0	0	1	—	—	—	—
Asian-Chinese	—	—	—	—	—	—	—	100	—	—
Asian-Vietnamese	—	—	—	—	—	—	—	—	—	100
Asian-Cambodian	—	—	—	—	—	—	—	—	100	—
Female (%)	52	47	39	58	56	52	52	56	64	59
Age (%)										
18–44 yrs	68	75	78	63	54	50	39	29	49	29
45–64 yrs	24	22	19	30	30	39	41	34	33	46
65+ yrs	8	3	3	7	16	12	21	37	17	26

Annual household income (%)									
<$30,000	65	47	70	73	53	5	14	69	60	81
$30,000–69,999	31	37	27	26	35	50	38	31[c]	40[c]	19[c]
≥$70,000	4	16	3	1	11	46	47	—	—	49
High school graduate or higher (%)	60	75	44	74	78	96	99	46	45	49
Unemployed (%)	47	33	38	49	53	34	40[d]	18	38	59
Foreign-born (%)	34	31	71	1	1	20	20	93	80	100

Sources: Total Population estimates come from the 2000 U.S. Census; Sinai's Improving Community Health Survey 2002–2003; Jewish Community Health Survey 2003; Chicago Asian Health Surveys, 2006–2008.

Notes: All data are weighted for the probability of selection to account for the complex survey design. The Sinai Survey also includes poststratification weights based on the 2000 U.S. Census.
Sinai survey respondents had a maximum age of 75 years.
Percentages may not add up to 100 because of rounding.
Race/Ethnicity categories do not include other Hispanic, Hispanic Origin Unknown, or Other from the Sinai Survey.
Race/Ethnicity was self-reported as part of the screener to determine eligibility for the *Jewish and Asian Surveys*.
[a]Approximate number of Jews in the Chicago metropolitan area.
[b]Estimates for Asians from 2000 U.S. Census.
[c]Estimates include those making ≥ $70,000; Only data above and below $30,000 are available.
[d]Estimate for unemployed does not distinguish retired persons.

redevelopment and gentrification, along with the influx of immigrants, resulting in a change in population demographics. A greater proportion of households in Humboldt Park had an annual household income of less than $30,000 compared to its contiguous community of West Town. West Town has already gentrified, with about half of its population being younger White adults with an annual household income greater than $30,000.

The following four communities shown in Table 6-3 are racially and ethnically homogenous. These include South Lawndale (mostly Mexican), North Lawndale and Roseland (mostly Black), and Norwood Park (mostly White). To distinguish the two Black communities, North Lawndale is on the west side of the city, where SUHI is located, and is one of the poorest communities surveyed. Roseland is on the south side of Chicago, older, and has a higher socio-economic status than North Lawndale.

Norwood Park is on the north side of Chicago and has the one of the highest proportions of adults in Chicago with an average household income greater than $70,000. The other mostly White group is the Jewish community that includes portions of two officially designated CAs: North Park and West Ridge, often referred to as "West Rogers Park and Peterson Park" among local residents. This community is also older than the other minority (non-White) communities, like Norwood Park. Jewish residents surveyed in North Park and West Ridge are similar in income and education to residents of Norwood Park. However, although not shown here, because the majority of the Jewish residents surveyed were Orthodox Jews, the households tended to have a larger-than-average family size. Thus almost half reported having insufficient funds for several basic needs, such as health care and education (Benjamins, 2007). The overall socio-economic status of the Jewish community, when taking the household composition into consideration, may not be as high as assumed at first glance, especially when compared to Norwood Park.

Finally, the three Asian communities are shown (Table 6-3). The Chinese population surveyed had the greatest proportion of older adults compared with any other community, and the Cambodian population tended to be younger than the other Asian populations. The Vietnamese population was by far the poorest of all 10 communities, with 81% of the population reporting an annual household income of less than $30,000. In addition, they reported the highest proportion of adults who were unemployed (59%) and foreign-born (100%).

Five Key Health Measures

Although there were literally hundreds of different health measures on the surveys, five key health outcomes were selected for illustrative examination and comparison: health insurance, obesity, diabetes, smoking, and breast cancer screening. These were selected to represent common measures of chronic diseases, health behaviors, and access to services. Health data are presented for each community surveyed and compared to Chicago or U.S. estimates, depending on what was available.

Health Insurance Coverage

Individuals without health insurance are less likely to have a usual source of care, to use preventive or specialty services, to obtain needed prescription medications, or to receive high-quality services. As a result, they are at increased risk of poor health outcomes and death. There were several questions included on the community surveys about access to health services. For these analyses, data on health insurance coverage were examined. All respondents were asked, "Do you currently have any type of health insurance or medical coverage?" This is a standard question used in national surveys (e.g., BRFSS, NHIS, and Medical Expenditure Panel Survey [MEPS]). Figure 6-2 presents the proportions of individuals ages 18 to 64 years who reported that they currently had any type of insurance coverage for each of the 10 communities.

The proportion of non-elderly residents (ages 65 years and younger) with health insurance ranged from 50% among Mexicans in South Lawndale to 95% among Jews in North Park/West Ridge. In fact, the proportion with health insurance coverage in the two White communities was significantly

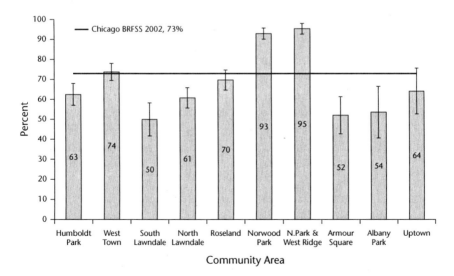

Figure 6-2 Proportion of Non-Elderly Adults with Insurance in Ten Chicago Communities

higher than all of the other non-White communities and the Chicago estimate (73%, $p < 0.05$) (Shah, Whitman, and Silva, 2006). Communities with
the largest immigrant population had the lowest insurance coverage—that
is, a little more than half of the residents in Asian communities, who were
primarily foreign-born (Table 6-3), had insurance coverage (52%–64%, Fig.
6-2). These data are comparable to the other immigrant communities of
South Lawndale (50%) and Humboldt Park (63%).

Racial and ethnic disparities in insurance coverage also exist nationally.
The factors that influence disparities nationally are likely to be contributing
to disparities observed between these Chicago communities. For example,
cost is a major barrier to insurance coverage. Many minority populations
who cannot afford private insurance may make too much money or may be
without appropriate immigration paperwork to be eligible for public insurance programs. Another important factor is that non-Whites are less likely to
have employee-sponsored insurance. For example, although more than half
of the adults in South Lawndale are employed, only half had some form
of insurance coverage. These results on insurance coverage have important
implications for interpreting data on health outcomes, as described below.

Obesity

Obesity is a risk factor for adult-onset diabetes, coronary heart disease,
and several other serious medical conditions that can lead to poor health and
premature death (Must et al., 1999; Kenchaiah et al., 2002; Fontaine et al.,
2003; American Obesity Association, 2005). To assess the prevalence of
obesity for these communities, all of the health surveys asked respondents to
report their height and weight. Data were used to calculate body mass index
(BMI), a measure of weight-for-height commonly applied to classify underweight, overweight, and obesity in adults (Centers for Disease Control and
Prevention [CDC], 1998). For these analyses, adults with a BMI of 30 kg/m^2
or greater are categorized as being obese and are presented in Figure 6-3.

About one-fourth of adults in the United States are obese, and these estimates vary by racial and ethnic group and geographic region (Ford et al.,
2005; CDC, 2006). The prevalence of obesity in the 10 surveyed communities
in Chicago ranged from 2% to 41% (Fig. 6-3), with several significant differences among communities. Over one-third of the population was found to be
obese in five of the communities, which were predominantly low-income and
African American or Hispanic. These percentages were significantly higher
than the obesity prevalence in the three Asian communities and the White
community of Norwood Park ($p < 0.05$), and higher than the Chicago average (22%). Specifically, residents in North Lawndale reported the highest
prevalence of obesity (41%), followed closely by residents in Roseland (39%).
The two predominantly White communities (Norwood Park [21%] and North

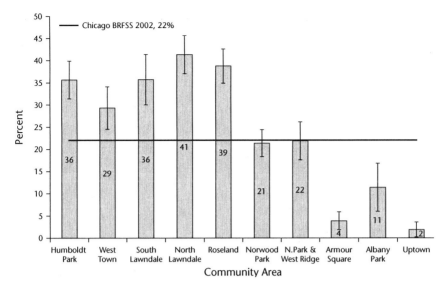

Figure 6-3   Obesity Prevalence in Ten Chicago Communities

Park/West Ridge [22%]) revealed obesity prevalence that was about half as high as this, similar to Chicago and national survey estimates.

Obesity rates also varied among the three Asian communities. The lowest proportion of individuals classified as obese were in the Vietnamese and Chinese communities, with proportions of 2% and 4%, respectively. Nationally, Asians report lower BMI estimates. However, there is evidence that cardiovascular disease, diabetes, and mortality associated with increased weight-for-height are far greater at lower BMI cut-offs for some Asian groups (Bell, Adair, and Popkin, 2002; McNeely and Boyko, 2004; Shai et al., 2006; Wen et al., 2008). The standard BMI cut-off for obesity (BMI $\geq$ 30 kg/m^2) may underestimate the risk for increased morbidity and mortality and thus have been recommended to be revised (World Health Organization Expert Consultation, 2004; Razak et al., 2007). Note that these revisions are in need of further study as it is still unclear whether all Asians or only some Asian subgroups are affected by the higher health risks associated with lower BMI cut-offs. This is certainly an important consideration in interpreting obesity data and health risks for the residents of these Chicago Asian communities (Magee et al., 2010).

Diabetes

Diabetes is one of the major causes of premature death in the United States and disproportionately affects some racial and ethnic minority populations. Consistent with several national health surveys, respondents were

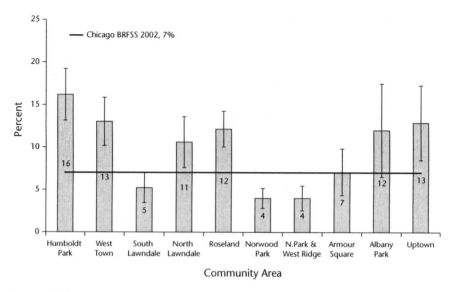

Figure 6-4 Diabetes Prevalence in Ten Chicago Communities

asked, "Have you ever been told by a doctor that you have diabetes or sugar diabetes?" to measure the prevalence of diabetes. Figure 6-4 presents the proportion of individuals who responded positively to this question in the 10 selected Chicago communities and illustrates substantial variation.

Six non-White communities reported diabetes rates that were three times higher than the predominantly non-Hispanic (NH) White communities of Norwood Park and West Rogers Park, and almost two times higher than the Chicago average (Fig. 6-4). The highest rates were found among residents of Humboldt Park and West Town (16% and 13%, respectively).

Because of the racial and ethnic diversity of these two communities, data were also examined by specific racial and ethnic groups. Results indicated that 21% of Puerto Ricans had diabetes compared to 15% of NH Blacks, 4% of Mexicans, and 3% of NH Whites. The Puerto Rican prevalence was significantly higher than the Mexican ($p = 0.025$) and NH White proportions ($p = 0.025$) (Whitman, Silva, and Shah, 2006). The prevalence of diabetes among Puerto Ricans from the Sinai Survey was also twice as high as estimates for Puerto Ricans from national surveys and the highest rate ever reported for any non-Native American population (Whitman, Silva, and Shah, 2006; Whitman et al., 2010).

The diabetes prevalence among residents in the Mexican immigrant community of South Lawndale was unusually low. It was 5% compared to 12% among Mexicans nationally (NDIC, 2008). This was in contrast to the diabetes mortality rate for this community, which in 2000 was higher than the overall Chicago estimate (40 per 100,000 individuals compared to 25 per 100,000;

Whitman, Williams, and Shah, 2004). On closer examination, the local survey offered some clarification and a greater understanding of how residents in South Lawndale experienced health. Low insurance coverage among this immigrant population likely explains the low diabetes prevalence found by the Sinai Survey in contrast to the high diabetes mortality. This discovery provides some insight on how to intervene. Residents in this community were dying from diabetes but had never been diagnosed with it. The survey data indicated that future community-based interventions would first need to make sure individuals were appropriately screened to obtain a more accurate estimate of prevalence; second, they would need to ensure that necessary services to manage and treat diabetes were available. This lack of screening is, of course, a result of the lack of health insurance coverage and thus access to primary care and the opportunity for diagnosis (Whitman, Williams, and Shah, 2004).

Asian Americans have also been found to be at high risk of diabetes compared to NH Whites (McNeely and Boyko, 2004). In Chicago, the Asian Surveys revealed dangerously high rates of diabetes in the Vietnamese (13%) and Cambodian (12%) populations, despite low obesity rates (Fig. 6-3). Such estimates of diabetes can be compared to 9% prevalence among U.S. Asians (Magee et al., 2010).

Similarly to the experiences of Mexicans in South Lawndale, the two Asian populations most affected by diabetes were predominantly foreign born (Fig. 6-4). As a result, it is possible that these proportions actually underestimate the true prevalence of diabetes because they rely on individuals having the opportunity to be screened for diabetes and presupposes that they present to the health-care system for preventive services (Southeast Asian Subcommittee of Asian American/Pacific Islander Work Group, 2006, p. 23). Unfortunately, diabetes mortality data for Asian subgroups are not so readily available for comparisons. It is thus difficult to understand these high diabetes prevalence estimates. However, the health survey data offer evidence that variation between different racial and ethnic populations in Chicago exists and only begins to unveil how specific social and historical factors influence the way different communities experience health.

Smoking

Smoking is known to be one of the leading preventable causes of disease and premature mortality. Individuals who smoke have a greater risk of death from many causes compared to individuals who do not smoke. Two questions, which are often asked on national surveys, were used to assess whether an individual was a current smoker. These were: "Have you smoked at least 100 cigarettes in your entire life?" and "Do you currently smoke cigarettes?"

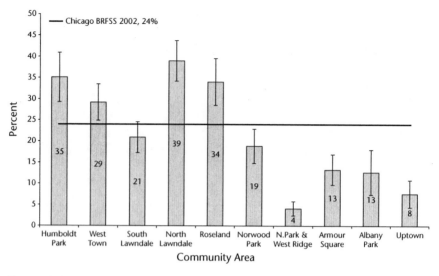

Figure 6-5   Smoking Prevalence in Ten Chicago Communities

The greatest proportions of current smokers were documented in three of the poorest, non-White communities: 39% in North Lawndale, 35% in Humboldt Park, and 34% in Roseland (Fig. 6-5). The smoking prevalences in these communities, which are mostly Black, are significantly higher than smoking estimates in the Mexican, White, and Asian communities. These proportions are also higher than the Chicago estimate of 24% (Shah, Whitman, and Silva, 2006). To further put these rates in context, the proportion of current smokers reported by the Sinai Survey for these three communities are comparable to the smoking rates documented before the U.S. Surgeon General first underscored the dangers of smoking. These Black communities are thus 40 years behind the smoking cessation curve of the country as a whole (Dell et al., 2005).

The lowest rate of smoking was observed among the Jewish population in North Park/West Ridge (4%). This proportion is much lower than 2007 national averages for NH Whites (21%; CDC, 2008) and reflects strong cultural norms against substance abuse including cigarettes, alcohol, and drugs.

Among the Asian communities, smoking prevalence ranged from 8% to 13%, compared to 10% among U.S. NH Asians in 2007 (CDC, 2008). Previous studies have found that factors associated with risk of smoking among Asian Americans include gender (Ma et al., 2002), unfair treatment (Chae et al., 2008), and neighborhood context (Kandula et al., 2009). Examining these local data by such risk factors indicate that among Chinese residents, 31% of male adults smoked compared to only 1% of females. This male proportion is comparable to some of the highest rates from other communities. These rates are similar to other studies that have examined smoking prevalence among specific Asian subgroups in other areas and offer insight on where and how to target smoking cessation efforts in Chicago and even within individual communities.

Breast Cancer Screening

Another measure of access to health care is the utilization of preventive services such as breast cancer screening. A mammogram is the best tool for early detection of breast cancer, and it is recommended by several organizations that women age 40 years and older obtain a mammogram every year. Two questions were asked in concert to measure routine mammography utilization: "Have you ever had a mammogram or breast X-ray?" and "How long ago did you have your most recent mammogram? Was it ... in the last 12 months, 2 years ago, 3 years ago, or more than 3 years ago?" To compare with existing data, survey data were analyzed to measure the proportion of women age 40 years and older who had a mammogram in the past 2 years, and Figure 6-6 presents these proportions.

Results show some variability in the utilization of mammography services among age-eligible women from the 10 different racial and ethnic communities surveyed in Chicago. In particular, Chinese and Cambodian women had the lowest proportion accessing breast cancer screening within the last 2 years (46% in Armour Square and 43% in Albany Park, respectively) compared to 90% of Mexican women in South Lawndale. Given the low

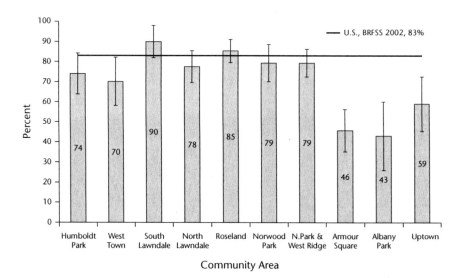

Figure 6-6   Proportion of Women (≥ 40 years) Who Had a Mammogram in the Last 2 Years in Ten Chicago Communities

coverage of insurance in the Mexican community, this finding was surprising. However, in examining the proportion who had a mammogram in the last year, only half of the women living in South Lawndale reported that they had obtained a mammogram (38%), which was significantly lower than the Chicago estimate of 67% (Shah, Whitman, and Silva, 2006).

Although there was limited variation reported in mammography history among women living in White, Black, and Hispanic communities, some caution should be taken in interpreting these findings. Biases exist for all self-report surveys (this is a given). Consistent with this finding, some studies have found that all women tend to over-report mammography history and that the degree of accuracy varies by racial and ethnic group (Lawrence, Moor, and Glenn, 1999; Rauscher et al., 2008) and other socio-economic variables (e.g., age, income, and education levels) (Holt et al., 2006). Thus, although the Chicago community survey data do not vary among the Hispanic, Black, and White communities, the true prevalence is likely underestimated. The extent to which reporting of mammography screening varies among the different racial and ethnic groups is unknown.

Conclusions

Variation in local level health outcomes is at the core of this chapter. The surveys conducted from 2002 to 2008 describe the health of 10 diverse communities in Chicago. For the first time, communities and researchers are able to quantify the health of local communities and racial and ethnic groups within an urban setting not only in absolute terms but also in relative terms.

Comparison of five key health measures described in this chapter indicate a wide range of measurements and substantiate how existing national and city level data mask important variations in health. Substantial disparities in health outcomes were documented by race and ethnicity and by geographic area. For example, 21% of adults in the United States smoke, and about the same is true for Chicago. However, in two adjacent Chicago communities, 21% of adults smoke in one and 39% in another (Dell et al., 2005; West and Gamboa, 2010). Another example is that of breast cancer screening. Nationally, about 83% of women age 40 years and older have had a mammogram in the last 2 years, with similar estimates for Chicago. However, less than 50% of the Chinese and Cambodian women reported that they had received a recent mammogram. This proportion is far less than that reported by Mexican, Black, and White women who were surveyed. Further survey data analyses found that several other indicators similarly vary across communities (Shah, Whitman, and Silva, 2006). Unless such differences are routinely measured and carefully understood, public health programs cannot optimally target interventions and resources at the community level.

In addition, survey data are important because they begin to offer explanations for the causes of disparities at the local level. For example, the survey instruments asked questions about individual behaviors and their social environment, which were specific to the Mexican or Asian communities surveyed. These uniquely local data inform and guide community groups, academic centers, and other stakeholders on how to find sustainable solutions to prioritize and take ownership of the health problems identified. Because individuals can more readily relate to the information gathered, there is greater potential to generate interest and even catalyze local communities to take action. This is the next step of the Sinai model (Whitman, Shah, and Benjamins, 2010).

Large urban centers in the United States have utilized health surveys to better document the health of their diverse populations. Analyses of these data have already shown substantial disparities in how racial and ethnic groups experience health (ARHQ, 2005). However, successful translation of such data to combat disparities has yet to be fully achieved. The local level survey data described here offer such pertinent information to enable communities in Chicago to prioritize health problems and design community-based solutions to address them. Utilizing local data to drive change is thus the essence of our vision for urban health improvement and the story of the chapters to follow. Findings from these local community health surveys will guide health interventions and shape where and how to intervene effectively. Furthermore, it has been our experience that survey data findings, when presented in the context of other neighboring communities, underscore disparities in health and push foundations, policymakers, and community leaders toward greater justice and fairness in their policies and programs. This strategy will lead to the greatest gains in the public's urban health and ultimately to eliminating racial and ethnic disparities in health.

Acknowledgments

I am indebted to Dr. Steve Whitman and my colleagues at the Sinai Urban Health Institute for 8 incredible years of learning how to transform the art of social epidemiology to improve community health. Sinai's public health practices inspired the Jewish Federation and the Asian Health Coalition of Illinois to gather similar local level data. It is because of their initiative and hard work in administering these additional surveys that we are able to examine the health of 10 Chicago communities presented here. To this end, I thank Maureen Benjamins and Matt Magee for managing this work so effectively. Generous funding was made possible to support my time for this work from The Robert Wood Johnson Foundation and The Chicago Community Trust.

Note

1. All data shown are adjusted using the same age categories for all 10 communities. Age categories used were: 18 to 44 years, 45 to 64 years, 65 years and older (or 65–75 years only for the Sinai Survey). Results from other published sources may have used different age categories and thus may result in estimates that vary slightly from the data presented here.

References

Agency for Healthcare Research and Quality (ARHQ). 2005. National healthcare disparities report. U.S. Department of Health and Human Services, ARHQ Publication No. 06-0017. Online. Available: http://www.ahrq.gov/qual/nhdr05/nhdr05.pdf. Accessed December 2, 2009.

American Obesity Association. 2005. Health effects of obesity. Online. Available: http://obesity1.tempdomainname.com/subs/fastfacts/Health_Effects.shtml. Accessed December 1, 2009.

Bell, A. Colin, Linda S. Adair, Barry M. Popkin. 2002. Ethnic differences in the association between body mass index and hypertention. *American Journal of Epidemiology* 155:346–353.

Benjamins, Maureen R. 2010. The Jewish Community Health Survey of Chicago: Methodology and key findings. In: *Urban Health: Combating Disparities with Local Data*, ed. Steve Whitman, Ami M. Shah, and Maureen R. Benjamins. New York, NY: Oxford University Press.

Centers for Disease Control and Prevention (CDC). 1998. *Clinical Guidelines on the Identification, Evaluation, and Treatment of Overweight and Obesity in Adults.* National Heart, Lung and Blood Institute. June 17.

Centers for Disease Control and Prevention (CDC). 2006. State-specific prevalence of obesity among adults—United States, 2005. *Morbidity and Mortality Weekly Report* 55:985–988.

Centers for Disease Control and Prevention (CDC). 2008. Cigarette Smoking Among Adults—United States, 2007. *Morbidity and Mortality Weekly Report* 57(45):1121–1226.

Chae, David H., David T. Takeuchi, Elizabeth M. Barbeau, Gary G. Bennett, Jane Lindsey, and Nancy Krieger. 2008. Unequal treatment, racial/ethnic discrimination, ethnic identification, and smoking among Asian Americans in the National Latino and Asian American Study. *American Journal of Public Health* 98(3):485–492.

Dell, Jade L., Steve Whitman, Ami M. Shah, Abigail Silva, and David Ansell. 2005. Smoking in 6 diverse Chicago communities—A population study. *American Journal of Public Health* 95(6):1036–1042.

Fontaine, Kevin R., David T. Redden, Chenxi Wang, Andrew O. Westfall, and David B. Allison. 2003. Years of life lost due to obesity. *Journal of American Medical Association* 289(2):187–193.

Ford, Earl S., Ali H. Mokdad, Wayne H. Giles, Deborah A. Galuska, and Mary K. Serdula. 2005. Geographic variation in the prevalence of obesity, diabetes, and obesity-related behaviors. *Obesity Research* 13(1):118–122.

Galea, Sandro, and Amy Schulz. 2006. Methodological considerations in the study of urban health: How do we best assess how cities affect health? In: *Cities and the Health of the Public*, ed. Nicholas Freudenberg, Sandro Galea, and David Vlahov. Nashville, TN: Vanderbilt University Press.

Holt, Kathleen, Peter Franks, Sean Meldrum, and Kevin Fiscella. 2006. *Mammography self-report and mammography claims: Racial, ethnic, and socioeconomic discrepancies among elderly women*. Medical Care 44(6):513–518.

Kandula, Namratha R., Ming Wen, Elizabeth A. Jacobs, and Diane S. Lauderdale. 2009. Association between neighborhood context and smoking prevalence among Asian Americans. *American Journal of Public Health* 99(5):885–892.

Kenchaiah, Satish, Jane C. Evans, Daniel Levy, Peter W. F. Wilson, Emelia J. Benjamin, Martin G. Larson, et al. 2002. Obesity and the risk of heart failure. *New England Journal of Medicine* 347:305–313.

Keyfitz, Nathan 1966. Sampling variance of standardized mortality rates. *Human Biology* 38:309–317.

Lawrence, Valerie A., Carl De Moor, and M. Elizabeth Glenn. 1999. Systematic differences in validity of self-reported mammography behavior: A problem for intergroup comparisons? *Preventive Medicine* 29:577–580.

Ma, Grace X., Steve Shive, Yin Tan, and Jamil Toubbeh. 2002. Prevalence and predictors of tobacco use among Asian Americans in the Delaware Valley Region. *American Journal of Public Health* 92(6):1013–1020.

Magee, Mathew J., Lucy Guo, Ami M. Shah, and Hong Liu. 2010. The Chicago Asian Community Surveys: Methodology and key findings. In: *Urban Health: Combating Disparities with Local Data*, ed. Steve Whitman, Ami M. Shah, and Maureen R. Benjamins. New York, NY: Oxford University Press.

McNeely, Marguerite J. and Edward J. Boyko. 2004. Type 2 diabetes prevalence in Asian Americans: Results from a national health survey. *Diabetes Care* 27(1):66–69.

Must, Aviva, Jennifer Spadano, Eugenie H. Coakley, Alison E. Field, Graham Colditz, and William H. Dietz. 1999. The disease burden associated with overweight and obesity. *Journal of the American Medical Association* 282:1523–1529.

National Diabetes Information Clearinghouse (NDIC). 2008. National Diabetes Statistics, 2007. National Institute of Diabetes and Digestive and Kidney Diseases, National Institutes of Health. Online. Available: http://diabetes.niddk.nih.gov/DM/PUBS/statistics/#race. Accessed December 1, 2009.

Rauscher, Garth H., Timothy P. Johnson, Young Ik Cho, and Jennifer Walk. 2008. Accuracy of self-reported cancer-screening histories: A meta-analysis. *Cancer Epidemiology, Biomarkers & Prevention* 17(4):748–757.

Razak, Fahad, Sonia S. Anand, Harry Shannon, Vladimir Vuksan, Bonnie Davis, Ruby Jacobs, et al. 2007. Defining obesity cut points in a multiethnic population. *Circulation* 115(16):2111–2118.

SAS Institute Inc. 2002-2003. SAS statistical software, version 9.1.3 for Windows@. Cary, NC: SAS Institute.

Simon, Paul A., Cheryl M. Wold, Michael R. Cousineau, and Jonathan E. Fielding. 2001. Meeting the data needs of a local health department: The Los Angeles County Health Survey. *American Journal of Public Health* 91(12):1950–1952.

Shah, Ami M., and Steven Whitman. 2010. Sinai's Improving Community Health Survey: Methodology and key findings. In: *Urban Health: Combating Disparities with Local Data*, ed. Steve Whitman, Ami M. Shah, and Maureen R. Benjamins. New York, NY: Oxford University Press.

Southeast Asian Subcommittee of Asian American/Pacific Islander Work Group. 2006. Silent trauma: Diabetes, health status, and the refugee, Southeast Asians in the United States. U.S. Department of Health and Human Services' National Diabetes Education Program (NDEP), June.

Stata Corporation. 2003. STATA statistical software, version 8.0 for Windows@. College Station, TX: Stata Corp.

The Chicago Fact Book Consortium. 1995. *Local Community Fact Book: Chicago Metropolitan Area, 1990*. Chicago: IL, Academy Chicago Publishers.

Volz, Erik., Cyprian Wejnert, Ismail Degani, and Douglas D. Heckathorn. 2007. Respondent Driven Sampling Analyses Tool (RDSAT), Version 5.6. Itasca, NY: Cornell University.

West, Joseph and Charlene Gamboa. 2010. Working Together to Live Tobacco Free: Community-Based Smoking Cessation in North Lawndale. In *Urban Health: Combating Disparities with Local Data*, ed. Steve Whitman, Ami M. Shah, and Maureen R. Benjamins. New York, NY: Oxford University Press.

Whitman, Steve, Abigail Silva, Ami M. Shah, and David Ansell. 2004. Diversity and disparity: GIS and small area analysis in six Chicago neighborhoods. *Journal of Medical Systems* 28(4):397–411.

Whitman, Steve, Abigail Silva, and Ami M. Shah. 2006. Disproportionate impact of diabetes in a Puerto Rican community of Chicago. *Journal of Community Health* 31(6):521–531.

Whitman, Steve, Cynthia Williams, and Ami M. Shah. 2004. *Sinai Health System's Improving Community Health Survey: Report 1*. Chicago, IL: Sinai Health System.

Whitman, Steven, Jose E. Lopez, Steven K. Rothschild, and Jaime Delgado. 2010. Disproportionate impact of diabetes in a Puerto Rican community of Chicago. In: *Urban Health: Combating Disparities with Local Data*, ed. Steve Whitman, Ami M. Shah, and Maureen R. Benjamins. New York, NY: Oxford University Press.

Whitman, Steve, Ami M. Shah, and Maureen R. Benjamins. 2010. Sinai model for reducing health disparities and improving health. In: *Urban Health: Combating Disparities with Local Data*, ed. Steve Whitman, Ami M. Shah, and Maureen R. Benjamins. New York, NY: Oxford University Press.

World Health Organization Expert Consultation. 2004. Appropriate body-mass index for Asian populations and its implications for policy and intervention strategies. *Lancet* 363(9403):157–163.

Section 3

Translating Data into Community Action

Steven Whitman, Ami M. Shah, and Maureen R. Benjamins

Section 3 contains six chapters that each describe specific efforts to improve health within vulnerable communities. Importantly, each of these case studies was motivated by data from *Sinai's Improving Community Health Survey*. These chapters provide a detailed account of efforts to improve health outcomes, including smoking, diabetes, obesity, and pediatric asthma (both of these latter outcomes were targeted in two different communities). Different approaches are illustrated, reflecting the diversity of the communities represented in these chapters. Although some of these projects are just getting started, some are well underway, and one has ended because of discontinued state funding, each description provides unique insight into how communities can translate data into action.

Similarly to all others working in the fields of health care and public health, the editors of this book would like to help all people be healthier and, in fact, to obtain optimal levels of health. Further, although we would like to improve health for all, we also believe that the first priority is improving health for those whose health is worst. (This is explicit in the "Sinai Model for Reducing Health Disparities and Improving Health," described in the Introduction to this book.) In this sense, this book is timely and enlightening but not unique in its desire to improve health. It is unique, however, in the sense that the central purpose of this book is to provide a feasible strategy for pursuing the goals of improved health and reduced disparities.

In each of these six chapters, survey data have identified a very important problem that exists in a specific community of color. The underlying schema delineated in the "Sinai Model" urges that once the community and the health issue are selected, potential solutions must be developed and resources obtained to improve the situation. In this way, researchers and practitioners can begin working to reduce disparities instead of simply documenting them.

The "Sinai Model" has been successfully followed in each of the six case studies presented here. Although these are not the only interventions that stemmed from the survey results, the selected case studies will provide examples of how different communities used the data to respond to their individual health problems. Specifically, each chapter describes what the survey data found, what interventions were selected, who was involved, and how funding was obtained. Importantly, each chapter provides detailed descriptions about the effectiveness of the intervention, the challenges confronted, and the lessons learned. Through these examples it is hoped that other communities will not only be motivated to undertake their own efforts, but that they will also benefit from the variety of experiences described in the following chapters.

7

WORKING TOGETHER TO LIVE TOBACCO-FREE: COMMUNITY-BASED SMOKING CESSATION IN NORTH LAWNDALE

Joseph F. West and Charlene J. Gamboa

Introduction

Chicago prides itself as a "City of Neighborhoods." There are 77 neighborhoods that define the rich diversity and history of the city. North Lawndale is one of these. Once a predominantly White middle-class neighborhood, the community is now predominantly Black, poor, and dilapidated.

North Lawndale was the point of entry for many Eastern European immigrants and became home to large numbers of Blacks as early as 1960 during what has become known as the Second Great Migration (Satter, 2009). North Lawndale is a part of the "West Side" in common Chicago parlance. This community is the former home to industrial giants such as Sears, International Harvester, and Western Electric. As industry, and employment, left the community, "White Flight" took place, and in a few short years the community fell into rapid economic and social decline.

In 1966, the neighborhood's poverty prompted Martin Luther King, Jr. to pick North Lawndale as the base for the northern civil rights movement. Following King's assassination, rioting, crime, unemployment, and physical deterioration led to further flight by residents and businesses (Abraham, 1994; Steans Family Foundation, 2009). In 1960, the community reached a height of 124,000 residents. Today, North Lawndale has 42,000 residents, with 44% living below the poverty level, 68% below twice the poverty level, and a median household income of $18,400.

Smoking is a pervasive public health issue for North Lawndale compounded by the deeply rooted issues of race and class. Although smoking rates in the United States and the city of Chicago have declined over the past four decades, smoking rates in North Lawndale have not. Nationally, about 47,000 Blacks die each year from smoking-related disease, a population approximately the same size as North Lawndale.

This chapter begins with an introduction to the data on smoking prevalence for North Lawndale gathered from a comprehensive community survey. This is followed by a discussion of a community-based intervention illustrating all of the features of its multifaceted design. The intervention features a collaboration that started with a few community partners and the state public health department and grew into substantial partnerships with local community groups, schools, churches, and outreach organizations—all focused on eliminating tobacco use in North Lawndale. Finally, the chapter discusses some key outcomes and lessons learned from the intervention.

Community Survey Data and Smoking in North Lawndale

Methods

Community Survey

Data were obtained from the Sinai Health System's Improving Community Health Survey (Dell et al., 2005). The survey is described in detail in Chapter 3. The questions analyzed in this report were those contained in the smoking module of the survey, which were taken from the Behavioral Risk Factor Surveillance System (BRFSS). A current smoker was defined as a person who answered yes to both of the following questions: *(1)* "Have you smoked at least 100 cigarettes in your life?" and *(2)* "Do you currently smoke cigarettes?"

Data Analysis

Data were weighted to account for the probability of selection (at the block, household, and respondent levels) and to ensure that the sample resembled the community area demographics. Data were analyzed with Stata (Stata Corp, College Station, Texas). A 95% confidence level was employed for all analyses. The significance among prevalence proportions was tested with the *t*-test. Trends among the results from the six community areas were tested for statistical significance.

Results

Table 7-1 presents smoking prevalence data. The proportion of self-reported current smokers ranged from 18% in a predominantly White community area (Norwood Park) to 39% in North Lawndale. The prevalence ratio between Norwood Park and North Lawndale was 2.11. Data presented in Table 7-1 also show that a majority of current smokers (ranging from 46% to 58% across community areas) reported that they tried to quit during the last year and that most of current smokers were still trying to stop.

The socio-economic correlates of smoking in the six communities surveyed were generally similar to those reported in previous studies (Northridge, Morabia, and Ganz, 1998; Nelson et al., 2003), although most of the associations found by the current study were not statistically significant. Demographic groups that were more likely to be current smokers included men, people living in households with lower incomes (<$30,000 per year) or without working telephones, and people without a high school diploma. Mean and median ages for smoking initiation fell in the range of approximately 15 to 17 years, and more than 90% of all current smokers started smoking while they were teenagers. Most current smokers smoked about half a pack a day.

Smoking prevalences for each community area, stratified by four social and demographic measures, were also analyzed (data not shown). In all six communities, men were more likely than women to smoke, but in none of the six communities was this difference statistically significant. However, this difference in smoking prevalence by gender among all six communities taken together was significant ($p = 0.02$). Income showed a generally nonsignificant negative association with smoking. In five of the communities (the exception being West Town), people living in households with an annual income below $30,000 smoked at a higher rate compared to those residents with a higher income. Only in Roseland was the association of a lower household income with current smoking significant ($p < 0.01$). In four of the six communities, the lowest proportion of smokers was found among people with more than a high school education.

The proportion of households without telephone service (excluding cellular phones) ranged from 2% to 21%. Because five of the six communities demonstrated higher smoking proportions among households without telephones, a telephone survey would have underestimated smoking prevalence in these communities. However, the inverse association of the presence of a telephone with smoking prevalence was statistically significant only in Roseland ($p < 0.025$).

TABLE 7-1   Current Smoking Prevalence Proportions, Associated Prevalence Ratios, and Two Measures of Smoking Cessation Efforts: Six Chicago Community Areas, 2002–2003

Chicago Community Area	No. of respondents	Smoking prevalence (95% CI)	Prevalence ratio	p	Tried to quit in past 12 months, %	Still trying to quit at interview (%)
Norwood Park	190	0.18 (0.16, 0.21)	Reference		54	57
Humboldt Park	298	0.35 (0.27, 0.44)	1.90	<0.001	58	68
West Town	303	0.32 (0.26, 0.39)	1.72	<0.001	46	49
South Lawndale	300	0.20 (0.15, 0.26)	1.09	NS	58	75
North Lawndale	303	0.39 (0.33, 0.45)	2.11	<0.001	46	70
Roseland	302	0.33 (0.25, 0.42)	1.78	<0.01	51	65

Source: Whitman S, Williams C, Shah AM. 2004. Sinai's Improving Community Health Survey: Report 1. Chicago, Illinois: Sinai Health System
CI= confidence interval; NS = not significant.

Working Together to Live Tobacco-Free: Community-Based Smoking Cessation Intervention in North Lawndale

This North Lawndale smoking proportion among adults of 39% was among the highest ever found in a U.S. community. As Sinai Urban Health Institute's (SUHI) members began disseminating overall findings from the survey, this was one of the highlighted observations. In addition, it was repeatedly pointed out that although Illinois was receiving $350 million a year from the Master Settlement Agreement (Illinois Department of Public Health, 2009), virtually none of that was going toward tobacco prevention or even health (General Accounting Office, 2001).

In this context, the Chicago Chapter of the American Lung Association asked SUHI researchers to participate in a press conference that would highlight the smoking results from the survey. That press conference was held on World No Tobacco Day 2005 at the State of Illinois Building in Chicago. The event was attended by most of the city's major media outlets. The coverage was substantial and on message. The *Chicago Defender*, the city's Black newspaper for more than a century, carried a banner front page headline that read "Racism Drives Smoking" (Fig. 7-1). An anti-smoking activist who spoke at the press conference noted, "First they made us pick it, now they want us to smoke it," and spoke about the disproportionate impact of the targeting of mentholated cigarettes to the Black community. The American Lung Association used the event to push for a city ordinance to require smoke-free workplaces, including restaurants and bars in Chicago. In 2007, the city passed this ordinance, and 1 year later the state passed a similar law making Illinois businesses and public venues smoke-free.

Finally, based on the survey findings, the attention brought forward by the dissemination efforts and the urging of the residents of North Lawndale, the Illinois Department of Public Health requested a proposal for smoking prevention in North Lawndale. SUHI submitted such a proposal in collaboration with the Sinai Community Institute (SCI) and the work was funded. It would be a 4-year multifaceted intervention for smoking cessation and prevention in North Lawndale. SCI has been working in North Lawndale for more than two decades as a service delivery agency of the Sinai Health System offering programs focused on health, education, training, leadership development, case management, intervention, and prevention. They also serve as the service agent for the county Women, Infants, and Children (WIC) program.

Breathing Freedom: Building the Community Intervention

The proposal was bolstered by an extensive literature review and 1 year of planning and community meetings. The literature suggested that the most

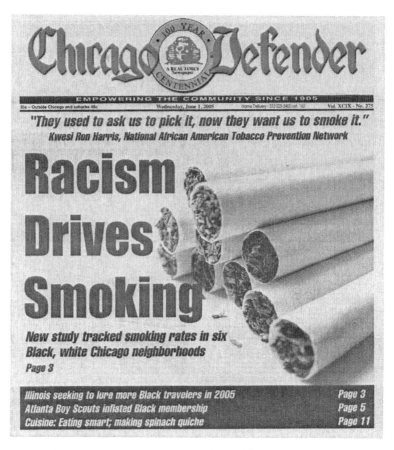

Figure 7-1 Local Newspaper Article Following World No Tobacco Day 2005 Event and Press Conference for "Smoking in 6 Diverse Chicago Communities—A Population Study" (Dell et al., 2005).

effective interventions are those that incorporate more than one type of program. For example, the most extensive interventions may include programs designed to educate or motivate individuals, address systematic changes in the health-care system, and change policies related to smoking (COMMITT I and COMMITT II 1995; Hopkins et al., 2001; Manske et al., 2004).

The proposed intervention, Breathing Freedom, emphasized a community-based approach, which had been shown as effective in other communities (Fisher et al, 1998; Andrews et al., 2007). The work also drew on the importance of integrating social support and faith in cessation programming for Blacks (Ahluwalia, Resnicow, and Clark, 1998; Nolen et al., 2005).

The first step to building an effective community-based program began with a series of meetings with community organizations to determine smoking-related issues specific to the North Lawndale community that could not be captured in the scientific literature. These early pre-implementation meetings were also important for establishing a baseline understanding of the kind of smoking cessation services or programs available up to that point and to what degree they had been successful.

Meetings were held with several community, health, and ministerial groups. The meetings emphasized the importance of having an identifiable name for the program, the importance of engaging neighborhood partners and collaborating with other organizations, and sharing information with the community about the program's progress. The importance of engaging community stakeholders, including businesses (e.g., barber shops, hair salons, and restaurants), churches, civic leaders, and community service organizations, was also highlighted.

Using this knowledge and building from the scientific literature, the program (aptly called Breathing Freedom) had the following 4-year intervention (2007–2011) goals: promote quitting and not starting among youth and adults, and reduce smoking prevalence in North Lawndale to 19% from 39%. The program was composed of numerous components, as discussed below.

Media Campaigns and Public Education

Breathing Freedom promoted smoking cessation and its free services using posters, flyers, billboards, classes, health fairs, and self-help kits. The media campaign also entailed the distribution of 2,000 *Pathways to Freedom* books to the community. *Pathways to Freedom* is a Centers for Disease Control and Prevention smoking cessation publication tailored to Blacks (CDC, 2003).

Quitline

Breathing Freedom partnered with the Illinois Tobacco Quitline (Quitline) for a focused promotion and data collection campaign. The Quitline offered telephone support and counseling, along with cessation materials. Both a proactive (provider-initiated) and reactive (smoker-initiated) approach were used. North Lawndale residents were referred to the Quitline by a health educator or physician, and the Quitline would follow-up the referral with a mailing of smoking cessation materials and a phone call.

Free Nicotine Replacement Therapies (Quit Kits)

Breathing Freedom offered program participants "Quits Kits." The kits were packaged in 32-ounce reusable plastic mugs with the program name, logo, phone number, and Quitline number printed on the mugs. Inside the mugs were cessation support materials, including instructions that encouraged increased water consumption as a part of the cessation plan. Other instructions included breathing exercises, stress relief, and tips on gradually reducing nicotine dependence. Also included were stress balls, nicotine gum, and coupons for nicotine replacement therapy (NRT) purchases. The program also offered participants free 7-, 14-, and 21-milligram nicotine patches (provided by the Chicago Department of Public Health). Participants wanting patches signed a consent form describing patch use and potential side effects.

Group and Individual Counseling

North Lawndale residents wanting to quit were offered group counseling provided by either Breathing Freedom or another smoking cessation group in North Lawndale or elsewhere in Chicago. Breathing Freedom offered one 90-minute group session each week that was open to the public and one 90-minute group session each week that was open to new and expectant mothers. The group sessions were culturally modified workshops based on the Freedom from Smoking model of the American Lung Association (ALA, 2009). The modifications entailed incorporating pictures of Blacks and messages and life examples to which the health educators believed participants could relate.

Residents could also receive individual physician-assisted smoking cessation counseling. Twice a month a dedicated physician with more than two decades of smoking cessation experience was available for a 4-hour period to meet with patients and residents interested in quitting smoking. The physician provided behavioral counseling and pharmacotherapy support to patients. The physician was accompanied by a health educator who shared smoking cessation materials with patients and offered them the group counseling option. The visits could be covered by Medicaid.

Provider Education and Provider Reminder Systems

Breathing Freedom encouraged physicians to take a more active role in encouraging patients to quit. The program provided clinician-specific smoking cessation materials and Quitline referrals. Breathing Freedom's Program Director and Project Coordinator held grand-rounds with hospital clinicians talking about the program and smoking cessation. The program also provided information regarding reminder systems and pharmacotherapy. In addition the program employed the Ask, Advise, Refer strategy (Fiore et al., 2000) with clinicians and health professionals working in the Sinai Health System. This strategy allows clinicians and health professionals to:

- Ask patients about their smoking behavior;
- Advise patients on the importance of quitting smoking; and
- Refer patients to appropriate counseling services, which included Breathing Freedom group sessions, the Illinois Tobacco Quitline, and a physician dedicated to smoking cessation.

Ruth M. Rothstein Core Center

Breathing Freedom successfully piloted an intervention at the Ruth M. Rothstein CORE Center. The CORE Center, a part of the Cook County health system, is one of the largest HIV/AIDS clinics in the United States. Breathing Freedom and the CORE Center implemented a center-wide smoking cessation intervention that included pharmacy services. Eligible patients receiving their Highly Active AntiRetroviral (anti-HIV) Therapy (HAART) prescriptions at the CORE Center pharmacy who were trying to quit smoking could also receive free NRT. The intervention also included a weekly 60-minute support group meeting and weekly clinician follow-up.

This collaboration was the result of a ground-breaking study showing cigarette smoking diminishes important benefits provided by HAART therapy in the treatment of HIV/AIDS, resulting in elevated viral loads and diminished T-cell counts (Feldman et al., 2006). In addition, the work was driven by knowledge that smoking increases the risks for HIV-associated pulmonary infections and oropharyngeal lesions and higher incidences of AIDS-defining and non-AIDS defining malignancies. Smoking is also an established risk factor for atherosclerosis and has been associated with coronary events in patients receiving protease inhibitor therapy. In fact, as people who are HIV-positive continue to live longer, they are dying from many smoking-related causes (Lavolé et al., 2006; Gillison, 2009).

Women, Infants, and Children

Breathing Freedom provided smoking cessation to new and expectant mothers enrolled in WIC. Cigarette smoking has been associated with increased risk of ectopic pregnancy, placenta complications, and stillbirth (U.S. Department of Health and Human Services, 2001). The decision to focus on new and expectant mothers was driven by data on pregnant women who smoke in Chicago. Table 7-2 presents the percent of births in Chicago to mothers who smoke. Between 1989 and 2006, the percent of births to mothers who smoke declined sharply for non-Hispanic Whites and Hispanics but less so for non-Hispanic Blacks. North Lawndale in particular had a couple of years where the percentages actually increased, and as of 2006 the rate was more than three times the rate for White women in Chicago and was 11 times as high as the predominantly Hispanic neighborhood of South Lawndale. Most importantly, the smoking proportion was higher in 2006 than it had been in 1990 and had only declined 23% in the 18-year interval.

Analysis of the WIC alcohol and tobacco assessment used by SCI during enrollment showed WIC clients from North Lawndale smoked at a rate that was more than twice that of other clients (Table 7-3). Literature suggests that these rates may well be underestimations given that disclosing smoking behavior during pregnancy may be looked upon unfavorably (Mullen et al., 1991). Also, research suggests that smoking prevalence among WIC clients is more likely to decline if smoking cessation is offered throughout

TABLE 7-2   Percent of Women Who Smoked During Pregnancy in Chicago by Race/Ethnicity, and Two Community Areas

Year	All Chicago	Non-Hispanic Black	Non-Hispanic White	North Lawndale	South Lawndale
1989	15.3	19.4	19.2	14.2	6.2
1990	12.4	16.3	15.6	9.7	4.0
1991	12.0	16.2	14.2	13.6	3.8
1992	12.8	18.0	14.7	12.1	3.5
1993	11.7	16.8	13.6	13.4	2.7
1994	10.2	14.9	12.1	10.4	2.5
1995	9.9	16.0	11.0	12.9	2.3
1996	9.9	16.7	10.1	12.8	1.9
1997	9.5	16.1	9.3	17.4	2.0
1998	8.8	15.0	8.7	18.2	2.0
1999	8.5	14.8	8.8	16.4	1.2
2000	7.8	14.3	7.4	15.7	1.5
2001	7.2	14.0	6.0	19.7	1.2
2002	6.8	13.6	6.1	16.5	1.3
2003	6.2	12.9	5.1	15.3	1.2
2004	5.6	11.7	4.7	15.6	1.4
2005	4.7	10.5	3.6	12.7	0.6
2006	4.5	9.9	3.1	11.0	1.0
% change 1989–2006	−70.6%	−49.0%	−83.9%	−22.5%	−83.9%

Source: Illinois Department of Public Health, Vital Records Data.

TABLE 7-3   Number of WIC Clients Living in Cook County and North Lawndale who Smoke

Location	No. of WIC clients	No. currently smoke
County-wide	3658	198 (5.4%)
North Lawndale	344	42 (12.2%)
n	4,002	240

the course of pregnancy (Windsor et al., 1993; Yunzal-Butler, Joyce, and Racine, 2009). There were two components for this intervention: *(1)* smoking cessation group meetings were designed and scheduled exclusively for WIC clients; and *(2)* the program trained WIC case managers and nutritionists using a smoking cessation teaching guide specifically designed for them. WIC case managers and nutritionists were then expected to work with their clients to establish a quit plan. The guide, "Helping Mothers and Caregivers

Stop Smoking: A Client Service Guide for Case Managers and Nutritionists," contained some simple tools. They were:

- Pregnancy and Smoking Newsletter
- Refresh Yourself! Stop Smoking—worksheet
- My Declaration of Self-Esteem—worksheet
- Positive Self-Talk to Stop Smoking—worksheet
- This is it—My Quit Day Plan—planning activity
- Ready to Quit and Ready to Plan—planning activity
- I Quit Contract—planning activity
- Illinois Tobacco Quitline Referral Form

Logic Model: Theory of Change

The underlying behavioral change model was based on the Stages of Change Model (DiClement and Prochaska, 1982; Prochaska et al., 1988). The program developed measures to assess changes in attitudes and willingness to quit. Smoking assessments, outreach materials, and workshops assessments each had tools that measured where patients were located on the Stages of Change Model (Prochaska and DiClemente, 1983): Precontemplation (not thinking of quitting); Contemplation (thinking of quitting); Preparation (making an intent to quit—e.g., reducing number smoked per day); Action (having quit at least 7 days); and Maintenance (having quit at least 30 or more days). From these pieces we developed a logic model that outlines our delivery plan for the entire program (see Figure 7-2).

This model was used to maintain focus on specific program outcomes and impact related to our program goals. Breathing Freedom's short-term outcomes were to *(1)* increase awareness, knowledge, and intention to quit; *(2)* provide direct cessation services to the North Lawndale community; *(3)* train WIC case managers and nutritionists in smoking cessation outreach; and *(4)* increase calls and referrals to Quitline. The program's long-term outcomes were measured as a participant having quit at three follow-up periods (3, 6, and 12 months); increased calls and referrals to the Quitline and knowledge of telephone counseling; increased number of physicians and hospitals encouraging patients to quit and referring patients to smoking cessation programs.

Program Results

Breathing Freedom was developed as a 24-month intervention that involved a number of community-centered activities. The program was initially designed to be a 4-year initiative that would have included a follow-up survey to assess the intervention's impact on changing smoking prevalence in the

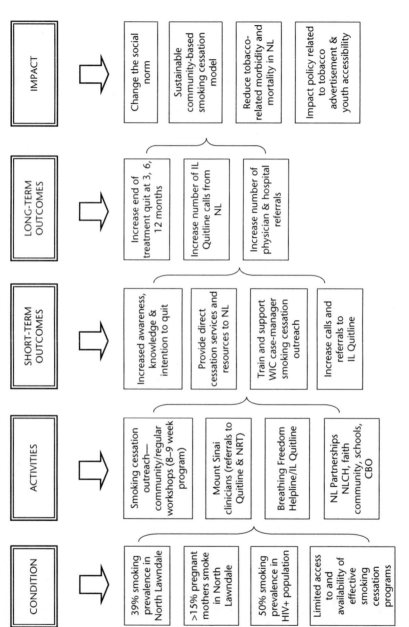

Figure 7-2 Breathing Freedom Program Logic Model Excerpt

neighborhood. The program's funding was abruptly suspended midway through the intervention because of state budgetary shortfalls and the follow-up survey was not implemented. However, over the 24-month period, data were collected for the number of North Lawndale residents that attended one of the program's workshops, received a clinical referral, or called either the program's helpline or Quitline and as a result made a cessation attempt. A program participant was defined as a North Lawndale resident, Core Center patient, or WIC client that received a quit plan, attended one or more counseling session, or called either the program helpline or Illinois Tobacco Quitline.

The program conducted 46 education workshops, 16 partnership trainings, and 12 community events (Table 7-4). The program also distributed 600 "Quit Kits," received 80 incoming calls, received 33 fax referrals, and scheduled 53 clinical appointments. A total of 1,823 residents attended program events of which 1,313 (72%) requested cessation plans. Using the Stages of Change Model, the program was able to capture how many program participants moved from the Precontemplative to Action stages. Intensive follow-up measured cessation progress by whether the participant quit *(1)* less than 30 days; *(2)* 30 to 60 days; *(3)* 61 to 90 days; or *(4)* greater than 90 days.

A quit attempt was counted when a participant either stopped smoking for a day (24 hours) or reduced the amount of smoking by half (e.g., from a full pack a day to half a pack a day). Eighty-five percent of participants made at least one or more attempt to quit during the first 7 days of their cessation plan. The program recorded that 467 of the 1,313 (35.6%) receiving cessation plans quit for less than 30 days, 62 quit between 30 and 60 days (4.7%), 33 quit between 60 and 90 days (2.5%), and 2 reported having quit

TABLE 7-4   Breathing Freedom Outreach Activities, Cessation Plans Requested, 24-Hour Quit Attempts, and Quit Results 2008-2009

Type	No. of participants	No. of cessation plans requested	24-hr quit attempts	Quit <30 days	Quit 30-60 days	Quit >60 days
Education workshops	886	642 (72%)	563 (88%)	232	33	16
Partnership trainings	278	199 (72%)	167 (84%)	105	12	7
Community events	372	273 (73%)	143 (52%)	19	0	0
Cessation clinic	46	13 (28%)	11 (85%)	0	0	0
Breathing freedom helpline/Fax referrals	241	186 (77%)	164 (88%)	111	17	10
n	1,823	1,313	1,048	467	62	33

after more than 90 days (0.15%). The remaining 57% were not able to quit at all. These results are comparable to similar community-based programs that offer incentives to quit, culturally sensitive materials, or free NRT to low-income Black communities like North Lawndale. For example, "quit and win" contests may have initial 3-month quit rates ranging from 8% to 20%, then have 6- and 12-month follow-up rates as low as 3% and 0.2%, respectively (Cahill and Perera, 2008). Like other cessation programs targeted toward a disadvantaged community, Breathing Freedom realized a high initial participation of 70% to 80%, and then saw a gradual decline in participation and smoking abstinence (King et al., 2008).

In addition to providing residents with cessation plans, the program was featured in four Chicago-area news stories and distributed 1,000 anti-smoking church fans, 1,000 anti-smoking bags, 500 anti-smoking backpacks to community youth, and 2,000 Pathways to Freedom booklets. The neighborhood city councilwoman distributed program contact information to 5,000 constituents in a newsletter dedicated to anti-smoking in the community and was a featured part of five community-wide health forums.

A total of 80 businesses, churches, community organizations, health centers, and schools in the community received anti-smoking promotional materials. Twenty-seven neighborhood placements of three anti-smoking and Quitline promotional billboards also ran during the 24-month period (see Figure 7-3). An appreciable mark of success is that prior to the program the Quitline had received zero calls from the North Lawndale community since the line's inception. Over the 2-year period, the Quitline received 173 calls from the North Lawndale community. Each caller received a packet of smoking cessation and lung health education materials from the ALA, and if the caller left an accurate phone number, then they received a follow-up call from a smoking cessation counselor. We were unable to discern with any accuracy how many smokers quit as a result of calling the Quitline.

A majority of the smokers identified by this program were men (55%). However, women made up the greater proportion of those making a quit attempt. Also, adults that started smoking later in life (after age 18 years) were more likely to make a quit attempt and try to stay quit longer than those that started at a younger age. Persons that smoked half a pack a day or less, had some education beyond high school, or were employed on a consistent basis were more likely to make a quit attempt.

The program's collaboration with the CORE center delivered 231 nicotine patch prescriptions to 83 HIV-positive patients and 60 nicotine gum prescriptions to 25 HIV-positive patients. There were also 55 reactive Quitline contacts by HIV-positive patients. Twelve HIV-positive patients consistently attended the once-a-week smoking cessation class. One person from this group stayed smoke-free beyond 6 months. Breathing Freedom's collaboration with SCI delivered 16 smoking cessation workshops at designated WIC sites and four

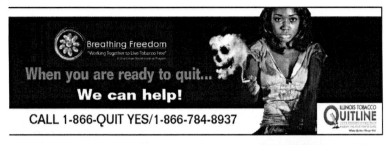

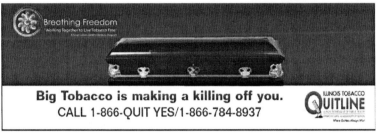

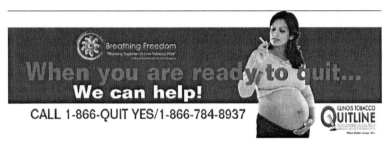

Figure 7-3   Breathing Freedom Illinois Tobacco Quitline Promotion Ads

90-minute smoking cessation trainings for 61 WIC case managers and nutritionists. There were 122 WIC clients participating in the workshops: 71 (58%) requested cessation plans and 32% of these reported making a quit attempt.

Finally, because it seemed important to program success, Mount Sinai Hospital, a 90-year-old hospital located in North Lawndale, became a smoke-free campus. Facilitated by Breathing Freedom, hospital administration and caregivers sought to set an example for North Lawndale residents. Twenty-five non-smoking caregivers completed a half-day certified smoking cessation class and 31 smoking caregivers received cessation plans, with all making a quit attempt in the first week.

Breathing Freedom's Community Impact and Lessons Learned

Breathing Freedom, a multifaceted community-based program, established several different types of free services and education outreach for helping the residents of North Lawndale quit smoking. Unlike a national or even city-wide intervention,

Breathing Freedom was focused on a specific community area and worked with a number of community organizations, churches, businesses, and civic groups in the area to raise awareness about smoking risks. Breathing Freedom was guided by what the epidemiological data provided about the dimensions of smoking in North Lawndale and also by what the literature said about evidence-based effectiveness of interventions across several areas. The program was culturally relevant using materials and creating messages that were oriented for a predominantly Black audience. From all indications, these messages were well-received.

Although an experimental design would have been ideal for this work, our budget and timeline did not make this possible. The program, however, successfully tracked participant readiness to quit and number of quit attempts. Some strong evidence of the impact of the services and outreach is reflected in the consistent number of residents the program found that were trying to quit. The Sinai Survey, which demonstrated the urgent need for the program, showed that 7 out of 10 North Lawndale smokers said they were trying to quit at the time of the survey, and 46% of those surveyed had tried to quit in the previous year leading up to the survey. Breathing Freedom found that 72% of persons attending a workshop, contacted by a health educator, or encouraged by their physician requested a cessation plan, and just over 8 out of 10 of them made a quit attempt in the first week.

The program also engaged new and expectant mothers involved in the WIC program, which had not been done before in Chicago. A tool to be used by WIC case managers specifically designed to help new and expectant mothers quit was developed by this program.

A comprehensive smoking cessation model for HIV-positive and AIDS patients was also developed by this program. Feedback from clinicians involved in directly treating HIV-positive patients stated that based on work from this program, they have learned to follow patient smoking behavior as a cue to changes in compliance with anti-retroviral medication and/or drug treatment program. HIV-positive and AIDS patients who consistently attended the smoking cessation classes or requested a NRT prescription were also seen as patients most likely to comply with treatment regimens.

The Ruth M. Rothstein Core Center and WIC program components were unique features as they were intervention efforts that focused on specialized populations and extended beyond the general North Lawndale community. Another particularly unique feature of Breathing Freedom was the physician-assisted counseling. Prior to our program we were not able to identify any other community-based smoking cessation effort that featured 8 hours of physician-dedicated time each month to smoking cessation.

There were also some clear failures to the program that other planned interventions can learn from. One such failure was that the program was unable to establish a consistent weekly group intervention in the community.

Although the program was able to hold workshops on a regular basis, it was very difficult to get residents to commit to attend a group session on a regular basis. Instead the program collaborated with a faith-based smoking cessation counselor that prior to the program's implementation held sparsely attended group meetings. The combined efforts were only marginally successful.

Another weak area for the program was the physician-assisted clinic component. Several logistic challenges hampered the start of the clinic, including securing adequate space for patient visits, identifying appropriate times in the physician's schedule to consistently schedule the visits, and establishing a subcontract and reimbursement schedule for the physician. One advantage for establishing the clinic was having a dedicated physician be a part of the planning process and engaged in the smoking cessation efforts throughout. However, of the 53 clinical appointments made, only one-fourth of the patients kept their appointments. Also none of the patients attending the clinic returned for follow-up visits or quit. Patients making their first appointment were clearly demonstrating a stage of change. On the other hand, retention was dismal and there was no evidence that the clinic helped patients quit.

The actual work of the program revealed that helping residents to quit smoking is a monumental undertaking that is both labor- and resource-intensive. It also revealed that in an area of concentrated poverty like North Lawndale, smoking cessation was not a subject that enlisted a significant amount of excitement. In fact, given the magnitude of the social and domestic issues such as poverty, social isolation, community violence, and joblessness that many of the residents faced on a day-to-day basis, smoking seemed to be, for many, a means of escape or self-medication. This much was voiced by residents who would willingly admit to knowing the risks associated with smoking but felt the risks did not outweigh the effects that smoking had on helping them cope with anxiety and stress.

Therefore, a clear message that can be drawn from Breathing Freedom seems to be that although such programs are desperately needed and can have some measurable impact in raising awareness and helping people work toward quitting, more needs to be done to help residents cope with their daily lives as well as with the nicotine addiction itself.

Acknowledgments

This innovative initiative was made possible by several community partners, including our funders the Illinois Department of Public Health and the American Lung Association.

The authors would like to acknowledge the Sinai Health System, Sinai Community Institute, Ruth M. Rothstein CORE Center, Respiratory Health of

Metropolitan Chicago, Lawndale Christian Health Center and Cook County Health System. We would also like to thank the supportive churches, social service organizations, civic groups and community residents of North Lawndale.

References

Abraham, Laurie Kaye. 1994. *Mama Might Be Better Off Dead: The Failure of Health Care in Urban America.* Chicago, IL: University Of Chicago Press.

American Lung Association. Freedom from Smoking Online. American Lung Association website. Online. Available: www.ffsonline.org. Accessed June 1, 2009.

Andrews, Jeannette O., Gwen Felton, Mary Ellen Wewers, Jennifer Waller, and Martha Tingen. 2007. The effect of a multi-component smoking cessation intervention in African-American women residing in public housing. *Research in Nursing and Health* 30:45–60.

Ahluwalia, Jasjit S., Ken Resnicow, and W. Scott Clark. 1998. Knowledge about smoking, reasons for smoking and reasons for wishing to quit in inner-city African-Americans. *Ethnicity & Disease* 8:385–393.

Cahill, Kate and Rafael Perera. 2008. Quit and win contests for smoking cessation. *Cochrane Database System Review* 8(4):CD004986.

Centers for Disease Control and Prevention (CDC). 2003. Behavioral Risk Factor Surveillance System Survey Data. Atlanta, Georgia: U.S. Department of Health and Human Services, Centers for Disease Control and Prevention.

Centers for Disease Control and Prevention (CDC). 2003. Pathways to Freedom: winning the fight against tobacco. Atlanta, Georgia: U.S. Department of Health and Human Services, Centers for Disease Control and Prevention. Online. Available: www.cdc.gov/TOBACCO/quit_smoking/how_to_quit/pathways/pdfs/pathways.pdf.   Accessed August 17, 2009.

COMMIT Research Group. 1995. Community Intervention Trial for Smoking Cessation (COMMIT), I. Cohort Results from a Four-Year Community Intervention. *American Journal of Public Health* 85(2):183–192.

COMMIT Research Group. 1995. Community Intervention Trial for Smoking Cessation (COMMIT), II. Changes in adult cigarette smoking prevalence. *American Journal of Public Health* 85:193–200.

Dell, Jade L., Steven Whitman, Ami M. Shah, Abigail Silva, and David Ansell. 2005. Smoking in 6 diverse Chicago communities—A population study. *American Journal of Public Health* 95(6):1036–1042.

DiClemente, Carlo C. and James O. Prochaska. 1982. Self-change and therapy change of smoking behavior: A comparison of processes of change in cessation and maintenance. *Addictive Behaviors* 7:133–142.

Feldman, Joseph G., Howard Minkoff, Michael F. Schneider, Stephen J. Gange, Mardge Cohen, D. Heather Watts, et al. 2006. Association of cigarette smoking with HIV prognosis among women in the HAART era: A report from the women's interagency HIV study. *American Journal of Public Health* 96(6):1060–1065.

Fiore, Michael C., William C. Bailey, Stuart J. Cohen, Sally Faith Dorfman, Michael G. Goldstein, Ellen R. Gritz, et al. 2000. *Treating Tobacco Use and Dependence: Clinical Practical Guideline.* Rockville, MD: Department of Health and Human Services (June).

Fisher, Edwin B., Wendy F. Auslander, Janice F. Munro, Cynthia L. Arfken, Ross C. Brownson, and Nancy W. Owens. 1998. Neighbors for a smoke free north side: Evaluation of a community organization approach to promoting smoking cessation among African Americans. *American Journal of Public Health* 88(11):1658–1663.

General Accounting Office. 2001. Tobacco settlement: States' use of master settlement agreement payments. Washington, DC. (June).

Gillison, Maura L. 2009. Oropharyngeal cancer: A potential consequence of concomitant HPV and HIV infection. *Current Opinion in Oncology* 21(5):439–444.

Hopkins, David P., Peter A. Briss, Connie J. Ricard, Corinne G. Husten, Vilma G. Carande-Kulis, Jonathan E. Fielding, et al, 2001. Reviews of evidence regarding interventions to reduce tobacco use and exposure to environmental tobacco smoke. *American Journal of Preventive Medicine* 20(2S):16–66.

Illinois Department of Public Health. Illinois tobacco free communities: Master settlement agreement. Online. Available: http://www.idph.state.il.us/TobaccoWebSite/msa. htm. Accessed October 1, 2009.

Johnson, Timothy and Linda Owens. 2003. Survey response rate reporting in the professional literature. Paper presented at the 58th Annual Meeting of the American Association for Public Opinion Research, Nashville (May). Online. Available: http://www.srl.uic.edu/publist/confpres.htm. Accessed August 17, 2009.

King, Andrea, Lisa Sánchez-Johnsen, Sarah Van Orman, Dingcai Cao, and Alicia Matthews. 2008. A pilot community-based intensive smoking cessation intervention in African Americans: Feasibility, acceptability and early outcome indicators. *Journal of National Medical Association* 100(2):208–217.

Lavoléa, Armelle Marie Wislezab, Martine Antoinebc, Charles Mayaudab, Bernard Milleronab, and Jacques Cadranelab. 2006. Lung cancer, a new challenge in the HIV infected population. *Journal of Lung Cancer* 51(1):1–11. Epub 2005 Nov 21.

Manske, Steve, Susan Miller, Cheryl Moyer, Marie Rose Phaneuf, and Roy Cameron. 2004. Best practice in group-based smoking cessation. Results of a literature review applying effectiveness, plausibility, and practicality criteria. *American Journal of Health Promotion* 18:409–423.

Mullen, Patricia Dolan, Joseph P. Carbonari, Ellen R. Tabak, and Marianna C. Glenday. 1991. Improving disclosure of smoking by pregnant women. *American Journal of Obstetrics and Gynecology* 165(2):409–413.

National Center for Health Statistics. 2001. *National Health Interview Survey.* Hyattsville, MD: U.S. Department of Health and Human Services, CDC, NCHS. Online. Available: www.cdc.gov/nchs/nhis.htm. Accessed June 1, 2009.

Nelson, David E., Eve Powell-Griner, Machell Town, and Mary Grace Kovar. 2003. A comparison of national estimates from the National Health Interview Survey and the Behavioral Risk Factor Surveillance System. *American Journal of Public Health* 93:1335–1341.

Nollen, Nicole L., Delwyn Catley, Gwen Davies, Matthew Hall, and Jasjit S. Ahluwalia. 2005. Religiosity, social support and smoking cessation among urban African-American smokers. *Addictive Behaviors* 30:1225–1229.

Northridge, Mary E., Alfredo, Morabia, Michael L. Ganz, Mary T. Bassett, Donald Gemson, Holly Andrews, and Colin McCord 1998. Contribution of smoking to excess mortality in Harlem. *American Journal of Epidemiology* 147:250–258.

Prochaska, James O. and Carlo C. DiClemente. 1983. Stages and processes of self-change of smoking: Toward an integrative model of change. *Journal of Consulting and Clinical Psychology* 51(3):390–395.

Prochaska, James O., Wayne F. Velicer, Carlo C DiClemente, and Joseph Fava, 1988. Measuring processes of change: Applications to the cessation of smoking. *Journal of Consulting and Clinical Psychology* 56:520–528.

Satter, Beryl. 2009. *Family Properties: Race, Real Estate, and the Exploitation of Black Urban America.* New York, NY: Metropolitan Books.

Standard Definitions: Final Dispositions of Case Codes and Outcome Rates for Surveys. 2004. Ann Arbor, MI: American Association for Public Opinion Research.

Steans Family Foundation. Online. Available: www.steansfamilyfoundation.org/lawn-dale_history.shtml. Accessed August 17, 2009.

Troldahl, Verling C. and Ray E. Carter. 1964. Random selection of respondents within households in phone surveys. *Journal of Marketing Research* 1:71–76.

U.S. Department of Health and Human Services. Public Health Services, Office of the Surgeon General. 2001. Women and Smoking; A report of the Surgeon General. Rockville, MD: U.S.D.H.H.S.

U.S. Census Bureau. *2000 Census of Population and Housing, Summary File 3.* Washington, DC: US Census Bureau; 2002: Table DP-3. Online. Available: http://www.nipc.org/test/dp234_CA_2000.htm. Accessed June 1, 2009.

Whitman, Steven, Cynthia Williams, and Ami M. Shah. 2004. *Sinai's Improving Community Health Survey: Report 1.* Chicago, IL: Sinai Health System.

Windsor, Richard A., John B. Lowe, Laura L. Perkins, Dianne Smith-Yoder, Lynn Artz, Myra Crawford, et al. 1993. Health education for pregnant smokers: Its behavioral impact and cost benefit. *American Journal of Public Health* 83(2):201–206.

Yunzal-Butler, Cristina, Ted Joyce, and Andrew D. Racine. 2009. Maternal smoking and the timing of WIC enrollment. *Maternal and Child Health Journal* (Feb): EPub, 21.

8

COMBATING CHILDHOOD OBESITY THROUGH A NEIGHBORHOOD COALITION: COMMUNITY ORGANIZING FOR OBESITY PREVENTION IN HUMBOLDT PARK

Adam B. Becker, Katherine Kaufer Christoffel, Miguel Angel Morales, José Luis Rodríguez, José E. López, and Matt Longjohn

Data and the Origins of a Community Approach to Obesity Prevention

Prior to 2003, very little data existed to describe childhood obesity in Chicago and its neighborhoods. National data indicated that prevalence rates were alarmingly high across the country and that children and families of color experienced a higher burden than their White counterparts. Then, as now, few data existed to describe how these disparities were reflected across specific states, cities, or neighborhoods. In Chicago, researchers and practitioners relied largely on national data until three studies were conducted to further describe the epidemiology of childhood obesity in the city. Beginning in 2003, epidemiologists and researchers from three institutions conducted studies to further define childhood obesity prevalence (Fig. 8-1). The Illinois Department of Public Health's Healthy Smiles Initiative conducted a study

171

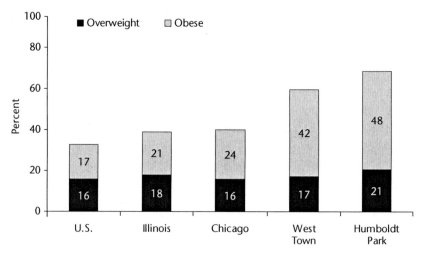

Figure 8-1 Existing Data on the Prevalence of Childhood Overweight Obesity

Sources: [a]U.S. data: Prevalence presented as a weighted estimate from National Health and Nutrition Examination Survey 2003–2004 obesity data for children age 2–5 (13.9%) and 6–11 (18.9%).
[b]Illinois data: Third graders across the state of Illinois with BMI between 85th and 94th percentiles (18%) and >95th percentile (21%) (IDPH, 2006).
[c]Chicago data: Prevalence of 3- to 5-year-olds in Chicago with BMI percentiles between 85th and 94th percentiles (16%) and >95th percentile (24%) (Mason et al., 2006).
[d]Children 2–12 years based on caregiver reported height and weight (Margellos-Anast, Shah, and Whitman, 2008).

among third graders across the state and found that approximately one in five students was overweight or obese (IDPH, 2006). The Consortium to Lower Obesity in Chicago Children (CLOCC; www.clocc.net) conducted an analysis of data submitted to schools for children entering kindergarten in Chicago and found that approximately one in four children began school overweight or obese (Mason et al., 2006).

Although these studies helped make the case for childhood obesity prevention in Illinois and Chicago, it was the Sinai Urban Health Institute's (SUHI) study of health and wellness in six Chicago communities that helped to guide local practitioners to the city's neighborhoods that were in high need of initiatives to support healthy lifestyles and reduce childhood obesity (Whitman, Williams, and Shah, 2004). The SUHI study found that childhood obesity rates in some of Chicago's neighborhoods were as high as 60%. Low-income communities of color had the highest rates. Among these communities were Humboldt Park—a community that is 47% Black and 48% Hispanic—and the adjacent West Town—a quickly gentrifying community that is 47% Latino. More than 60% of children in these two neighborhoods were found to be either overweight or obese (Margellos-Anast, Shah, and Whitman, 2008). Presentations of these data were a catalyst to action that sparked a number of neighborhood initiatives.

The information resonated with CLOCC's mission to protect the city's children from the obesity epidemic. CLOCC's founding funder, The Otho S. A. Sprague Memorial Institute, challenged SUHI and CLOCC to find a way to translate the SUHI data and CLOCC's momentum into a model, action-oriented, community-level effort to foster healthy lifestyles. SUHI and CLOCC identified Humboldt Park and the western part of West Town (identified by its Latino residents as part of Humboldt Park, although it lies outside of that community area's official boundaries) as an ideal site for this undertaking. The result was Community Organizing for Obesity Prevention in Humboldt Park (CO-OP HP). CO-OP HP was established in August 2004 with the Puerto Rican Cultural Center (PRCC; http://prcc-chgo.org/) as its anchor organization. CO-OP HP adopted the motto: *"Con familias saludables, nuestra comunidad echa pa'lante"* ("With healthy families, our community can move ahead").

The PRCC has led progressive work in the Puerto Rican section of the Humboldt Park community for more than 40 years. A hallmark of the PRCC's work is fostering a culture of citizen involvement and commitment, providing a rich context for community organizing. A variety of organizations in the community had a long-standing history of working together to improve quality of life for residents. The SUHI study had led separately to an emerging effort to create a "community of wellness" in Humboldt Park, which was envisioned as an interorganizational collaboration with a broad health-centered focus that would include healthy lifestyle promotion for obesity prevention and reduction. The relationships among the key organizations, the emerging focus on health in the community, and the history of rich community engagement enabled Humboldt Park to begin to build a model for community engagement in the creation of community support systems for healthy lifestyles, and so for reducing obesity.

Several other community characteristics made Humboldt Park fertile ground for innovation and incubation of intervention strategies that could be disseminated and replicated throughout the city. In addition to a concentration of Chicago's Puerto Rican residents, the area also includes large Mexican-American and Black populations and thus represents a cross-section of the dominant racial and ethnic minority groups in the city. The racial and ethnic diversity of Humboldt Park held out the possibility that interventions developed there would likely be culturally appropriate in other parts of the city. In addition, the population median income is low, representing the socio-economic class most disproportionately burdened by obesity and related chronic diseases.

One of CO-OP HP's first strategies was to collect more data about obesity and health in Humboldt Park. The project steering committee used focus groups to elicit qualitative information about local obstacles to healthier living and opportunities to increase healthy habits. CO-OP HP staff and volunteers with experience in the method conducted nine focus groups among Puerto Rican caregivers of children ages 2 to 18 years, community leaders, and adolescents; five focus groups among Mexican caregivers of children ages 2 to 18 years; and three focus groups among Black caregivers. These focus groups, conducted in both English and Spanish, explored behaviors and attitudes regarding nutrition and physical activity in the neighborhood.

CO-OP HP staff and volunteers also conducted surveys in which body mass index (BMI) and perceptions of overweight were measured during an annual festival along the community's main business corridor, *Fiesta Boricua on Paseo Boricua*, in 2004 and 2005. Five hundred surveys were conducted each year. Finally, a more comprehensive survey, the Community Wellness survey, was conducted among 100 Puerto Rican and 100 Mexican-American families concerning behaviors, attitudes, and knowledge of physical activity and nutrition. The survey was developed by SUHI, so that the content was tied to the larger multicommunity survey that had been done. Community members were trained in how to conduct the survey. The survey identified some clear problems. For example, only one in four area residents ate the recommended five servings of fruits and vegetables a day, and one in four children drank at least two cans of soda a day. Nearly half of area children watched at least three hours of television a day. Two-thirds of area residents felt unsafe walking in the community (Estarziau et al., 2006). The initial data collection was envisioned as a first phase in an ongoing series of data collections that would document gradual changes in lifestyle in the area and how these changes related to CO-OP HP efforts. Data from a second wave of the Community Wellness Study in Humboldt Park are currently being analyzed for presentation to CO-OP HP partners to use in refining intervention approaches. Data have been shared with CO-OP HP leadership and plans are underway for community-wide dissemination.

The resulting data from all of these collection strategies helped the emerging CO-OP HP Steering Committee to define initiatives to promote healthy eating and physical activity for children and families in Humboldt Park. The data revealed many barriers community members faced when making choices about food and activity (Table 8-1).

Evolution of CO-OP HP

In response to some of the data described above, PRCC, SUHI, and CLOCC initiated CO-OP HP in 2004. The Sprague Institute provided funding for a full-time coordinator. PRCC brought to the group its programs, community

TABLE 8-1   Barriers to Eating Healthy and Being Physically Active Reported by Community Members in One Latino Community in Chicago

- Limited access to affordable produce
- Community retail outlets carry an abundance of high-sugar and high-fat foods
- Families have limited time to shop for healthy foods
- Little knowledge about nutrition
- No time to engage in physical activity with family
- Safety issues that prevent families from going outside or allowing children outside to play
- Preference for devoting leisure time to watching television and playing video games

leadership role, and social and political connections. SUHI brought its understanding of HP's health and related survey data. CLOCC brought obesity content expertise and city-wide connections to relevant programs and policymakers. This starting group envisioned the creation of a coalition of local organizations, with the goal of identifying obstacles to healthy eating and active lifestyles in Humboldt Park as well as the development of a plan to reduce those obstacles and encourage a culture of healthy living. Over time, several organizations were added to the emerging CO-OP HP Steering Committee.

Steering Committee Membership

Bickerdike Redevelopment Corporation (Bickerdike; http://www.bickerdike.org/) was the first to join the founding partners. Bickerdike's mission is to redevelop West Town, Humboldt Park, and two neighboring communities for the benefit of and control by the lower and moderate-income residents of those areas. The organization began by developing affordable single-family homes and has evolved into a multifaceted driver of community development. Bickerdike is the anchor organization for the New Communities Program of the Local Initiatives Support Corporation (LISC; www.lisc.org). In that role, Bickerdike was charged with developing and implementing a "Quality-of-Life Plan" through a participatory planning process, making it a likely partner in the CO-OP HP endeavor. The second group to join was Centro Sin Fronteras, a local grassroots organization in the Mexican-American community with a track record for reaching thousands of constituents at a time for varied initiatives. A third member was Association House, established in 1899 with a continued mission to offer services to economically disadvantaged individuals and families in Humboldt Park and West Town. Association House carries out its mission currently through providing human services, child welfare activities, behavioral health services, and a continuing education center.

With each addition to the Steering Committee, there was a period of adjustment for CO-OP HP, which had to incorporate new perspectives and priorities.

Over time some of these partners have needed to focus on community issues that were more directly aligned with their original missions (e.g., immigration policy, housing development, health more broadly) and have shifted out of CO-OP HP leadership roles. Other partners have joined as well. Some have stayed, others have left. Table 8-2 presents the primary partners in the CO-OP HP initiative, their roles, and the evolution of their engagement over time. The key partnership between CLOCC and PRCC remains the central partnership that sustains CO-OP HP.

CO-OP HP Structure and Partnerships

Since its inception in 2004, CO-OP HP's structure has evolved and grown. Currently, the CO-OP HP Steering Committee receives reports and provides input to a food subcommittee that develops strategies to improve fruit and vegetable consumption in the neighborhood. At one time, the CO-OP HP Steering Committee also had subcommittees focused on physical activity and evaluation. As CO-OP HP partners who are not formally part of the Steering Committee have become increasingly interested in these areas, steering committee members influence these efforts through partnerships rather than lead them through subcommittees. For example, physical activity interventions are influenced by CO-OP HP Steering Committee members through participation on the Active Lifestyles Task Force of The Greater Humboldt Park Community of Wellness (CoW; http://www.ghpcommunityofwellness.org/home.aspx). Multiple community organization leaders (including PRCC's Executive Director) formed the CoW in response to the SUHI study about Humboldt Park. The involvement of CLOCC and CO-OP HP staff ensures that strategies are aligned with the work of CO-OP HP. Similarly, a number of research and evaluation activities are carried out in Humboldt Park by the Steans Center for Community-Based Service Learning at DePaul University in Chicago. Although Steans Center staff and students do not participate on the CO-OP HP Steering Committee, they frequently partner with CO-OP HP to conduct research to support or evaluate CO-OP's approaches.

CO-OP HP staffing has changed over time as well. CO-OP HP began with one full-time manager and a part-time CLOCC Community Networker in West Town provided early support. When full funding was available for both positions, the CO-OP HP Manager became the CLOCC networker and the current CO-OP HP Manager was hired. CO-OP HP has also added two project coordinators. One coordinator oversees food strategies. The other coordinates a physical activity program with modest beginnings that has grown into a large-scale, multisite initiative. Numerous volunteers and student interns also have contributed to the success of CO-OP HP strategies (each of these strategies is described in more detail below). Although CO-OP

TABLE 8-2 Partners Within Community Organizing for Obesity Prevention in Humboldt Park (CO-OP HP)

Partner Organization	Mission/Purpose	Historical Role	Current Status
Puerto Rican Cultural Center	To serve the social/cultural needs of Chicago's Puerto Rican/Latino community; based on a philosophy of self-determination, a methodology of self-actualization and critical thought, and an ethic of self-reliance	Originating Partner	Anchor Organization, houses staff, coordinates all programs, provides primary linkage to community
Sinai Urban Health Institute	To develop and implement effective approaches that improve the health of urban communities through data-driven research, evaluation, and community engagement	Originating Partner	Supports surveillance and evaluation efforts on *ad hoc* basis
Consortium to Lower Obesity in Chicago Children	To confront the childhood obesity epidemic by promoting healthy and active lifestyles for children throughout the Chicago metropolitan area; to foster and facilitate connections between childhood obesity prevention researchers, public health advocates and practitioners, and the children, families, and communities of Chicagoland	Originating Partner	Provides funding, participates in steering committee and all subcommittees, provides public health expertise
Otho S. A. Sprague Memorial Institute	To pursue the investigation of the cause of disease and the prevention and relief of human suffering in the City of Chicago, County of Cook, State of Illinois	Originating Partner and Funder	Provides funding through CLOCC, serves as catalyst for new intervention models
Bickerdike Redevelopment Corporation	To redevelop the West Town, Humboldt Park, Logan Square and Hermosa communities for the benefit of and control by the lower and moderate-income residents of those areas	Joined in first expansion	Provides staff and programmatic support as needed; links to LISC for funding as needed
Centro Sin Fronteras	To advocate for immigrants' rights in Chicago	Joined in first expansion; link to Mexican American community	No longer involved
Association House	To offer services to economically disadvantaged individuals and families in Humboldt Park and West Town	Joined after first expansion	Member of steering committee
Norwegian American Hospital	To promote wellness within the family and to be dynamic partners in health with the communities we serve	Joined after first expansion	No longer involved

HP is managed and staffed by the Puerto Rican Cultural Center and guided by a partnership between CLOCC and the PRCC, a variety of community partners also participate in CO-OP HP meetings and initiatives. Although the participation of these partners ebbs and flows, their contributions to the work of CO-OP HP are critical elements of its success.

CO-OP HP Funding

A guiding principal of CO-OP HP is that initiatives should be community-driven and sustainable. To ensure both local ownership and longevity, CO-OP HP strategies are not highly dependent on external funding. However, staff and some of the strategies do require financial support. The Sprague Institute provided original funding to SUHI for CO-OP HP. In subsequent years, CLOCC has raised funds to provide subcontracts to the PRCC for CO-OP HP staff, projects, and promotional materials. PRCC contributes in kind, adding resources to CO-OP HP intervention approaches, hosting meetings, and providing or supplementing staff salaries. More recently, PRCC has begun to include CO-OP HP funding in its fundraising strategies to sustain the effort directly. Over the years, a variety of funders, in addition to the Sprague Institute, have invested in CO-OP HP to support CO-OP HP management, programming, environmental change strategies, and evaluation. In addition, local partners have contributed time, money, and other resources to support CO-OP HP initiatives. As CO-OP HP enters its sixth year, full ownership and control, as well as fundraising responsibility, will shift to the PRCC.

CO-OP HP Intervention Strategies

Based on the data gathered through the multiple methods described above, CO-OP HP leadership determined that in addition to supporting a coalition of community-based organizations, it would pilot and implement a variety of intervention approaches that would ultimately increase healthy eating and physical activity in the community and strengthen health-related resources that could support healthy lifestyles. These interventions are described below.

Increasing Access to Produce

To address low levels of fruit and vegetable consumption, local leaders identified both nutrition education and access to fresh produce as priorities. The issue of local food access is understood by the PRCC as central to broader issues of community identity, sustainability, and redevelopment. As gentrification moves toward the community, the PRCC and its partners work to assert community ownership of strategic spaces to protect the history and culture of the Puerto Rican community in Chicago. In this context, assuring food access is important in a number of ways. First, food production in the community (including gardening and urban agriculture) can help develop an indigenous commercial base, creating local wealth that can help people to become property owners or afford increasing rents and stay in the community. Second, fostering local demand for produce can help keep local businesses operating while also changing peoples' diets to become healthier. Healthier residents are, in turn, more able to gain and maintain wealth. Thus, CO-OP HP's food goals embody the broader objectives of local business development and wealth creation, establishing a consumer base for these new business endeavors and using community public space to provide goods and services that will ultimately improve the health of the community as well as demonstrate positive uses of these spaces by and for the community.

Farmers' Market

One of the multifaceted produce access endeavors has been the Humboldt Park Farmers' Market. In the early years of CO-OP HP, numerous organizations met to develop a farmers' market in Humboldt Park. The group was comprised of local and external organizations. Some had the protection of green space as a mission, some had organic food production and consumption as a mission, some had missions related to protecting the health and well-being of the community, and a few aimed to provide new goods and services to the increasing population of Chicagoans moving into Humboldt Park from other areas of the city. As CO-OP HP got established in 2004, staff met with this farmers' market interest group to discuss the role that CO-OP HP could play, with a goal of ensuring that this market was primarily by and for the people of Humboldt Park who had been in the neighborhood for generations. Members of the group agreed to move the market from its original location off the beaten path to a spot on the main business thoroughfare that was particularly important to the Puerto Rican community. The PRCC became the host of the market in 2005 and renamed it *El Conuco Farmers' Market on Paseo Boricua*. The CO-OP HP manager took over logistics for the relocated market, got the necessary buy-in from businesses that owned or rented near the new location, took on the responsibility of advertising, arranged for the supply of electricity and water from a nearby business, and arranged for storage between market days. A partner organization, which had been involved with the market at its previous location, managed the newly organized market. Over time, and as CO-OP HP evolved, interest grew among some of the original stakeholders in shifting increasing management responsibility to the PRCC and CO-OP HP staff.

Throughout its 4-year history, as is the case with many small, locally driven markets, *El Conuco* has struggled to sustain sufficient numbers of shoppers and producers. Some days, a sufficient number of shoppers would come but not find a sufficient number of producers. The next week, after heroic efforts, sufficient numbers of producers would arrive, but dubious shoppers did not show up because of their experience the week prior. A great deal of staff time went into attempts to break this "vicious cycle." CO-OP HP leadership began to question the wisdom of managing the market and a number of criteria were set by the steering committee to determine how long CO-OP HP should devote energy and resources to the market. The success of the market, however, was important enough to the local leaders that they persisted.

Today, the market is in a new, more visible location in the local park at a busy intersection. CO-OP HP staff manages the market entirely. They have shifted the market's focus so that it is now a community market that includes locally grown produce, flowers grown in the community and on nearby farms, local crafts, and prepared foods. Some small, local grocery stores also attend and sell their inventory. To align the market with CO-OP HP's obesity prevention goals, partners (e.g., the Chicago Partnership for Health Promotion, University of Illinois Extension) periodically provide nutrition education and healthy recipes at the market. Although the market continues to struggle, it continues to survive as well. Local leaders' commitment to the multiple goals of the *El Conuco* provides the motivation to persist, even in the face of difficult challenges.

Produce Purchase and Delivery Programs

Another food intervention of CO-OP HP is a food basket dissemination program called *La Cosecha* (The Harvest). This program too has evolved over time and meets multiple goals of local leadership. The market basket program began as a product established by a partner organization, similarly to community-supported agriculture programs that have emerged in other places. Consumers ordered bags of produce weekly, and these bags were delivered to the PRCC for local pickup. Sometimes, a local business or clinic would order enough to justify direct delivery to that site. CO-OP HP's involvement in the original version of the program was to manage the ordering process and staff the distribution. CLOCC research staff conducted an evaluation of the program and identified a number of challenges. For example, consumers were not always pleased with the bags they received, which often contained produce with which they were unfamiliar. CO-OP HP staff tried to provide recipes, but lack of familiarity with the bags' contents could not be overcome by recipes alone. Attempts to change the contents of the bags were not successful because of the logistics of the providing agency.

Eventually, it became clear that a locally run program might do better at meeting consumer needs.

In 2009, CO-OP HP relaunched the program as *La Cosecha*, built on a relationship that has been developed with a local grocer who sells culturally appropriate produce to CO-OP HP at wholesale prices. CO-OP HP staff members bag the produce and customers pick them up weekly. CO-OP HP charges $1 per bag above cost, so that as orders increase, supplemental staff can be brought in to help with bagging and distribution. CO-OP HP staff has sometimes been able to arrange for bag distribution to take place inside local bodegas/corner stores. Local leaders see *La Cosecha* as having two important results: expanding local demand for produce and stimulating local business owners to get involved in produce retail. It is hoped that ultimately local production will supply a significant portion of local demand for fresh produce.

Producemobile

A third food intervention in which CO-OP HP has been involved is the Producemobile. This service is provided by the Greater Chicago Food Depository (GCFD; http://www.chicagosfoodbank.org), a part of the national Feed America network. In this program, GCFD sends a truck full of contributed produce to community settings for free distribution by local organizations. The local organizations organize the distribution site, manage the often long lines of consumers, get the produce off the truck and into bags, and clean up the location after delivery is complete. CO-OP HP staff members coordinate one of several monthly Producemobile days in Humboldt Park and ensure that members of the local community have continuing access to this emergency food service.

CO-OP HP staff has also worked with CLOCC partners to provide nutrition education and sample recipes to consumers during Producemobile. In an effort to identify additional opportunities to provide services during Producemobile delivery, CLOCC did a survey to assess if additional health-related services would be well-received. The results indicated that consumers were interested in information that would help them make the best use of the produce they received. Other services (such as health screenings and immunizations) were not welcomed because of long waits for produce and a reluctance to bring children to the produce distribution site.

CO-OP HP staff and leadership continue to innovate to increase the availability of healthy food for community residents. Staff has identified three local store owners who are willing to house a CO-OP HP produce cooler on their premises. The coolers will be used to store surplus produce from *La Cosecha* and will also make it feasible for those stores to begin to stock produce. Staff is also working with local restaurateurs to develop a program that will publicize participating restaurants that are willing to feature items on their menus that contain fresh produce. The PRCC has an ongoing program at a partner high school that engages students in community gardening and urban agriculture. CO-OP HP leadership and staff remain committed to the idea that the combination of local supply and demand enhancement will help to attain community goals for the use and occupation of community space while also improving the diets, and ultimately the health, of community members.

Physical Activity Interventions

CO-OP HP has initiated a number of strategies related to increasing physical activity for community members. These efforts range from the delivery of specific programs to changing the physical activity environment and working with government agencies to implement policy and systems changes.

¡Muévete!

A cornerstone of CO-OP HP's physical activity work is the *¡Muévete!* intervention model. *¡Muévete!* (Move!) began with one woman recognizing her own urgent need for more physical activity and has become an intervention strategy that is implemented in numerous settings in and around Humboldt Park and serving hundreds of women and their children. Leony Calderón, *¡Muévete!* founder, is a young obese woman who was told by her physician that she had elevated cholesterol and borderline hypertension. She was told that she needed to lose weight to get these problems under control, or she would face a lifetime of medications to control them. She began a physical activity regime by walking around Humboldt Park, the 200-plus-acre park after which the community is named. Soon, friends and even strangers started walking with her.

When the cold winter weather set in, Ms. Calderón took her walking group inside. To adapt to the indoor setting, she took an aerobic instruction class at the Chicago Park District and turned the activity into an aerobic dance program, using Latin and other culturally relevant music to inspire the growing number of women, and their children, participating in the program. Since its humble beginnings in 2004, *¡Muévete!* has expanded to include two additional park-based programs, several new community- and school-based programs, and a variety of appearances and special sessions at community events all over Chicago.

Promoting Cycling in Humboldt Park

Increasing the numbers of community members who cycle in the community has been another physical activity initiative of CO-OP HP. The first

CO-OP HP Manager expressed this goal as a desire to "make cycling sexy for Puerto Ricans." Efforts began with organized bike rides that included a bike tour of murals that depict Puerto Rican history and culture. CO-OP HP's partner, Bickerdike, received a grant to develop a map of these local murals that could be used in bike rides and walking tours. With the relocation of the farmers' market, the bike tours expanded to include the market and local gardens. Soon other partner organizations joined in. As interest in cycling grew, Bickerdike developed "Bickerbikes." In 2004, this bicycle safety and repair program for youth became West Town Bikes (http://westtownbikes. org/), a nonprofit organization whose mission is to promote bicycling, educate youth with a focus on underserved populations, and foster and serve Humboldt Park's growing bicycling community. Although it maintains headquarters and a workspace in Chicago's West Town neighborhood, West Town Bikes has become a city-wide service provider for youth programs in the city of Chicago. In a shining example of how CO-OP HP initiatives become sustainable entities, the leaders of West Town Bikes, in collaboration with CO-OP HP and PRCC staff, developed a for-profit business called Ciclo Urbano. This full service community bicycle shop supports the Humboldt Park and West Town neighborhoods. The shop focuses on affordable and reliable transportation, offering bicycle sales, service, new and used bike parts, and accessories. All sales from the shop support West Town Bikes' larger mission of providing bicycle education to Chicago youth.

Skateboarding Programming and Infrastructure

CO-OP HP staff and partners have also begun to examine skateboarding as a strategy for engaging youth in physical activity. A space behind the PRCC was opened for skateboarders during the summer of 2008. Also in 2008, CO-OP HP staff integrated the participants in the skateboarding group into Open Streets, a five-community strategy to encourage active transportation by closing major streets to motorized vehicles (described below). Although skateboarding has yet to become a formal intervention strategy, CO-OP HP staff continue to consider its role in physical activity programming. As of this writing, CO-OP HP staff is monitoring the potential development of a city skate park nearby. This park would replicate a successful skate park built by the City of Chicago in a neighboring community.

Open Streets and Humboldt Park in Motion

As CO-OP HP physical activity programming evolved, the Greater Humboldt Park CoW established its Active Lifestyles Task Force. The activities of the task force promote active lifestyles for adults and youth to combat obesity and related health problems, including diabetes and heart disease. The task force organizes events and programs focused on making the community more active. Most recently, the task force has been the primary Humboldt Park partner in Chicago's Open Streets initiative (http://www.activetrans. org/openstreets). Open Streets is a day-long event during which 8 miles of Chicago boulevards on the city's west side are opened to nonvehicular traffic so that community members can ride bikes, walk, rollerblade, and engage in other forms of active transportation while enjoying the streets in their neighborhoods without the usual congestion of cars, trucks, and buses. CO-OP HP staff and partners helped to organize events along the route, including skateboarding clinics and a bike repair station. Motivated by the Open Streets initiative, Humboldt Park organizations developed a series of activities to engage participants in the park and along the route. The partners called this series of activities "Humboldt Park in Motion" and soon agreed that this would be a theme of their work year-round in the community.

Marketing, Publicity, and Communications

CO-OP HP staff and partners see the promotion of their many intervention strategies and programmatic activities as an important element of their work. Such activities can increase participation and also help to change community norms around healthy lifestyles through visual reminders that Humboldt Park is a community in which residents can be healthy and active. Starting early in CO-OP HP's history, staff used the local newspaper, *La Voz del Paseo Boricua* (*La Voz*), to educate the community about the importance of healthy lifestyles. *La Voz* is operated as a separate business by the PRCC. Each month, 10,000 copies of the paper are distributed throughout the community, and revenue is generated through advertising. The CO-OP HP manager wrote regular articles for *La Voz* on health and health-related events, covering topics such as obesity, metabolic syndrome, diabetes, hypertension, and the evolving CO-OP HP strategies that could help community residents to confront these problems.

CO-OP HP continues to promote its activities in this local newspaper and also buys space periodically to advertise its healthy lifestyle message (Fig. 8-2). Developed by CLOCC, the *5-4-3-2-1 Go!*™ message (http:// www.clocc.net/partners/54321Go/index.html) promotes daily steps toward a healthy lifestyle: 5 servings of fruits and vegetables, 4 servings of water, 3 servings of low-fat dairy, 2 hours or less of screen-time (e.g., television, computer, video games), and 1 hour or more of physical activity. In addition to these public education ads, CO-OP HP staff and partners have made sure that community events, study results, political initiatives, and other activities related to health are also included in *La Voz*. CO-OP HP has also pursued other outlets to promote activities and the healthy lifestyle message, including spots on Univision, the local NPR satellite station, NBC news, and community radio feeds.

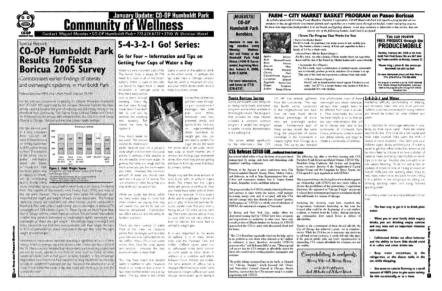

Figure 8-2   Public Education Advertisement in a Local Newspaper
Source: *La Voz*, January 2006 Issue.

From Programs to Systems and Environmental Change Approaches

As public health, medical, and community practitioners increase their understanding of the causes and effects of the childhood obesity epidemic, intervention strategies have evolved. Initial strategies focused on individual-level factors such as knowledge and attitudes and their impact on diet and activity behaviors. Over time, however, as the complexity of the childhood obesity problem has emerged, interventions are increasingly based on a social ecological model of public health problems (Becker, Longjohn, and Christoffel, 2008; Davison and Birch, 2001; McElroy et al., 1988). This model recognizes the importance of the built and social environment and its role in individual behavior. Childhood obesity prevention approaches based on social ecology consider risk and protective factors beyond the individual to focus on family, community, and institutional and public policy. For example, creating and sustaining the local farmers' market, opening Ciclo Urbano on Division Street, and regular *5-4-3-2-1 Go!* and CO-OP HP ads in *La Voz* all foster access to healthy food and physical activity, change the social environment through frequent cues to healthy living that are highly visible, and, in some cases, create enduring changes in the community landscape.

Most recently, CO-OP HP staff and partners have been involved in developing a community garden on Humboldt Park grounds with the co-located

Institute for Puerto Rican Arts and Culture. Students from the Dr. Pedro Albizu Campus Puerto Rican High School, an affiliate of PRCC, will manage the garden. Produce grown in this garden will be sold in the *El Conuco* market. As a sign of their commitment to the project's development, landscape architects from the Chicago Botanic Garden have produced design renderings of the garden to ensure that it is in keeping with the architectural style of the surrounding facilities, as required. The community garden is one of a few strategies being developed by the PRCC to sustain CO-OP HP activities through its approach to urban agriculture (described in the "Next Steps" section below).

Evaluating CO-OP HP

Humboldt Park Organizations and CO-OP HP staff develop programs, engage in activities, and institute policies that increase access and educational opportunities related to healthy food and safe opportunities for physical activity in the community. CO-OP HP partners work together to enhance relationships and expand resources in clinical settings and in interorganizational collaborative efforts. Each of these programmatic arenas is comprised of an ever-changing number of interventions and strategies. These interventions and strategies are expected to result in intermediate outcomes related to individual, family, and organizational behavior. These outcomes, over time, are expected to result in long-term changes in health status. Evaluating these anticipated changes is one of the most challenging aspects of the CO-OP HP effort.

The Challenges of CO-OP HP Evaluation

A combination of factors makes understanding the impact of CO-OP HP a complex endeavor. First and foremost is that CO-OP HP does not have sufficient funds to mount a comprehensive evaluation strategy. Intervention approaches such as CO-OP HP require a multimethod, multidimensional approach to evaluation to assess change at multiple levels. Multiple strategies are needed to measure influence on individual behavior, community environmental conditions, and institutional and local policy (Baker, Metzler, and Galea, 2005). Evaluation at any one of these levels is expensive. Evaluation across all of the levels requires significant time and money.

A second factor is the fluid nature of the interventions and strategies implemented under the CO-OP HP umbrella. CO-OP HP strategies emerge and take shape as local opportunities become available rather than as prospectively planned actions that roll out in predetermined ways. Initiatives focus on food, physical activity, or both. Standardized evaluation involves standardized methods and instruments to measure both of these complicated human behaviors. In addition, CO-OP HP interventions occur in varied and multiple settings (e.g., childcare settings, health-care settings, within business and retail, in parks and schools). These settings open and close their doors as funding dictates, sometimes welcome and sometimes prohibit external programming, and change their emphases from time to time. Participation in specific programs is highly variable, making the measurement of participation a challenge. With the exception of *La Cosecha*, in which people submit contact information with their produce order, program staff do not have ways of contacting participants in CO-OP HP interventions. Participation fluctuates week-to-week. People come to a *¡Muévete!* class, shop at the farmers' market, or receive free produce from Producemobile when they need to and when their schedules allow. The CO-OP HP Steering Committee has made the conscious choice not to collect contact information from participants on an ongoing basis because of the time that registration might take, the confidentiality needs of people who have to avail themselves of free produce programs, and concerns with immigrant status. Measuring participation alone is challenging. Measuring *change* among participants is even more difficult. Previous efforts have even interfered with participation, as when women avoided *¡Muévete!* when staff sought to weigh them in an effort to track change in BMI.

Within each of the programmatic arenas (e.g., food, physical activity), the specific interventions are in constant flux and evolution. As opportunities arise (e.g., funding, political will, a new partner-driven initiative) CO-OP HP staff and leadership look for ways to connect, enhance, and leverage these opportunities to make them stronger and more available to Humboldt Park residents. As certain opportunities end, others emerge. Documenting and monitoring this ever-fluctuating landscape is difficult. Evaluating the impact of the various components on community members is even more challenging. To date, CO-OP HP leadership has chosen to monitor only those intervention strategies over which they have the most influence and control and for which the tracking of participants would not require an added dimension to the program itself or burden on participants.

Evaluation Strategies

Tracking Change Among Participants and Partners

CO-OP HP leadership has established a number of ways to document progress and understand the impact the CO-OP HP initiatives have in the Humboldt Park community. In the summer of 2009, the CO-OP HP Steering Committee revised the original CO-OP HP survey developed by SUHI (described above) and administered it again to 200 residents in Humboldt

Park. As of press time, the results have been shared with the steering committee and plans are under way to release them to the community. CO-OP HP leadership will host a Town Hall meeting to disseminate the results of the second wave of the survey and to share any changes that have occurred as measured through the survey. In addition, CLOCC staff is conducting interviews with CO-OP HP partners and other organizations in Humboldt Park to learn about the ways that CO-OP HP facilitates interorganizational collaboration on issues related to healthy lifestyles.

Several CO-OP HP interventions have also been evaluated as stand-alone strategies. As described above, a survey of Market Basket consumers helped to identify strengths and weaknesses of the intervention and led to the development of the locally managed *La Cosecha*. The one-time survey among Producemobile participants (described above) clarified the additional services that participants would welcome and utilize. CO-OP HP staff monitors attendance and participation in *¡Muévete!*, Producemobile, and *La Cosecha* to understand the reach of these interventions. The trends in participation help CO-OP HP leadership to problem-solve and make adjustments in programming to ensure that programs are used to their maximum potential. The tables below present trends in participation in the two key intervention strategies that involve individual community residents.

Table 8-3 presents average monthly participation in the Produce Purchase Program each year from 2005 when Market Basket was initiated to the middle of 2009. Table 8-4 presents average monthly participation in Producemobile from 2005 to 2009. Table 8-5 presents data on *¡Muevete!* participation. This table includes the total number of participant sessions (participants are counted each time they participate, as opposed to only the first time) and the average number of participants per class each year between the start of the program in 2006 and the middle of 2009. Overall, these tables show that the CO-OP HP programs that are free-of-charge experienced an increase in participation each year, whereas the produce purchasing programs may be leveling or even tapering off.

Tracking Change in the Social, Physical, and Institutional Environment

Equally important to describing the effects of CO-OP HP programs is documenting the changes that have occurred in the physical and institutional environments in Humboldt Park. CO-OP HP has served as a catalyst that encourages partner organizations to increase their focus on healthy lifestyle promotion and programming. Changes are new enough that they are best seen as promising trends. For example, more local organizations now include healthy lifestyle promotion among their top priorities. Funders increasingly view Humboldt Park as an appropriate community in which to invest

TABLE 8-3   Annual Average Monthly Participation in Produce Purchase Program

Period	Average orders per month
October 1, 2005–June 30, 2006	63
July 1, 2006–June 30, 2007	77
July 1, 2007–June 30, 2008	70
February 1, 2009[a]–August 30, 2009	51

[a]*La Cosecha,* a separate food basket distribution program, was initiated in February 2009.

TABLE 8-4   Annual Average Monthly Participation in Producemobile

Period	Average Orders per Month
August 2005–June 2006	180
July 2006–June 2007	93
July 2007–Jun 2008	184
July 2008–June 2009	212

TABLE 8-5   Muévete Participation

Period	Number of participant sessions[a]	Average participants per class
January 9, 2006–June 30, 2006	916	18
July 1, 2006–June 30, 2007	2,776	20
July 1, 2007–June 30, 2008	5,717	40
July 1, 2008–June 30, 2009	7,174	51

[a]Numbers reflect the total number of people in each session, not unique individuals who participated.

because of the synergy created by CO-OP HP and its partner organizations. For example, the Sprague Institute has funded other initiatives in the area to support and/or reinforce CO-OP HP goals. These initiatives include nutrition counseling and a fitness center for those with chronic conditions who visit the local health department clinic as well as school nurse aids in Humboldt Park schools to help with administrative functions, freeing the nurses to conduct more prevention and disease management activities. Other CLOCC funders have been increasingly willing to fund initiatives in Humboldt Park because of the demonstrated commitment of local organizations to obesity prevention strategies.

Participating organizations, the PRCC chief among them, have expanded initiatives to increase food access or physical activity beyond the CO-OP HP partnership structure. Small businesses with products and services related to healthy eating and physical activity are opening up or relocating within the CO-OP HP boundaries, and existing businesses are beginning to integrate new products or services into their business model—in particular, local restaurants are adding more healthy items to their menus (e.g., reducing sugar, eliminating trans fat, introducing salads and fresh produce). Such changes are indicators of the potential long-term sustainability of CO-OP HP's goals, whether or not the current structure of CO-OP HP endures. Systems for documenting these changes over time remain both a goal and a challenge for CO-OP HP leadership and staff.

Understanding CO-OP HP: Some Lessons Learned

Over the last 5 years, CO-OP HP staff and partners have learned a number of lessons that have helped them to refine obesity prevention strategies. CLOCC has disseminated these lessons through a number of technical assistance initiatives locally and across the country; these lessons have been especially useful as CLOCC expands the CO-OP HP strategy to two new communities in Chicago. These lessons are presented here in the hopes that they can support readers who are interested in established similarly holistic and locally driven initiatives.

Maintaining a Focus on the Entire Community

Inclusivity in a racially and ethnically diverse community is a constant goal and a constant challenge. As originally envisioned, CO-OP HP was to cut across racial and ethnic divisions in HP, involving multiple organizations based in various demographically defined communities in the leadership, and fielding programs that served all who might benefit. Although some progress was made, this remains a vision that has not been fully realized. The involvement of Centro Sin Fronteras (CSF) as a partner in the CO-OP HP steering committee, and the organization's legitimacy among Mexican-Americans, made it possible to conduct the Community Wellness survey (Estarziau et al., 2006) and obtain equal samples of Puerto Rican and Mexican residents. CSF's involvement resulted in shared management of some programs and wide publicity of CO-OP HP work in the Mexican community. But over 1 or 2 years, immigration activism increasingly absorbed the CSF leaders, who eventually dropped out of CO-OP HP. One of the factors that contributed to this was sparse funding, which made it impossible to keep CSF leaders in paid roles.

Several efforts were made early on to bring on Black organizers to identify and engage groups in CO-OP HP. None of these efforts worked. After several years, when CLOCC was able to hire a full-time networker for the Black community just west of the Puerto Rican one, he became an active participant in CO-OP HP. This allowed some activities to cross communities (e.g., the Producemobile). But for others—for example, *¡Muévete!*—strong informal boundaries required the creation of parallel activities in the Black community. Again, limitations in funding made it impossible to offer incentives that might have helped to bridge the divide.

Forging Connections

Embedding neighborhood activities within a broader city-based network can enhance local efforts. As described above, many CO-OP HP programs benefitted from the involvement of organizations that were part of the CLOCC network but not based in Humboldt Park. For example, nutrition education was provided by organizations outside of the community. *¡Muévete!* faced challenges from time-to-time when Chicago Park District policies set at the central-office level did not fit with the agreements made locally (e.g., the use of free space, programming for participants' children). CLOCC's links to central office staff were beneficial in ironing out these challenges.

Similarly, there are other organizations located within Humboldt Park or serving the community that are not formal partners of CO-OP HP or of CLOCC. CO-OP HP's staffing model and budget are modest. As such, CO-OP HP is not envisioned as the sole agent of change. One of CO-OP HP's goals, then, is to increase awareness of and attention to the multidimensional factors that contribute to childhood obesity so that local programs, services, and the environment will be more conducive to healthy eating and physical activity for children and families.

Encouraging Participation and Expanding Reach

Linking action at the organizational level to benefits for community residents is a continuing challenge. Ensuring that community residents are connected to available programs and services and take advantage of positive environmental changes remains a challenge reflected in the participation rates described earlier. Significant resources are put toward promoting programs (e.g., distributing flyers door-to-door, purchasing advertising space in local newspapers, "tabling" at community events), yet CO-OP HP leadership continues to work to increase community participation.

Phases of Development

Community-driven strategies with minimal funding must be flexible enough to take advantage of opportunities as they arise and include new partners as they emerge. Although intervention strategies with significant funding for planning, implementation, and evaluation over long periods of time can be predetermined, those with minimal funding must rely on the opportunities that arise as organizational resources, focus, and capacity shifts over time. Programs that evolve organically are likely to experience distinct phases of development. CO-OP HP was 5 years old in 2009, and those who have been involved since its start can now see relatively clear but unplanned phases in its development. The start-up phase took it from conception to a steering committee of five or six organizations and through the wellness survey and focus groups. The work was funded, and optimism prevailed. Funding was obtained by all three of the leadership groups. This period was filled with the energy of novelty and creation.

The program development phase was a more sober one. The steering committee became smaller, and the focus of work became more clearly the Puerto Rican community. Food initiatives—including the market basket program, Producemobile, and the farmers' market—got off to strong starts but then hit challenges. It is daunting to create new food distribution systems, even when they are clearly needed. Chicago's short growing season and dense city traffic made it hard to draw a critical mass of produce growers to the farmers' market, where prices were high for many residents. The logistics of helping area residents to use public assistance benefits (e.g., Women, Infants, and Children [WIC], Food Stamps) to buy produce were challenging. Area resident participation was inconsistent. The idea of backyard community gardening did not catch on as widely as once hoped.

One physical activity program, *¡Muévete!*, grew steadily under the charismatic leadership of its founder. But it, too, faced serious obstacles. Its attendees counted on it being a free program, so it generated no income and depended on Chicago Park District willingness to provide free space. Childcare was not available, and this proved to be a disruptive issue. Other physical activity programs, mostly related to biking, were slow to grow. Sprague funding shifted to CLOCC, and most of the fundraising came through CLOCC. Sustainability became a real worry.

CO-OP HP is currently in its third phase of development. This is a phase of maturation and long-term planning and, with these, of renewed energy and momentum. Interest in the CO-OP strategy has grown in Chicago. Two new CO-OPs have been established by CLOCC and key community partners in other neighborhoods (one Mexican-American, one Black). Funders are increasingly willing to invest in the model and its evaluation. Each CO-OP, although similar to the others in structure and focus, has unique characteristics relevant to the local community context. Clearly, CO-OP HP has had an impact on the organizations involved. Environmental changes are also beginning to occur as all the CO-OPs seek to create long-term, sustainable change.

Measurement of impact on community residents remains to be done and will be a long-term challenge. Yet there is growing national consensus that improved community health status only becomes possible when locally based, respected organizations make long-term commitments to creating the multicomponent environment that is needed for sustained changes in lifestyle. CO-OP HP is shining a light on how that can be done.

Engaging Organizational Staff

Program success is tied to how well the vision, mission, and goals are articulated to the entire staff of the host organization, beyond those who are working on the particular initiative. If organizational staff members do not see programs and the behaviors promoted through them as important, then their participation may be limited. Lack of participation among organizational staff may also result in the lack of translation within the community at large. More buy-in among organizational staff will likely lead to those staff members promoting the programs within their own social networks. Conversely, lack of such participation can dissuade the community at large—even if staff members are not explicitly discouraging such participation. Community members may be well-aware that organization staff are not participating in the organization's own programs and interpret that as a lack of confidence in the program or an indication that the recommended behaviors are not that important.

The PRCC has taken a number of steps to ensure that increasing numbers of staff participate in the programs so that the broader community can see the shared commitment across the organization. During monthly all-staff meetings, CO-OP HP staff members promote the various healthy lifestyle interventions. At biweekly directors' meetings, the CO-OP HP manager reports in more detail on successes and challenges faced by CO-OP HP, and the team discusses methods for increasing organizational involvement in CO-OP HP programs. Data on levels of participation by PRCC staff are used to help CO-OP HP staff identify opportunities to increase staff participation.

Although these strategies have helped, they have not fully solved the problems. CO-OP HP staff is looking to more innovative approaches to promoting CO-OP HP programs and the importance of healthy lifestyles. These include the use of social networking media and implementing program demonstrations at PRCC events.

Next Steps and the Sustainability of CO-OP HP Strategies and Philosophy

Although fund-raising for CO-OP HP has been challenging, PRCC continues to develop new ideas and plans for future projects. As previously stated, the Urban Agricultural Initiative is a community-wide effort developed to address the priority problems of availability and accessibility of fresh produce in the community. The future role of CO-OP HP will be to support urban farming endeavors by providing marketing services and through the distribution of the produce. Of the initiative's many components, the central goal is to engage community residents to take ownership and begin growing the produce they consume. CO-OP HP, through the distribution mechanisms already in place, hopes to make the produce available for sale to community residents at the farmers' market, through *La Cosecha*, to local restaurants, and to grocery stores. As the Urban Agricultural Initiative develops, PRCC and CO-OP HP staff hopes to rely less on the large commercial produce suppliers to meet the growing demands of community consumption. Current efforts will be expanded as funding allows, and new opportunities will be leveraged as they emerge.

CO-OP HP staff envisions an intersection between the local produce growing initiatives and the cycling programs it has helped establish. CO-OP HP and Ciclo Urbano staff have begun discussions centered on the construction of bicycle trailers specifically designed to carry and distribute locally grown produce to retail outlets and the farmers' market. These same produce trailers could circulate throughout the community offering produce for sale, as was traditionally common in towns in Puerto Rico with the "*Pregoneros*" (fruit and vegetable peddlers who traveled on foot) and is currently common in Latino communities in Chicago with produce trucks and street vendors. This envisioned strategy would not only employ community residents but encourage them to take up bicycle riding as an alternative mode of transportation and reducing the community's carbon footprint in the end.

Although cycling as physical activity is seen as an important distribution component of the Urban Agricultural Initiative, CO-OP HP staff is also developing ideas for sustaining and expanding the successful ¡*Muévete!* initiative. Increasingly, CO-OP HP staff describes ¡*Muévete!* as a comprehensive physical activity promotion strategy that includes not only the current dance aerobics program but also cycling, walking, and other forms of active transportation. For example, in collaboration with Ciclo Urbano, CO-OP HP staff has returned to the concept of weekly bicycle rides, now named Boricua Bikes. Building on the original model, the rides will be organized to incorporate tours of significant historical/cultural markers in the community (i.e., Mural Tours, Garden Tours).

The original idea for *¡Muévete!* was based on walking, and Ms. Calderón has re-introduced walking into her personal regime as well as into the *¡Muévete!* initiative, with a *¡Muévete!* walking session in the morning. She is currently exploring the possibility of a walking club during the lunch hour. Many agencies in the community employ community residents, making local worksites a promising context for healthy lifestyle promotion among community members. Many of these residents, in the various methods of data collection, cite lack of time as a barrier to regular physical activity once they get home. Organizing walking clubs during the lunch hour would help to address that barrier. CO-OP HP staff also envisions healthy competitions among teams of workers, with awards at the end of a defined period of time for combined weight lost, miles walked, or other outcomes of interest.

The CO-OP HP experience, with all of its challenges, has inspired PRCC staff and partner organizations to support CO-OP HP strategies and develop new strategies. A primary element of this inspiration is the fact that these strategies were not developed with large amounts of funding and were not imported by external organizations. Instead, CO-OP HP's successes almost solely result from the most important resources that Humboldt Park has: human capital and rich cultural tradition.

As described earlier, the data collected initially by SUHI and then later by CO-OP HP staff and partners clearly described the needs of the Humboldt Park community relative to nutrition and physical activity. Few residents met daily recommendations for healthy behaviors. A plethora of environmental and access barriers made healthy lifestyles difficult for community members to achieve. Although CO-OP HP strategies to address these needs constantly evolve as opportunities arise and dissipate, early data provide a constant "goalpost" on which to focus. The data also provide a rationale that CO-OP HP staff and leadership use to engage partners, funders, and the community at large in innovative approaches to facilitate healthy eating and physical activity for Humboldt Park residents. New data will provide an indication of whether CO-OP HP has helped to move Humboldt Park closer to the goal and whether additional goals must be set.

Acknowledgments

Staff and leadership of Community Organizing for Obesity Prevention in Humboldt Park (CO-OP HP) would like to acknowledge the following organizations who have provided financial support: The Otho S. A. Sprague Memorial Institute, Kraft Foods, the Chicago Tribune Charities, the Michael and Susan Dell Foundation, the Chicago Community Trust, Local Initiatives to Support Communities (LISC) Chicago, and the Administration for

Children and Families of the Department of Health and Human Services. The authors would also like to thank the staff and partners of the Puerto Rican Cultural Center who have volunteered for and participated in CO-OP HP events and programs. This chapter is dedicated to the children and families of the Greater Humboldt Park community. Their strength in the face of adversity is a constant inspiration.

References

Baker, Elizabeth A., Marilyn M. Metzler, and Sandro Galea. 2005. Addressing social determinants of health inequities: Learning from doing. *American Journal of Public Health* 95(4):553–555.

Becker, Adam B., Matt Longjohn, and Katherine Kaufer Christoffel. 2008. Taking on obesity in a big city: Consortium to Lower Obesity in Chicago Children (CLOCC). *Progress in Pediatric Cardiology* 25:199–206.

Davison, Kirsten K. and Leann L. Birch. 2001. Childhood overweight: A contextual model and recommendations for future research. *Obesity Review* 2(3):159–171.

Estarziau, Melanie, Miguel Morales, Anita Rico, Helen Margellos-Anast, Steven Whitman, and Katherine Kaufer Christoffel. 2006. Report on the findings and recommendations of the Community Survey in Humboldt Park: Preventing obesity and improving our health. Online. Available: www.suhichicago.org/files/publications/K. pdf. Accessed November 30, 2009.

Illinois Department of Public Health (IDPH), Healthy Smiles Healthy Growth, 2003–2004. Springfield, IL, 2006.

Mason, Maryann, Patricia Meleedy-Rey, Katherine Kaufer Christoffel, Matt Longjohn, Myrna P. Garcia, and Catherine Ashlaw. 2006. Prevalence of overweight and risk of overweight among 3- to 5-year-old Chicago children, 2002–2003. *Journal of School Health* 76(3):104–110.

Margellos-Anast, Helen, Ami M. Shah, and Steven Whitman. 2008. Prevalence of obesity among children in six Chicago communities: Findings from a health survey. *Public Health Reports* 123:117–125.

McLeroy, Kenneth R., Daniel Bibeau, Alan Steckler, and Karen Glanz. 1988. An ecological perspective on health promotion programs. *Health Education Quarterly* 15:351–377.

Whitman, Steven, Cynthia Williams, Ami M. Shah. 2004. Sinai Health System's Community Health Survey: Report 1. Chicago, IL: Sinai Health System. Online. Available: www.suhichicago.org/files/publications/P.pdf. Accessed September 25, 2009.

9

FIGHTING CHILDHOOD OBESITY IN A JEWISH COMMUNITY

Maureen R. Benjamins

Introduction

Inspired by the power of having specific health data for one's own community, leaders of the Jewish community in Chicago undertook the steps necessary to conduct a similar survey within the most densely populated Jewish neighborhoods (discussed in Chapter 4; Benjamins, 2010). This unique survey, the *Jewish Community Health Survey of West Rogers Park and Peterson Park*, was able to identify many health issues within the community. Of these, childhood obesity was selected by community members as the most important problem to address because it was found to affect a large percentage of children and because it foreshadowed serious health consequences for the future. Specifically, the community survey revealed that over half of all children in this Jewish community were overweight or obese. Unfortunately, the consequences of being overweight are considerable, including being at higher risk for a wide variety of health outcomes such as lowered life expectancy, diabetes, heart disease, stroke, and impaired mobility, as well as social and emotional problems (Must et al., 1999; Mokdad et al., 2003).

This chapter presents additional details about childhood obesity in this community, including age and gender differences and possible determinants. Following this is a detailed description of the development, implementation, and evaluation of a school-based intervention designed to reduce obesity rates among children in Jewish day schools in Chicago. This intervention, the Jewish Day School Wellness Initiative, has produced substantial changes within the schools and students of the Associated Talmud Torah school system over a 4-year intervention period (2006–2010). These results will be shared, as will information on how the model has been disseminated to other Jewish communities across the country.

Data

The survey data showed that among Jewish children ages 2 to 12 years living in this community, 28% were overweight and an additional 26% were obese. In other words, less than half were an appropriate weight for their height. Children were classified as overweight or obese based on their body mass index (BMI). BMI is calculated with a formula that uses an individual's weight and height (703 * [weight in pounds]/[height in inches] * [height in inches]). The categorization for children was done according to the Center for Disease Control and Prevention's (CDC's) "BMI-for-age" gender-specific charts (CDC, 2009a). Specifically, the following guidelines were used: *Underweight* = BMI for age < 5th percentile, *Normal weight* = 5th percentile ≤ BMI for age < 85th percentile, *Overweight* = 85th percentile ≤ BMI for age < 95th percentile, and *Obese* = BMI for age ≥ 95th percentile.

The height and weight data were obtained from each child's primary caregiver. It is important to note that only 58 interviews were conducted for children. and of these, only 50 were older than age 2 years (and thus old enough to use the BMI measures). Furthermore, valid height and weight data were only available for 43 of these children. The community survey results discussed here are based on this small sample, and these data are unweighted.

Distribution of Weight Status

Figure 9-1 shows the percent of children in each BMI category by gender. Boys were more likely to be normal/underweight or overweight, whereas girls were disproportionately in the obese category. In fact, more than one-third of girls included in this survey were obese. As a result, there were almost as many obese children as overweight ones. It is also helpful to examine BMI status by age group. As seen in Figure 9-2, older children (those ages 6–12 years) were more likely to be overweight in both the Jewish survey and in a national sample compared to children ages 2 to 5 years. This trend is also seen in national data for obesity. In contrast, the younger Jewish children were significantly more likely to be obese. Remarkably, more than one-third of children ages 2 to 5 years were obese in this Jewish community according to the survey.

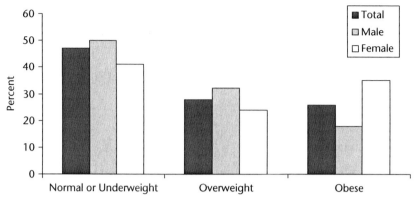

Figure 9-1   Children's Weight Status by Gender

Source: Jewish Community Health Survey, 2003.
Notes: Data represents children 2–12 years of age; $N = 43$.

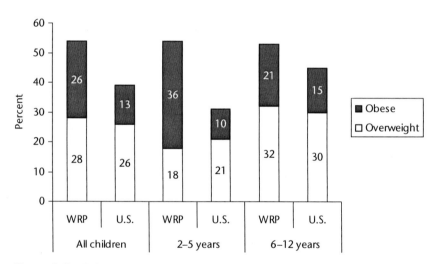

Figure 9-2   Children's Weight Status by Age

Source: Jewish Community Health Survey, 2003; NHANES, 1999–2000.
Notes: U.S. data is for children 2–5 years and 6–11 years of age. WRP = West Rogers Park.

Perceived Weight Status

To better understand factors influencing childhood obesity, the primary caregiver for each child (who was almost exclusively a parent) was asked to describe their child's weight. These questions showed a large discrepancy

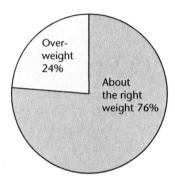

Figure 9-3   How Parents of Overweight and Obese Children Perceive Their Child's Weight

Source: Jewish Community Health Survey, 2003.

between the parent's perceptions and the child's actual weight status. Overall, nearly half of the parents did not correctly classify their children. This is particularly problematic for those with overweight or obese children, where less than one-fourth of parents of an overweight child correctly perceived that their child had weight problems (Fig. 9-3). These results are similar to those found in other populations (Jeffery et al., 2005). If parents cannot adequately identify weight problems in their children, it is increasingly important for physicians to do so. Unfortunately, the data from our survey showed that only 24% of overweight or obese children had been advised to lose weight by their doctor in the previous year (data not shown).

Eating Habits

The community survey also provided insight into the eating habits of children living in this community. Several questions identified promising targets for possible intervention. For example, more than two-thirds of all children failed to eat the recommended number of servings of fruits and vegetables each day (Table 9-1). Unfortunately, this percentage would be even higher if fruit juices were not included in the question. In addition, nearly one-third of children ate fast food at least once a week. This percentage was higher for overweight and obese children compared to non-overweight children (38% vs 28%, not shown). Other unhealthy eating habits were also seen. For example, one-third of children reported eating baked goods four or more times a week and approximately one-fourth ate chips at least this often. These findings indicated that any intervention would need to focus on improving nutritional habits by both increasing the amounts of healthy foods consumed and limiting the amount of unhealthy foods that children eat on a regular basis.

TABLE 9-1 Goals and Objectives of the Jewish Day School Wellness Initiative

- Students and staff will demonstrate improved knowledge, attitudes, and beliefs about nutrition and physical activity.
  - Students and staff will report better dietary choices.
  - Soft drinks and candy will be eliminated from school vending machines.
  - All school events for students, staff, or parents will offer healthier options.
  - Foods served during breakfast or lunch programs will have improved nutritional content (such as less calories and fat, or more vitamins or minerals).
  - Students will consume less baked goods, candy, and soda through classroom-sponsored parties and other school events.
  - The percentage of students who reach recommended levels of physical activity will increase.
  - The percentage of students reporting disordered eating behaviors will decrease.

Levels of Physical Activity

Several questions were also asked about the children's physical activity levels. The findings showed that about half of the children (48%) watched TV for at least an hour every day (Table 9-1). About the same percentage reported levels of activity below the recommended amount of 1 hour or more per day. Specifically, only 51% reported being active 1 hour or more a day. Despite the barriers to being involved in organized sports (such as the fact that many Jewish day schools do not have any sports teams and that observant Jews do not participate in such activities on Saturdays), approximately 68% of children played in some type of organized activity (such as a sports team).

Intervention

Process, Partners, and Funding

Process

The findings discussed above, along with the rest of the survey results, were presented to all interested organizations and individuals within the Jewish community of Chicago. Specifically, the project director from the Sinai Urban Health Institute (SUHI) and a member of the local Jewish Federation held open meetings with local rabbis, social service providers, health-care providers, educators, lay leadership, and other community members and groups. These sessions were designed to share information about the surveys and its findings, as well as to elicit feedback about how to translate this data into actual changes within the community. Individuals attending these sessions were asked two questions after being told about the survey findings: *(1)* What is the most important issue to address first? and *(2)* Who should we partner with to address that issue? Almost without exception, the community members said that childhood obesity was the health problem that should be addressed first. The most frequently suggested partner was the Jewish school system, the Associated Talmud Torahs (ATT), although synagogues, summer camps, and childcare sites were also mentioned.

Partners

Since the initial data collection effort in 2003 to 2004, the strong partnership between the Jewish Federation and SUHI has continued. In particular, members of the Jewish Federation were instrumental in finding financial support for the proposed intervention and in helping to establish SUHI as a trustworthy partner for the Jewish community. This latter task was especially important for this project given the inclusive nature of the Orthodox community and SUHI's lack of experience working with this community in the past. For the school initiative, these two partners reached out to the ATT, which is the only Jewish school system within the Chicago region. It includes approximately 20 elementary, middle, and high schools. Not all Jewish day schools in the city or metropolitan region are members of ATT, although most of the Orthodox ones are.

The steering committee that was convened to oversee the first two phases of the initiative (data collection and analysis) was also used to lead the school-based obesity prevention intervention. Specifically, members came from the Jewish Federation, SUHI (the institute's director and the epidemiologist who served as project director), and the ATT school system (the director of student services). One member of the committee was from the local Orthodox community. This committee met quarterly during the first years of the intervention and as necessary afterward.

Funding

The first 3 years of the school-based intervention, the Jewish Day School Wellness Initiative, were primarily funded by two local foundations, the Michael Reese Health Trust and the Polk Bros. Foundation. These foundations were also supporters of the data collection efforts, and both were interested in building on their initial investments by being involved with subsequent steps to address the health issues revealed by the survey. A small amount of additional funding for the first year came from the Washington Square Health Foundation, another local organization. Funding for the fourth year came exclusively from the Michael Reese Health Trust. This foundation funded the project as a "proactive" grant, which means that they sought out the project and were actively involved in its development and direction.

Jewish Day School Wellness Initiative

Even before funding was received, it was necessary to find individual schools that would be willing to serve as pilot schools for the proposed intervention. This step was facilitated by a meeting with all ATT principals during which the survey data were presented. At the conclusion of this meeting, the principals were asked if they would be interested in participating in a pilot study, should funding be received. All principals present (approximately 15) indicated that they would like to participate. Two elementary schools (grades K–8) were chosen by the grant steering committee, with input from the ATT administration. These schools, Joan Dachs Bais Yaakov and Yeshivas Tiferes Tzvi, were selected because they were in the geographic region of the original community survey, their administrators were motivated to make changes, and the schools (and school families) were considered to have fewer resources than others within the system. Joan Dachs Bais Yaakov had approximately 400 female students, and Yeshivas Tiferes Tzvi had approximately 250 male students.

Need for Culturally Appropriate Model

Once funded, the first challenge faced by the project staff was that interventions developed for public schools would likely be inappropriate or ineffective in a Jewish school system because there are specific dietary, behavioral, and belief systems that differentiate Jewish individuals from other populations. This is particularly true for Orthodox Jews, for whom the current initiative was developed. For example, Jews who keep kosher do not eat pork, shellfish, or dairy and meat at the same meal. As an example of behavioral differences, observant Jews follow modesty guidelines (Tzniut) that affect their speech, interpersonal conduct, and mode of dressing. For example, observant women wear skirts that fall below the knee (no pants or shorts) and their shirts must cover their collarbone and elbows. These rules must be followed at all times, even when exercising. Furthermore, observant women are restricted from swimming, biking, hiking, or jogging in public or in mixed company. These are just a few examples of the many guidelines that distinguish observant Jews from other individuals. However, even among Orthodox Jews, interpretation of or adherence to these rules and norms may vary by community, family, or individual.

In addition, numerous relatively unique characteristics of Orthodox day schools made addressing childhood obesity a challenge. The most obvious limitation was the lack of culturally appropriate health materials. Perhaps because of the difficulty of finding acceptable materials, the pilot schools (and most other schools in the school system) had no existing health education curriculum. In addition, day schools generally taught a "dual curriculum" in which half of the day was reserved for secular subjects (such as math, science, English, and social studies) and the other half was used for religious studies. Thus, the shortage of time for health education that public schools face was doubled because health classes needed to fit into one half of the day along with all other secular subjects.

Several other school-related factors also hindered efforts in this area. Specifically, most of the schools did not have federally funded meal programs and, as such, were not required to follow the recently established federal policies requiring school districts to have a wellness policy and a wellness council. In addition, the pilot schools belong to a network of schools, not a formal school district. This means that policies have to be made by each school instead of by a district superintendent, so no single mandate to include health curriculum, for example, can be declared. Finally, one cultural factor that plays a role in any programming or educational efforts is that Orthodox families are unusually large. For example, the student surveys found that students in the pilot schools had 6.4 siblings, on average. This is in contrast to the average American household with children, which includes just under two children (U.S. Census, 2008). Correspondingly, the families within this school community were on limited budgets, and the parents had greatly restricted amounts of time to attend meetings or educational events or even to read materials sent home.

Intervention Design

For the reasons noted above, it was clear that a culturally appropriate model of school wellness was necessary. After researching existing models, the Coordinated School Health Program (CSHP) model developed by the CDC was selected to guide the development of the Jewish day school intervention (CDC, 2008). Primary focus was placed on five of the original eight components of the CSHP model: health education, physical education, school environment, family involvement, and staff wellness. The remaining components (health services; nutrition services; and counseling, psychological, and social services) were deemed to be less relevant to these schools because of their lack of formal positions or programming in these areas. However, throughout the course of the intervention, these remaining areas were addressed to varying degrees.

During the first year of the 2-year pilot, project staff developed or adapted health materials to make them culturally acceptable. This included reviewing entire health curriculum guides and adapting each lesson to remove all

TABLE 9-2 Weight-Related Issues Among Children in the Jewish Community Health Survey

Eating Habits	
Eats ≥ 5 fruits or vegetables a day	30%
Eats fast food weekly	32%
Eats baked goods 4+ times per week	26%
Eats chips 4+ times per week	
Activities	
Watches TV ≥ 1 hour per day	48%
Active play ≥ 1 hour per day	51%
Participates in organized sports	68%

Notes: Children 2–12 years of age; *n* = 44.

mentions of non-kosher foods, television viewing, and other topics deemed inappropriate or irrelevant by the school administrators. To meet the goals outlined in Table 9-2, each of the participating schools was required to form a health committee, write a school wellness policy, and implement at least one project from each of the five defined intervention areas. These areas are: health education, physical education, family involvement, school environment, and staff wellness, as described below.

Health Education   Project staff selected several health curriculum guides that had been empirically shown to improve health knowledge, behaviors, or outcomes for use in these schools. School administrators were then given all the choices to review and were allowed to pick the specific ones they wished to use in their school. All lessons that included culturally inappropriate materials were adapted, and the adapted lesson plans were given to the teachers, along with supplemental resources, in grade-specific binders. Teacher training sessions were held to familiarize staff with the materials once at the beginning of the year for each school. Schools were instructed to implement at least two lessons per month in all grades (K–8). In addition, special attention was given to mental and emotional health issues. Led by a mental health consultant from a local Jewish social service agency, this part of the program provided culturally appropriate education on body image, self-esteem, conflict resolution, eating disorders, and other related issues for middle school girls. Finally, an effective health education program needs to supplement the formal teaching of the curriculum with other related activities. The schools were allowed to select one or more other options to implement, such as a health tip of the day, health information in school newsletters, displays in the hallway or cafeteria, a health fair, or creating a health section of books in the library, among others. In all cases, the project staff was available to assist the schools in acquiring any additional materials; for example, schools were offered two different sets of short articles that could be included in school newsletters or given to parents or teachers throughout the year, one of which was religiously based.

Physical Education   A small grant was given to each school as part of the intervention to implement or improve their physical education programs or to otherwise increase the amount of physical activity that the students received during the school day. Each school determined how to best use this money. Uses of the money included initiating before- or after-school activities, purchasing physical education curriculum guides or activity kits, and purchasing fitness equipment (e.g., jump ropes, resistance bands, hand weights, pedometers, mats, and balls). An emphasis was placed on expenditures that would continue to support physical activity among students after the grant ended.

Family Involvement   The involvement of parents and other family members was an important component of this initiative. At least one parent had to be included on the health committee for each school, and, preferably, a parent was selected to chair each committee. Schools were also encouraged to make the wellness committee part of the existing parent organization to facilitate parent involvement and improve the project's sustainability. In addition, many other grant activities were focused on increasing parental knowledge concerning nutrition, physical activity, and eating disorders. For example, the health educator was available to provide information at school events (such as orientation or parent–teacher conferences), health fairs, and through school newsletters that were sent home to parents.

School Environment   To provide a supportive environment and to be consistent with the messages being taught through health and gym classes, the schools were expected to make changes to policies and structures related to health. Schools were specifically encouraged to provide ample opportunities for physical activity, allow students easy access to water, and limit exposure to unhealthy foods such as soda and candy. In addition, schools were asked to take steps toward the goal of prohibiting the use of foods as rewards. This is one commonly recommended policy designed to reduce children's exposure to unhealthy foods, as well as to prevent unhealthy eating habits caused by thinking of food as a reward instead of strictly as a source of nourishment.

Health Promotion for Staff   Because teachers are such important role models, a variety of health promotion seminars and activities were made available for school staff. Each school had a designated amount of the health educator's time to provide whatever education or training they deemed most important. The health educator was available to speak at staff meetings or other times. Staff were also invited to all educational sessions and activities offered to parents. Teachers were encouraged to participate on the wellness council, and ideas for other staff wellness changes were solicited. Several no-cost (or low-cost) ideas were implemented for the staff during the pilot project. For example, a bulletin board in the staff lounge was organized for staff members at one school to post healthy recipes, and walking groups before or after school were started.

Evaluation

The goals of the evaluation process were twofold. First, an initial assessment was needed to guide the development of the project. Second, the evaluation enabled project staff to determine if the changes being made in the schools resulted in any improvements in student knowledge, attitudes, behaviors, and/or BMI.

The evaluation involved numerous tools to best gauge the progress and outcomes of the interventions. First, student surveys were conducted during class to evaluate changes in self-reported behaviors, attitudes, and knowledge. The questionnaires included items on average intake of different foods, beverage intake, levels of physical activity, motivation to be healthy, body image, and perceived support for healthy behaviors. The survey for younger students (grades K–4) was adapted from the Hearts N' Parks Survey, which has been used extensively across the country to measure eating habits and nutritional knowledge of young children (NHLBI, 2009). The survey for older students (grades 5–8) was created using a variety of measures from existing surveys, particularly from the Youth Risk Behavior Surveillance System (YRBSS), which is one of the largest federal sources of information on adolescent and child health (CDC, 2009b). New questions tailored to the target population were also added. Surveys were also conducted for staff members and parents. These surveys measured health knowledge, opinions regarding health education, changes in school policies, and other related issues.

In addition, the School Health Index, a nationally used school-level assessment tool, was used to look at changes in school environment and policies (CDC, 2009c). This tool was filled out by a team of individuals from each school representing administration, staff, and parents. It offered summary scores for numerous areas and related suggestions for improvement. Although time-consuming, this tool was helpful for guiding the newly formed wellness councils and for making the schools aware of all of the various aspects of the school that are related to student health.

Finally, BMI was collected for all students in grades K through 8 at the two pilot schools. For these measurements (as well as the surveys), parents were able to "opt out" if they did not want their child or children to participate. Students were also required to give their assent as well. The height and

TABLE 9-3 Health-Related Outcomes from the Student Survey for Students in Grades 2–4

	Range	2006[a] Mean (S.D.)	2008 Mean (S.D.)	Significant Difference[b]
2nd Grade		$n = 61$	$n = 77$	
Nutrition Knowledge	0–7	5.11	6.09	***
Eating Healthy	0–7	4.51	3.54	***
Eating Intention	0–6	3.16	2.57	*
Confidence in Physical Abilities	4–12	9.21	9.73	
3rd Grade		$n = 66$	$n = 69$	
Nutrition Knowledge	0–7	5.36	6.19	***
Eating Healthy	0–7	3.86	4.14	
Eating Intention	0–6	2.65	3.07	
Confidence in Physical Abilities	4–12	10.05	9.62	
4th Grade		$n = 69$	$n = 44$	
Nutrition Knowledge	0–7	5.42	5.66	
Eating Healthy	0–7	3.46	3.09	
Eating Intention	0–6	2.22	1.84	
Confidence in Physical Abilities	4–12	10.19	10.56	

Note: *$p \leq 0.05$; **$p \leq 0.01$; ***$p \leq 0.001$.

[a]First graders were not included in the analyses since the 1st graders in year 2 did not participate in the intervention in year 1 as kindergartners.

[b]Wilcoxon-Mann-Whitney rank sum test used to determine significance of differences
S.D. = Standard Deviation.

weight measurements were taken in a private room by the part-time school nurse, who was a member of the community.

All schools completed the surveys and the School Health Index at their entry into the project (baseline) and then once at the end of each grant year (years 1–4). BMI screenings were performed three times (baseline of the pilot project, end of year 2, and end of year 3). Finally, for the process evaluation, all schools were required to submit quarterly reports that detailed all health-related activities and purchases. Only results from the 2-year pilot project are discussed here.

Selected Outcomes

Younger Student Surveys   Table 9-3 shows selected health-related outcomes for students in grades 2 to 4. The most notable change for these grades following the intervention period was seen for nutritional knowledge. Specifically, the percentage of students in grades 2 and 3 who could correctly identify the healthiest foods increased significantly between 2006

TABLE 9-4 Health-Related Outcomes for Students in Grades 5–8 ($n = 107$)

	2006[a] Percent	2008 Percent	Significant Difference[b]
Knowledge			
Knew fruit/vegetable recommendations	16	34	**
Knew dairy recommendations attitudes	24	51	***
Unhappy with body behavior	21	16	
Five fruits and/or vegetables daily	35	35	
Breakfast daily	52	49	
Soda daily	24	23	
Fast food weekly	25	27	
Hour of activity four times a week	41	62	***
Exercising or dieting to lose weight environment	47	55	
Class parties involve sweets	64	70	
Parents encourage exercise	31	37	
Parents limit sweets	50	51	
Parents limit soda	65	59	
Parents exercise with children	14	10	

Source: Table reprinted from Benjamins and Whitman, 2010.

Notes: $*p \leq 0.05$; $**p \leq 0.01$; $***p \leq 0.001$; all outcomes are dichotomous.

[a]2006 data includes students in grades 5–7. 2008 data includes those same students 1 year later, in grades 6–8.
[b]McNemar's chi-square tests used to determine significance of differences between proportions.

and 2008. These questions asked, for example, which food was healthier: whole wheat bread or white bread? By the end of the pilot project, 82% of students answered all six knowledge questions correctly compared to only 57% at baseline. Seeing a change in knowledge first is common for new health behavior interventions that often aim to improve knowledge first, which then drives changes in intentions, and finally changes in behaviors. Table 9-3 also reveals two other findings pointing in the opposite direction. Specifically, second graders reported eating more unhealthy foods and that they would select less healthy foods if given a choice. Fortunately, these negative findings were not seen for the other grades. For the rest of the outcomes, there were no significant differences during the 2-year pilot project.

Older Student Surveys   Table 9-4 shows results for the older students (grades 5–8). Selected measures related to knowledge, attitudes, behaviors, and environmental factors are displayed. To measure nutrition-related knowledge, students were asked how many servings of fruits and vegetables health experts recommend eating every day. They were also asked how many servings of dairy children should consume each day. The results show that only 16% of students at baseline knew that they should eat five or more servings of fruits and vegetables daily. By 2008, this number had increased to 34% ($p < 0.01$). A significant improvement was also seen for knowledge of dairy recommendations. Specifically, the percentage who answered correctly increased from 24% to 51%, which is significant at $p < 0.001$. In analyses not shown, it was discovered that the significant increase in knowledge for the fruit and vegetable recommendation entirely resulted from increases by female students. Similarly, increases in knowledge for the dairy recommendation were also more significant for females. Overall differences in the percent of students who knew this recommendation also favored girls.

To look for improvements related to mental and emotional health, students were asked whether they were happy with their body and physical appearance. Although the percentage reporting that they were slightly or very unhappy with their body decreased from 21% to 16%, this difference did not attain statistical significance.

Numerous questions were asked to measure intake of fruits and vegetables, breakfast, various beverages, and fast food, among other items (Table 9-4). Questions related to physical activity and possible signs of disordered eating were also asked. The one significant change observed was that the percentage getting the recommended amount of daily activity (≥ 1 hour) 4 days or more of the week increased. Overall, less than half of students reported this level of activity before the intervention, but almost two-thirds reported it at the end (41% to 62%, $p < 0.001$). Gender differences were found (not shown). Specifically, the percentage of girls reaching this level of activity started off lower and saw a less significant increase (36% to 53%, $p < 0.01$, for girls; 55% to 84%, $p < 0.01$, for boys).

Finally, students were asked a series of questions regarding the availability of healthy and unhealthy foods at home and at school, as well as the extent to which their parents encouraged physical activity. Unfortunately, no significant changes were seen in the number of class parties that included candy, cookies, cakes, or other sweets, nor in the limits that parents place on the children regarding intake of sweets or soda. Similarly, the percentage reporting that their parents encouraged them to exercise or play sports increased but not significantly. A question about how often parents actually exercised with their children also showed a lack of improvement as well as overall low initial numbers.

Staff Surveys   All teachers were also given surveys at the beginning and end of the 2-year pilot project. The survey for staff measured eating habits, nutritional knowledge, physical activity, and attitudes related to nutrition. In addition, questions were asked about classroom policies, teaching attitudes and training, support for wellness initiatives, and participation in wellness programming. The overall response rates were 68% (Fall 2006) and 52% (Spring 2008). Some results are summarized below.

The percentage of staff who knew how many servings of fruits and vegetables children need each day did not significantly increase. New knowledge questions in the second year showed that 61% of teachers knew the recommended daily dairy intake for children and 81% knew that reduced fat milk was healthier for children older than age 2 years. However, less than 30% knew how much activity children should get each day.

In 2008, 59% of teachers felt that their eating behaviors influenced the eating behaviors of students. Also, 75% strongly agreed that the food students eat during the school day affects their readiness to learn. Almost two-thirds of responding staff members (62%) reported that they attended one or more health education session in the last year (and 100% found these sessions to be somewhat or very helpful). The average amount of physical activity reported increased, whereas the percentage of staff who ate fast food two or more times a week was cut in half. Many teachers reported improved overall eating habits. For example, the percentage reporting fair or poor eating habits decreased from 36% to 25%. Furthermore, the average amount of regular physical activity increased. This is probably related to the fact that 68% of responding staff members were currently trying to lose weight (compared to 57% at baseline). Significantly, of those trying to lose weight, 77% reported that they were now exercising and eating healthier, compared to baseline when only 42% were doing both.

The percentage reporting that they taught health lessons increased from 7% to 88%, with an average of six lessons taught the past year (range: 0–20). Overall, the perceived barriers to teaching decreased. Not having enough time and health having a lower priority than other subjects remained the top barriers. Of the responding staff, 40% had policies on the nutritional content of snacks brought into their class compared to only 24% at baseline (32% at the boys' school, 17% at the girls' school). More than 80% reported that the types of foods served at their class parties improved in the prior year. In 2008, only 29% reported that they never used food as a reward in their classroom, whereas 10% did it once a week or more. Only half of the teachers would support a school-wide ban on this practice. Staff were more supportive of other policies, such as banning all soda on school grounds (84% support), having a list of approved healthy snacks (81% support), and banning the sale of unhealthy foods for fundraisers (66% support).

Parent Surveys   Baseline and final surveys were mailed to all parents. These surveys briefly measured eating habits, nutritional knowledge, physical activity, and attitudes related to nutrition. In addition, questions were asked about the importance of health and physical education, support for wellness policies, and participation in wellness programming. The overall response rates were 26% (Fall 2006) and 22% (Spring 2008). Because of the low response rates, the results reported below cannot be considered representative of the entire parent body. It is likely that those who felt most strongly about the wellness program (either positively or negatively) were more apt to respond.

The percentage of parents who knew how much exercise children need each day increased from 28% to 38%. Those reporting that they know and understand current nutrition guidelines increased from 72% to 86%. The percentage of parents who think it is very important for schools to teach about health increased from 65% to 79%. The percentage of parents who think it is very important for schools to offer physical education increased marginally from 71% to 78%. The percentage reporting that they eat fast food once a week or more decreased from 25% to 19%. The average number of days that parents get 20 to 30 minutes of moderate and/or vigorous exercise increased slightly. The majority of parents responding to our survey were supportive of healthy policies, such as a ban on soda on school grounds (90% support), restrictions on unhealthy snacks (75% support), or a ban on using food as a reward (80% support).

Nearly one-third of responding parents had been to a wellness council meeting, 22% went to a nutrition workshop during orientation, 14% went to the body image talk, and 6% had consulted individually with the dietitian. The primary reason given for not attending each of these events was not being able to (i.e., too busy or had something else to do). Almost everyone knew when the council meetings were held and only small percentages reported not knowing about the other activities. Finally, 92% of parents reporting reading the health column in the school newsletter, and 89% found it to be somewhat or very useful.

School Environment Changes   As noted above, the School Health Index (SHI) was completed by schools to assess school-level factors such as environment, policies, organization, and curriculum. The ideal score for each area is 100%. Results from the two pilot schools are described here.

Within the boys' school, the largest improvements were noted in the areas of health education, which increased from 0% to 71%, and staff wellness, which increased from 0% to 54%. Health education scores reflected not only having health education in each grade but also having professional development in this area, culturally appropriate examples and activities, and covering a range of topics such as nutrition, physical activity, asthma, and tobacco use. In addition, staff wellness improved greatly, especially in the areas of nutrition education and training in first aid and CPR. More work was needed for staff in the areas of health screenings and stress management and fitness programs. Family involvement improved from 28% to 67%. The boys' school improved their family education, involvement in programs, and involvement in planning meals. Work was needed to improve community access to school facilities during non-school hours. Finally, the category of school policies and the environment increased from 54% to 80%. A few improvements included better communication of health and safety policies to parents and staff, maintaining a safe physical environment, and the prohibition of using physical activity as a punishment or food as a reward.

The girls' school also showed the largest improvements in health education (from 0% to 86%). Specifically, health education was now taught in every grade, with appropriate staff training. The school administrators felt they needed to work on getting more culturally appropriate examples and activities, giving the students opportunities to practice their skills, and using more active learning strategies. Big improvements were also seen for the category of physical education (PE) (from 36% to 92%). Although the school was nowhere near the 150 minutes of weekly physical activity recommended by the National Association for Sport and Physical Education and other groups, or the daily PE required by Illinois state law, they improved greatly by hiring a trained and credentialed PE teacher who followed a sequential curriculum, kept students moving, and made the class more enjoyable. Of the other areas, staff wellness moved from the lowest category to the middle (17% to 54%), family involvement increased from 39% to 50%, and school policies and the environment improved from 63% to 83%. This latter increase was the result of greater restrictions on unhealthy foods, new written policies on health and safety, a safer physical environment, and professional development on health risks like asthma.

Prevalence of Overweight and Obese Students   The impetus of this school-based initiative was the high level of childhood obesity in West Rogers Park/Peterson Park identified by the *Jewish Community Health Survey* (*see* Chapter 4; Benjamins, 2010). Although the results from this survey suggested that more than half of all children ages 2 to 12 years in this community were overweight or obese, these elevated rates were fortunately not found in the pilot schools. This discrepancy may result from differences between the community sample and the school population, the modes of data collection between the community survey and the school data (i.e., proxy report vs. measurement), or the individuals who declined to participate.

As noted above, BMI was collected for each student at the beginning of year 1 of the pilot study (2006), at the end of year 2 (2008), and at the end of

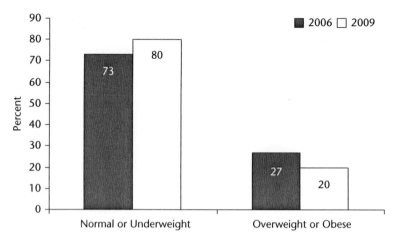

Figure 9-4 Overall Weight Status by Year: Results of the Jewish Day School Wellness Initiative Pilot Study

Note: Differences are significant at $p < .05$ based on McNemar chi-square tests.

year 3 (2009). BMI changes from the beginning of year 1 to the end of year 3 were examined. Participation rates at both time-points were high (88% and 84%, respectively, for boys; 91% and 88%, respectively, for girls), despite many vocal objections from parents and students when the screenings were announced. Those students who lacked parent consent or who declined screening themselves were more likely to be overweight (assessed observationally by the nurse or project director) than those who were screened. Thus, the estimates reported below likely underestimate rates of overweight and obesity in the schools.

Although measurements for one time or the other were available for more than 400 students, only 295 students had valid BMI data in both 2006 and 2009. The following findings are based on this sample. The results show that the percentage of students classified as overweight or obese was significantly lower at the end of year 3 than it was at the beginning of year 1 (Fig. 9-4). Specifically, 27% of students were classified as overweight or obese in 2006, whereas only 20% were in this category in 2009. When examining this difference more closely, the data show that 70 students were overweight or obese in 2006 but moved into the normal or underweight category by 2009. Conversely, only 35 students were in the normal or underweight category in 2006 but in the overweight or obese category in 2009. Analyses by gender show that this change was primarily driven by boys. (The decrease in percentage of overweight or obese girls was not significant.) Analyses by grades show that the change was seen more frequently in younger grades compared to older ones.

In addition to actually measuring students, the project staff originally planned to analyze height and weight data from existing surveillance systems required by the state. Data would come from child health examination forms for students entering the schools in kindergarten and those entering sixth grade. The goal of analyzing this data was twofold. First, establishing a system to collect and analyze the data would allow schools to begin their own surveillance of obesity and related health risks within their student body. Second, the data would provide baseline information for each school, which could then be used as a comparison for all future years. These data were not planned to measure changes in BMI over the intervention year (because they are only collected once per year). However, several problems arose with this plan. Most importantly, the schools were not interested in collecting this type of data, nor in setting up a system to do it in the future. In addition, they were concerned with the legal ramifications of using such data. Finally, several of the schools were also reluctant to do anything that would associate their wellness program with "obesity prevention" instead of maintaining a more pro-social and positive image promoting overall wellness. For these reasons, plans for setting up such a surveillance system were dropped.

Post-Pilot Activities

As alluded to above, the Jewish day school wellness project was able to continue past the 2-year pilot intervention. Specifically, following the completion of the pilot intervention, funding was obtained to expand the newly created model to three additional elementary schools (Akiba Schechter, Arie Crown, and Hillel Torah). Together, nearly 2,000 children in grades K through 8 participated during this phase of initiative. As with the pilot intervention, the expanded initiative focused on changes in the areas of health education, physical education, school environment, family involvement, staff wellness, and mental health. Subsequently, a fourth and final year was granted to the project (2009–2010) to expand to all of the remaining schools in the school system, including high schools.

In addition, a planning component was added to the project in this final year to begin coordinating the funding, management, and roles of all health-related services within the school system. Specifically, this component of the project entailed taking a comprehensive inventory of all social and mental health services, disability services, nursing services, and wellness-related programming within each school and system-wide. Project and school system staff also examined how the components work together (or do not) and how they are funded in an effort to assess efficiencies, collaboration, and sustainability. It was acknowledged that linking these services would enable the system to better continue the work started during the wellness initiative, as well as to identify other health-related gaps or overlaps in the system.

Sustainability

One of the main areas of focus of the project in the third and fourth years of the intervention was creating sustainable changes to continue benefiting students beyond the grant period. Several strategies were used to accomplish this, and examples are given here. To begin, schools were strongly encouraged to make the wellness council a subcommittee of their existing parent organization. Beyond facilitating the sustainability of the mission, this was considered useful for increasing parent familiarity with the program and providing a natural means by which to find volunteers for wellness activities and events. Schools were also encouraged to focus on making policy changes that would set standards for years to come. Some policies that were promoted included prohibiting the use of foods as rewards, establishing guidelines for appropriate snacks, making school campuses soda-free, and prohibiting the sale of candy for fundraisers. To further encourage the continuation of school changes, the project staff worked with school administrators and parents to share information about available grants related to school wellness. Practice writing grants was facilitated by making the schools write small grant applications to receive any grant funds from the project in the final year.

The schools were also left with a large amount of culturally appropriate educational materials that were collected, adapted, or created during the intervention. These resources included general materials for guiding schools in the implementation of a wellness program, as well as teaching resources and educational materials for parents. The teaching resources included the curriculum guides and grade-specific binders with adapted lessons and supplemental materials that all teachers were provided during the intervention. All of these materials (with the exception of the posters and copyrighted curricula) were put on a CD and given to each school.

Finally, during the final year of the intervention, the project partners embarked on a planning process to determine how to best maintain and extend the critical *infrastructure* to sustain health-related activities and gains within the member schools. At the end of the planning period, strategic recommendations were developed to specifically address how to sustain this wellness initiative and how to effectively and efficiently leverage existing resources. The resulting plan also identified strategic new directions and funding needed to comprehensively address health and mental health needs in the Jewish day school system of Chicago.

Challenges and Lessons Learned

As with any intervention, many obstacles were faced during the development, implementation, and expansion of this initiative. Fortunately, many of the challenges that confronted the project during the initial years were addressed in later years. Some of the bigger issues are described below, along with resolutions whenever they existed.

Creating a Positive First Impression

A critical challenge faced by this initiative was building support within each school as the project got underway. Creating a good first impression was difficult because of the intervention's goal of reducing childhood obesity, a notoriously sensitive topic and one many parents found threatening. To make it even more difficult, the first grant activity visible to parents and students was the BMI measurements. This led people (primarily female students and their parents) to hastily conclude that our goal was to make all of the children "skinny," instead of focusing on eating healthy and being active. This was despite the project's name being the "Jewish Day School Wellness Initiative" and no explicit mention of obesity in any project materials or activities. In addition, several schools had bad experiences in the past with well-intentioned but poorly executed parent groups addressing nutrition or other health issues. For example, one school's "nutrition committee" was poorly received by other parents at that school because of its progressive ideas and aggressive strategies. These parents did not want anyone, especially outsiders, coming to be the "food police." Overcoming these obstacles was a slow process. Fortunately, positively received events, such as family activities and the purchase of new gym equipment, increased both parent and student satisfaction and, thus, receptiveness to subsequent changes. Offering education for the students, parents, and staff also improved perceptions of the program.

In addition, the whole concept of school wellness was new to many members of the Orthodox school communities. At the beginning of the grant, almost none of the schools in the school system had a health curriculum, health-care professionals on staff, food service staff, trained PE teachers, or sports teams. In other words, they had no health-related resources within their schools. At the same time, the schools were isolated from existing external resources because of cultural issues, and they were exempt from recent federal school wellness mandates because of their lack of a school lunch program. As a result, many staff and parents lacked general health-related knowledge and had a limited understanding of the importance of school wellness programs. Working to first develop motivation and enthusiasm to achieve the project goals was necessary prior to providing any education or making any school changes. Initially focusing on the importance of wellness (as opposed to specific strategies) emerged as an important component of the project's success.

Importance of Being Culturally Sensitive

When working with any racial or ethnic minority community, it is obviously important to respect their rules, values, and customs. Being from outside of the community, the project staff was only able to achieve this by having an "insider" from the schools (and thus, from the community) to inform them of these important cultural guidelines. Having a liaison was critical throughout all 4 years of the initiative for familiarizing project staff with community norms and shaping grant goals and methods to be most beneficial for the community. Having organizational partnerships was also key to the acceptance of this initiative. Partnering with the local Jewish Federation brought credibility and greater opportunities for funding. Partnering with the school system (instead of just individual schools) also increased the project's credibility and sustainability.

Logistical Challenges

In addition to the broad challenges discussed above, the project also faced more specific obstacles related to the administration, implementation, and evaluation of the grant. For example, the project staff quickly realized that as the project expanded, they had increasingly little control of the health education component. It was difficult (and even impossible in some schools) to meet with all of the staff in charge of teaching health lessons to train them, answer questions, and get feedback. In addition, the requirement to teach at least two lessons a month was not always enforced by the administration, and teaching logs from teachers were completed erratically and perhaps not accurately. Thus, it was challenging to enforce and evaluate the health education component once the project expanded beyond in initial two pilot schools.

Project staff also had a difficult time ensuring that all of the project requirements were met by each school. This was important to know to approve school expenses and to document project activities. To address this after the first year, the schools were required to turn in a quarterly report that listed all project activities. This allowed the schools to keep a log of what they had accomplished and helped the project staff be aware of activities that were conceived and implemented by the individual schools. Grant funds were tied to these quarterly reports, so that the schools not only had to complete the required activities but also document them to receive any money.

School and Community Engagement

Finally, the importance (and difficulty) of engaging members of the community must be discussed. From the start, this was a community-driven project. To begin, the *Jewish Community Health Survey* was initiated by the

Jewish Federation and supported by local religious and lay community leaders in 2003. Moreover, a group of community leaders and key stakeholders defined the geographic boundaries of the community to be surveyed, helped to adapt the survey questionnaire for this community, and wrote introductory letters to respondents to encourage participation (more details in Chapter 5). An important indicator of community support was the fact that the survey cooperation rate was an impressive 75%. Following this, leaders from the local community were instrumental in interpreting the results of the empirical findings and determining which health concerns were most urgent. This communication took place through a series of meetings with over 100 community agency representatives and religious leaders in 2004 to 2005. Through these meetings, the project leaders were also able to identify individuals and groups who were interested in being involved in the intervention phase of the project. Finally, the day school intervention was initiated because of the community members' concern about problems related to childhood obesity. Within the intervention itself, all project activities were selected by each school's wellness council, which generally included school administration, staff, and parents.

In addition, changes to the intervention model and materials were made each year of the initiative, based on feedback from the administrators, staff, students, and parents of participating schools. The feedback, which came through meetings, surveys, calls, and other means, allowed the project staff to continually provide new or improved materials and activities. For example, one challenge was to engage teachers in the overall school efforts and help them understand the influence of nutrition and exercise on the students' classroom behavior and achievement. The principals maintained that staff meetings were too busy to allow for meaningful education, so a monthly newsletter for teachers was developed instead. In this way, health education, ideas, and resources were made available to all teachers at all schools every month. This process of continually improving the intervention also allowed the schools to implement changes or activities not originally envisioned. This served to not only improve the effectiveness of the intervention but also to increase the schools' buy-in for the overall project.

A related challenge was reaching parents to provide education to them and to seek their involvement in various aspects of the initiative. In this community in particular, the larger-than-average family sizes result in greater parent responsibilities for childcare. Financial constraints limited both the parents' and the school's ability to provide childcare for such events. To address this, a concerted effort was made to bring the health education messages to events that were already taking place (i.e., orientation and parent–teacher conferences). In addition, the monthly wellness updates that were developed for teachers were adapted to be relevant for parents as well. Many schools also included their own information, gathered by staff or the school nurse, in weekly parent newsletters. Furthermore, teachers were encouraged to make parental participation a requirement of homework assignments for the health lessons.

Finally, another one of the primary challenges to this initiative was something that is familiar to everyone who has worked in or with a school. Namely, the competing interests and limited resources (including staff time) of schools make any efforts to bring about changes difficult. After the pilot years (during which the model and materials were developed), the project staff purposefully adjusted their role to providing resources and advice, rather than implementing actual projects within any of the schools. This was both a matter of logistical necessity and an effort to increase the self-sufficiency of the schools. This was very challenging for the schools that were already taking steps outside of their comfort zone and now needed to solicit help from parents or other organizations within their community. This approach obviously required greater school initiative and independence. Although the schools professed a desire to address wellness issues, this goal is fairly long-term in nature and somewhat abstract and, therefore, is often a lower priority compared to test scores and other immediate demands. Furthermore, like many changes within schools, movement is often driven by one or two individuals. Identifying these individuals was a challenge for almost all of the participating schools.

Proof that the schools and communities were successfully engaged in the initiative was seen at an event sponsored by the project's funders and organized by the project staff at the beginning of year 4. Specifically, all 10 participating schools were invited to take part in a meeting to share success stories, discuss challenges, and provide an update for the funders, school system administrators, and other interested individuals. This 3-hour event included a presentation by the project director regarding the results of the first 3 years of the initiative, updates on specific components of the intervention, a panel of representatives from each of the schools that had participated in past years regarding their "success stories," and a presentation from the director of the Chicago public school system's school health department about what their schools were doing. Importantly, ample time was set aside for questions, comments, and discussion throughout the event. Each school was asked to send at least one administrator, teacher, and parent, and approximately 50 individuals attended.

The event was notable in several ways. To begin, all participating schools were represented, despite the challenges of setting aside that amount of time during a school day. More importantly, all individuals who attended were very interested in the issues discussed and motivated to continue making changes within their respective schools. Individuals took notes, requested more information, asked insightful questions, and generally demonstrated their engagement with issues related to children's wellness. Of particular interest was the panel of principals sharing their successes. For example, one principal discussed how Orthodox boys do not typically have the skills to play sports, so after-school activities run by volunteer parents were designed to teach them skills such as how to throw a football or catch a baseball. Another individual discussed how a family running event could be held at no cost to the school by getting local stores to donate T-shirts, refreshments, and advertising. As a final example, one principal explained how their school moved from almost exclusively using candy for rewards and fundraisers to the selling of vegetable peelers to fund the most recent eighth grade class trip.

One of the main themes that emerged from these discussions was that the intervention was helpful in bringing about a cultural shift within this community. Evidence for this change in community norms and practices was given through several examples. For example, all principals and teachers strongly agreed that they noticed students bringing in healthier snacks and lunches. In addition, many parents and teachers described improvements in the nutritional content of foods offered at both school and non-school events. As another sign of the spread of this initiative beyond school walls, one mother noted that the local kosher grocery store had greatly increased the amount of whole wheat products it offered. Although these changes are impressive (and not necessarily all a result of the project), many individuals noted that much work still needed to be done to spread the changes even further. For example, the possibility of working with local restaurants and caterers to provide healthier options was raised.

This event was a great opportunity for schools to interact with each other, for funders to better appreciate the achievements their support enabled, and for project staff to gather large amounts of feedback. The gathering of all interested parties for a structured event with built-in time for discussion could be a useful model for other intervention projects to follow.

Conclusions

This chapter describes how one religious community used data gathered by a population-based survey to motivate real changes within their community. The effort expended to make this school-based initiative culturally appropriate and community-driven was rewarded by signs of a cultural shift toward health seen at the end of the intervention. Although the various short-term evaluations showed that the intervention was successful in certain areas (such as lowering the percentage of overweight and obese students in the pilot schools and improving levels of nutritional knowledge), the overall effectiveness will be determined by how well the schools continue incorporating the wellness curricula, policy changes, and activities. Broader shifts in cultural norms within this inclusive community will also be critical to support changes within schools, families, and individuals. However, it is too early to know if the progress seen at the individual, organizational, and community levels will be sustained.

The success of this initiative can also be considered on a larger scale. Specifically, one of the primary goals of the project was to develop a model and materials that would be appropriate for Jewish day schools across the country. This represents more than 200,000 students in approximately 750 schools in the United States, and this number continues to rise (Schick, 2005; NCES, 2008). It is hoped that this wellness movement will not only be sustained within the day school system of Chicago but that the model created here will continue to be used for other Jewish schools. Based on responses to presentations made at national conferences and on the requests for information received by project staff, this is already beginning to happen. For example, another city with a large Jewish population has asked to use our survey data, model of day school wellness, school questionnaires, and other project information to replicate this project within their day school system. Funding is still being pursued for this new initiative, but it appears as if many other schools will benefit from the experiences of the current project. As the national attention to childhood obesity continues to swell, it is hoped that all day schools are likewise motivated to improve student health. If the model of school wellness and the culturally appropriate materials made available through this project can in any way assist these schools to overcome the many barriers to school wellness that exist, this initiative will be considered a success.

Finally, although the main outcomes of interest within this intervention were related to nutrition, physical activity, and body image, it is hoped that the structures left in place within this school system will allow other health-related issues to be addressed more effectively. Using day schools to educate children and reach their parents may be a worthwhile strategy for addressing other challenging problems identified by the community survey, such as depression and domestic violence.

This initiative has demonstrated that with adequate guidance and support, schools are willing to broaden their focus from a child's intellectual development to overall well-being that incorporates emotional, social, and physical dimensions. In accordance with the Jewish teaching to guard one's health, these schools can help students, staff, and families make healthier choices and, thus, improve their health now and in the future.

Acknowledgments

This ambitious initiative could have only been accomplished with the help of numerous individuals and organizations. To begin, I would like to acknowledge the funders again because of their consistent and generous support of the project. In particular, the Michael Reese Health Trust and the Polk Bros. Foundation have been invaluable for both their financial support as well as their overall guidance. Elizabeth Lee, Senior Program Officer at the Michael Reese Health Trust, was especially helpful throughout the four years of the project. I would also like to acknowledge assistance from colleagues at the Jewish Federation, Joel Carp, David Rubovits, and Dana Rhodes, as well as the director of the Sinai Urban Health Institute, Steven Whitman. Their input as members of the grant's steering committee helped to ensure that the project would be accepted by the community and that it was part of the broader agenda to improve well-being within the Jewish community of Chicago. I would also like to acknowledge two project staff members, Ashley Biscoe and Lindsay Weil, for their hard work and expertise in adapting or creating the culturally appropriate health education materials for this project and for their assistance with other logistical needs of the project. Finally, many thanks are due to the administrators, teachers, parents, and students of the Associated Talmud Torahs school system. The efforts of the principals and staff of the two pilot schools are especially appreciated. In addition, Debbie Cardash, Director of Student Services at Associated Talmud Torahs, cannot be thanked enough for her support of this project and her work with the schools and parents to facilitate community acceptance. The efforts and input of all of these individuals drove this initiative and deserve the credit for all of the positive changes seen.

References

Benjamins, Maureen R. 2010. The Jewish Community Health Survey of Chicago: Methodology and key findings. In: *Urban health: Combating disparities with local data*, eds. Steven Whitman, Ami M. Shah, and Maureen R. Benjamins. New York, NY: Oxford University Press.

Benjamins, Maureen R. and Steven Whitman. 2010. A culturally appropriate school wellness initiative: Results of a two-year pilot intervention in two Jewish schools. *Journal of School Health*. 80(8): 378–386.

Centers for Disease Control and Prevention (CDC). 2008. *Coordinated School Health Program*. Online. Available: http://www.cdc.gov/HealthyYouth/CSHP/. Accessed February 2, 2008.

Centers for Disease Control and Prevention (CDC). 2009a. *Clinical growth charts*. Online. Available: http://www.cdc.gov/growthcharts/clinical_charts.htm. Accessed October 7, 2009.

Centers for Disease Control and Health Promotion (CDC). 2009b. YRBSS: Youth Risk Behavior Surveillance System. Online. Available: http://www.cdc.gov/HealthyYouth/yrbs/index.htm. Accessed February 25, 2009.

Centers for Disease Control and Health Promotion (CDC). 2009c. Welcome to the School Health Index. online. Available: https://apps.nccd.cdc.gov/shi/Default.aspx. Accessed February 25, 2009.

Jeffery, Alison N., Linda D. Voss, Brad S. Metcalf, Sandra Alba, and Terence J. Wilkin. 2005. Parents' awareness of overweight in themselves and their children: Cross sectional study within a cohort (EarlyBird 21). *British Medical Journal* 330:23–24.

Mokdad, Ali H., Earl S. Ford, Barbara. A. Bowman, William H. Dietz, Frank Vinicor, Virginia S. Bales, and James S. Marks. 2003. Prevalence of obesity, diabetes, and obesity-related health risk factors, 2001. *Journal of the American Medical Association* 289(1):76–79.

Must, Aviva, Jennifer Spandano, Eugenie H. Coakley, Alison E. Field, Graham Colditz, and William H. Dietz. 1999. The disease burden associated with overweight and obesity. *Journal of the American Medical Association* 282(16):1523–1529.

National Center for Education Statistics (NCES). 2008. *Digest of Education Statistics, 2007* (NCES 2008-022), Chapter 1. U.S. Department of Education.

National Heart, Lung, and Blood Institute (NHLBI). 2009. Hearts-N-Parks Y2K training manual. Online. Available: http://www.nhlbi.nih.gov/health/prof/heart/obesity/hrt_n_pk/hnp_tm.pdf. Accessed February 2, 2009.

Schick, Marvin. 2005. *A Census of Jewish Day Schools in the United States, 2003–2004.* New York, NY: The AVI CHAI Foundation.

U.S. Census Bureau, Housing and Household Economic Statistics Division, Fertility & Family Statistics Branch. 2008. AVG3. Average number of people per family household with own children under 18, by race and Hispanic origin, marital status, age, and education of householder: 2008. Online. Available: http://www.census.gov/population/www/socdemo/hh-fam/cps2008.html. Accessed April 14, 2010.

10

DISPROPORTIONATE IMPACT OF DIABETES IN A PUERTO RICAN COMMUNITY OF CHICAGO

Steven Whitman, José E. López, Steven K. Rothschild, and Jaime Delgado

Introduction

The prevalence of diabetes in adults in the United States has been steadily increasing from 4.9% in 1990 to 6.1% in 2004 (Mokdad et al., 2000; Behavioral Risk Factor Surveillance System [BRFSS], 2005). Diabetes prevalence is higher in U.S. non-Hispanic Blacks and Hispanics compared to non-Hispanic Whites (Centers for Disease Control and Prevention [CDC], 2003a). Puerto Ricans have a particularly high prevalence of diabetes. One report, using a BRFSS methodology, produced a prevalence estimate of 9.6% for Puerto Rico, whereas a 2000 survey implemented with a similar methodology produced an estimate of 11.3% for Puerto Ricans living in New York City (Perez-Cardonna and Perez-Perdomo, 2001; Melnik et al., 2004).

Mortality from diabetes also exhibits substantial racial/ethnic disparities. In 2002, the age-adjusted mortality rates for diabetes were: 25.4 per 100,000 population for the entire United States, 22.2 for non-Hispanic Whites, 50.3 for non-Hispanic Blacks, and 35.6 for Hispanics. Furthermore, the diabetes mortality rate for people living in Puerto Rico was 69.5 (Kochanek et al., 2004), three times the mortality rate of the mainland United States.

225

Chicago is home to more Puerto Ricans than any U.S. city other than New York. *Sinai's Improving Community Health Survey* (Sinai Survey) (Whitman, Williams, and Shah, 2004), from which much of the data in this chapter are derived, included the largest Puerto Rican community in the city (Humboldt Park/West Town or HP/WT).

This chapter comprises three parts:

- First, data are presented describing the diabetes epidemic in the HP/WT area and the prevalence is stratified according to various demographic and risk factors. To better assess the impact of diabetes on this community, diabetes mortality rates are also calculated. In each of these cases, derived data are compared to local and national rates.
- The second part of this chapter discusses how the community took ownership of these data and their implications, disseminated them widely, and converted the bad news of the data and the energy of the community into funding for an intervention, which is now in place. This intervention offers an opportunity to reverse the terrible damage being wrought by diabetes in the community and also to shift the ideological manner in which community-based interventions are considered.
- The final part of this chapter offers some observations and implications.

The Data

Methods

Survey

The survey from which the prevalence data were obtained is described in detail in Chapter 3 (Shah and Whitman, 2010). As noted, West Town and Humboldt Park were among the six community areas surveyed in the Sinai Survey. These two areas are contiguous and are home to about 26,000 Puerto Ricans (23% of Chicago's total Puerto Rican population). These residents view themselves as being part of the same community and are treated as such (HP/WT) in this report. It is essential to note here that these two officially designated community areas were included in the survey both because they are among the most diverse in the city and also because previous work of the Sinai Urban Health Institute (SUHI) with this community suggested such placement might result in meaningful collaborations. As just one example, when SUHI was planning its survey, a Community Advisory Board was convened to select the topics and questions that would appear on the survey (Shah, Benjamins, and Whitman, 2010). One of the co-authors (JD), who has worked in HP/WT much of his life, was one of the leaders of the Board. He is also the director of the project that emerged out of all of this work and that is described below in some detail.

Data Collection

The race and ethnicity of survey respondents were measured by self-identification. Diagnosed diabetes was measured, consistent with the BRFSS survey, as those responding "yes" to the survey question, "Have you ever been told by a doctor that you have diabetes?" Women who had been told that they had diabetes only during a pregnancy were not included among those with diabetes. Body Mass Index (BMI) was calculated by using self-reported height and weight (BMI = kg/m^2). Respondents were categorized into: not overweight (BMI < 25.0), overweight (25.0–29.9), and obese ($\geq$30) (NIH, 1998).

Data Analysis

Data for denominators for mortality rates and prevalence proportions were drawn from the U.S. Census 2000 files. Mortality data were abstracted from Illinois Vital Records Death Files, which were provided to us by the Chicago Department of Public Health. Deaths from diabetes consisted of all deaths with an underlying cause coded as E10 through E14 under the International Classification of Diseases, 10th Revision (Hoyert and Lima, 2005). All mortality rates were age-adjusted to the U.S. standard 2000 population.

Consistent with other studies in this literature, the prevalence proportions in this analysis were not age-adjusted. The sampling weights employed in this analysis account for differential probabilities of selection and we employed post-stratification of the sample to resemble the 2000 Census distribution of the population for each of the community areas. Data were analyzed using STATA v8 to account for the sampling design effects (Stata Corporation, 2003).

The statistical significance between two prevalence proportions or two mortality rates was examined with a *t*-test. A 95% level of significance was employed for all analyses.

Results

Prevalence

Of the 603 people who were interviewed in HP/WT, 595 people had no missing study data, and 104 identified themselves as Puerto Rican. The Puerto Rican residents of this community tended to be young and female (57.3%), have more than an eighth-grade education (82.7%), and be born in Puerto Rico (58.6%) (Table 10-1).

TABLE 10-1   Non-Gestational Diabetes Prevalence by Risk Factors for Puerto Ricans in Humboldt Park-West Town ($n = 108$), 2002–2003

	Total (%)	Prevalence (%)	95% CI	P
Age (in years)				
18–44	65.0	13.1	(5.4, 28.4)	0.106
45–64	27.7	34.4	(12.2, 66.4)	
65+	7.3	34.5	(10.5, 70.2)	
Gender				
Male	42.7	12.5	(4.8, 28.9)	0.158
Female	57.3	27.1	(11.1, 52.5)	
Education				
≤ 8th Grade	17.3	33.6	(16.6, 56.3)	0.126
≥ 9th Grade	82.7	18.4	(7.7, 37.8)	
Nativity				
Puerto Rico	58.6	15.7	(9.4, 25.0)	0.383
United States	41.4	25.1	(9.2, 52.3)	
Weight Status				
Obese	33.2	33.4	(18.2, 54.1)	0.023
Non-Obese	66.8	14.8	(5.5, 34.3)	
Family History of Diabetes				
Yes	43.2	32.5	(12.9, 61.0)	0.064
No	56.8	12.3	(5.8, 24.0)	
Health Insurance				
Uninsured	23.3	10.8	(2.1, 40.3)	0.357
Insured	76.7	23.0	(10.3, 46.0)	
Total		20.8	(10.1, 38.0)	

Source: Sinai's Improving Community Health Survey, 2002–2003.

The risk for diabetes was also high in this community, as 33.2% of the residents were found to be obese and 43.2% had a family history of diabetes. The majority of the residents had health insurance (76.7%). A detailed summary of additional markers of socio-economic status may be found in Chapter 3 (Shah and Whitman, 2010).

The prevalence of physician-diagnosed diabetes in Puerto Ricans living in this community was 20.8%. The prevalence proportions for other people in these two communities were 3.1% for non-Hispanic White adults, 14.5% for non-Hispanic Black adults, and 4.1% for Mexican adults (Table 10-2). The Puerto Rican prevalence was significantly higher than both the Mexican ($p = 0.025$) and White proportions ($p = 0.025$).

Table 10-3 compares the diabetes prevalence found among Puerto Ricans in HP/WT to those found for Puerto Ricans living in other areas. Puerto Ricans in HP/WT (20.8%) report a prevalence about twice as high as Puerto Ricans

TABLE 10-2   Non-Gestational Diabetes Prevalence in Humboldt Park-West Town, by Race/Ethnicity, 2002–2003

Group	N	Prevalence (%)	95% CI
All	595	9.0	(6.4, 12.7)
Puerto Rican	104	20.8	(10.1, 38.0)
Mexican[a]	97	4.1	(1.4, 11.4)
Non-Hispanic White[a]	154	3.1	(0.7, 13.2)
Non-Hispanic Black	163	14.5	(9.4, 21.8)

Source: Sinai's Improving Community Health Survey, 2002–2003.

Note: [a]The Puerto Rican rate was significantly higher than Mexican (p = .025) and non-Hispanic White rates (p = .025)

TABLE 10-3   Non-Gestational Diabetes Prevalence Among Puerto Ricans in Recent Years, Various Reports

Humboldt Park-West Town, 2002–2003	20.8%
New York City, 2000	11.3%
Puerto Rico, 1999	9.6%
Puerto Rico, 1998–2002	9.3%

Source: Sinai's Improving Community Health Survey, 2002–2003.

living in New York City (11.3%) and Puerto Rico (9.6% and 9.3%) (Melnik et al., 2000; Perez-Cardonna and Perez-Perdomo, 2001; CDC, 2004).

Diabetes prevalence varied by associated risk factors (Table 10-1). Prevalence was significantly higher among obese people (p = 0.02) and marginally significantly higher among those with a family history of diabetes (p = 0.06). It was also higher (but not significantly) among older people, females, those with fewer years of education, those born in the United States, and those with insurance.

Mortality

Table 10-4 presents diabetes mortality rates by geographic area and race/ethnicity. Note that the diabetes mortality rate for Puerto Ricans (67.6 per 100,000 population) in HP/WT is consistent with the high prevalence. As can be expected, the Puerto Rican mortality rate caused by diabetes is significantly higher than the rate for Mexicans (p = 0.006) and non-Hispanic Whites (p = 0.002) and higher than for non-Hispanic Blacks (p = 0.11) in the same community. The rate is also more than twice the rate for all of Chicago (p = 0.006) and the United States (p = 0.002). Although the Puerto Rican rate in HP/WT is similar to that found among Puerto Ricans in the rest of Chicago and Puerto Rico, it is 50% higher than that found in Puerto Ricans living in the United States (p = 0.12).

TABLE 10-4   Age-adjusted Diabetes Mortality Rates by Race/Ethnicity in Recent Years[a]

	Total	NHW	NHB	Mexican	Puerto Rican
Humboldt Park-West Town, 1999–2001	36.1	22.0[†]	42.2	23.0[†]	67.6
Chicago 1999–2001	31.2[b]	23.8	37.9	41.7	70.9
United States[c] 2000	25.2[b]	22.0	53.4	39.0	45.4
Puerto Rico 2000	—	—	—	—	69.5

Source: Sinai's Improving Community Health Survey, 2002–2003.

Notes: [a]Rates are per 100,000 population
[b]Significantly different ($p < 0.05$) when compared to the Humboldt Park-West Town Puerto Rican mortality rate
[c]Excludes Puerto Rico
NHW = Non-Hispanic White; NHB = Non-Hispanic Black

TABLE 10-5   Age-adjusted Mortality Rates (per 100,000 Population) from Diabetes for Consecutive 3-Year Intervals for Humboldt Park-West Town Puerto Ricans, Chicago, and the United States

	1998–2000	2001–2003	Change
HP-WT Puerto Ricans	66.0	76.1	15.3%
Chicago	30.6	31.1	1.6%
United States	24.4	25.3	3.7%

Source: Sinai's Improving Community Health Survey, 2002–2003.

Note: HP-WT = Humboldt Park-West Town.

Table 10-5 presents the mortality rates from diabetes for consecutive 3-year intervals (slightly different from the interval employed in Table 10–4) surrounding the 2000 census for HP/WT, Chicago, and the United States. Note that although the rates for Chicago and the United States increased by small but notable amounts, the rates among Puerto Ricans in the community increased by 15.3% during this interval.

Discussion

Although the prevalence of diabetes is consistently found to be much higher for Hispanics than for non-Hispanic Whites, the prevalence observed in this community of Puerto Ricans in Chicago (20.8%) is the highest reported diabetes prevalence we have been able to locate for Puerto Ricans. This prevalence is twice as high as findings for Puerto Ricans living on the island or in New York City (Table 10-3).

It is relevant to note that the relationship to virtually every risk factor examined in this report (Table 10-1) is consistent with findings from other studies showing increased prevalence among older people, females, those with fewer years of education, those born in the United States, obese people, those with a family history of diabetes, and those with health insurance (Lethbridge-Cejku, Schiller, and Bernadel, 2004; BRFSS, 2005). The direction of the relationships of these risk factors to diabetes prevalence is also identical to other studies of diabetes among Puerto Ricans (Perez-Cardonna and Perez-Perdomo, 2001; Melnik et al., 2004). Of particular note is the high prevalence of obesity (33.2%) and family history of diabetes (43.2%), both important risk factors for diabetes, found in this community. The prevalence of obesity among Puerto Ricans in this study is higher than that of the United States (25%) and may thus be contributing to the increased diabetes prevalence rate (CDC, 2003b).

It is compelling that this elevated prevalence corresponds to a greatly elevated diabetes mortality rate of 67.6 (per 100,000 population). This is more than twice as high as the rate for Chicago (31.2) and almost three times as high as the rate for Illinois (25.4) and the United States (25.2). It is also noteworthy that this Puerto Rican mortality rate is virtually identical to that found in Puerto Rico, but studies there have found the prevalence to be only about half what has been found in this community (Perez-Cardonna and Perez-Perdomo, 2001; BRFSS, 2004; Kochanek et al., 2004). One plausible hypothesis for the lower prevalence on the island, despite the elevated mortality rate, is disproportionate underdiagnosis. However, we are not aware of evidence to support or contradict this.

This elevated diabetes mortality carries with it an alarming observation. For example, if this mortality rate of 67.6 prevailed for the United States as a whole, then diabetes would be the second-leading cause of death in the country, trailing only heart disease but well ahead of all separate types of cancers (e.g., lung, breast, colorectal) and cerebrovascular diseases (Kochanek et al., 2004). Given the already extraordinary—and growing—burden of diabetes in this country, it is a sobering thought that in this Puerto Rican community, the impact may already be three times greater than it is for the country as a whole (Saydah et al., 2002; Black, 2002).

Methodological Issues

There are important methodological issues to consider when examining the results from this study. First, consistent with virtually all the other literature in this field, we did not age-adjust our prevalence estimates. Our own data, along with that from the CDC, suggest that such adjustments generally increase prevalence by about 10%, although this estimate is quite variable (CDC, 2003b). For example, if we had age-adjusted our estimates (to the 2000 standard U.S. population), the prevalence for Puerto Ricans would have risen from 20.8% to 22.6%, an increase of 8.7%.

Second, our sample did not include residents over the age of 75. Because diabetes generally increases with age, this may bias the prevalence estimates. However national data show that the prevalence is similar for those ages 65 through 74 and those ages 75 and older (CDC, 1999). Therefore, the bias may be minimal.

Third, it is well-established that self-reporting of physician diagnosis underestimates the true prevalence of diabetes by 33% to 40% (Harris et al., 1998; CDC, 2003a; CDC. 2003b). Using the 33% adjustment, an estimate of the *actual prevalence* of diabetes among Puerto Ricans in this Chicago community could be as high as 31% for adults between the ages of 18 and 75.

Fourth, because one must see a physician to obtain a physician diagnosis of diabetes, lack of insurance would tend to minimize the prevalence estimates derived in this study. Indeed, 24% of the Puerto Ricans in the survey were without insurance, and these uninsured individuals had a reported diabetes prevalence that was less than one-third of those with insurance. This dynamic would serve to even further elevate the estimate of the *actual prevalence* of diabetes among Puerto Ricans in this community.

Finally, because of the small sample size ($n = 104$), the confidence limits around our estimates were wide. However, to determine statistical significance, we did not employ overlapping confidence intervals because this technique is more conservative (i.e., rejects the null hypothesis less often). Rather, we used the z-test in testing all the comparisons in this analysis (Schenker and Gentleman, 2001). Despite this effort, because of a small sample size, we failed to see some statistically significant differences that we otherwise may have obtained.

Implications

The continuing disparities in diabetes prevalence and mortality demonstrated here are inconsistent with the (at least) 25-year-old national initiatives to reduce disparities in general and for diabetes in particular (U.S. Department of Health and Human Services, 1991; U.S. Department of Health and Human Services, 2000). These disparities exist despite continued calls for improvement in screening and treatment for diabetes (Diabetes Control and Complications Research Group, 1993; Nathan and Herman, 2004). As the prevalence increases and more people become obese and acquire the disease earlier in life, diabetes-related complications and mortality will only increase. Of paramount concern would be the upstream issue of prevention. As McGinnis has aptly noted in his foreword to a supplementary issue of the *American Journal of Preventive Medicine* devoted to diabetes control: "...as perhaps with no other disease is the importance of the link between clinical and community interventions so clear. The potential for gain against the toll of diabetes is great, but only if we pair aggressive clinical interventions with equally aggressive community action fundamental to broad lifestyle changes" (McGinnis, 2002).

The elevated prevalence and mortality from diabetes in Puerto Ricans have largely gone unnoticed in the literature. Understanding why the diabetes prevalence and mortality rates for Puerto Ricans in HP/WT are twice as high as those of other communities is imperative. Almost certainly, the answer to this question will include reducing the prevalence of obesity, increasing diabetes education and early screening and diagnosis, and providing access to *effective* treatment.

This study revealed local level disparities in diabetes prevalence and mortality and thus offers an opportunity to improve the situation. Established guidelines and resources already exist that can improve the quality of diabetes care (Hu et al., 2001; Task Force on Community Preventive Services, 2002; Coffey, Matthews, and McDermott, 2004). One of our goals in conducting the six-community survey was to provide robust data that would empower researchers, service providers, and community members to work collectively to address health problems in Chicago's neighborhoods. In the HP/WT neighborhood, the findings of this study had exactly that impact, as described in the next section.

The Community Response

First Steps

As described in Chapter 3 (Shah and Whitman, 2010), the data from the survey were collected in 2002 and 2003. When the preliminary findings were developed, they were discussed with several community-based organizations that had helped implement the survey and with whom the researchers had working relationships. The response was most energetic. For example, the Puerto Rican Cultural Center (PRCC), which had been calling for the meaningful use of research data and community control of health interventions, started to informally disseminate and talk about the findings the same day the data became available. (The Executive Director of the PRCC (JEL) is one of the authors of this chapter.) Consistent with this effort was the establishment of the coalition called the Greater Humboldt Park Community of Wellness (COW), which contained several organizations (including the PRCC) working on health issues in the HP/WT community and which was dedicated to addressing both the medical as well as the social determinants of health. Soon the results from the survey became a guide for health improvement in the area, and several hundred copies of the report describing these results (Whitman, Williams, and Shah, 2004) were widely distributed.

Two community forums were held the by the COW in March and November of 2004 (one of which was sponsored by the City Council of Chicago) to discuss these reports. Over 200 community residents attended each event. There was wide community support and heated debate about which topics on the survey were most important and which were most amenable to effective action. Topics that were discussed included pediatric asthma, obesity, depression, and diabetes, among others (Figs. 10-1 and 10-2).

At the beginning of 2006, researchers from the Sinai Urban Health Institute learned that a paper submitted to a peer-reviewed journal about diabetes in HP/WT had been accepted for publication and would appear in the December 2006 issue. This is the paper that forms the basis for the first part of this chapter (Whitman, Silva, and Shah, 2006). Upon learning of the publication date, the study investigators realized that they did not want the paper to appear and bring only more bad news to the community. It was thus decided, with the leading participation of several other members of the community, to convene the "Humboldt Park Diabetes Task Force." Twenty-one people representing community-based organizations, medical institutions, and advocacy groups (e.g., the American Diabetes Association, the Illinois Kidney Foundation, the PRCC, the COW, Mount Sinai Hospital) served on the Task Force. One of the authors (SKR) chaired the Task Force. Data from the study were shared with faculty at a nearby academic health center with no prior significant engagement with the HP/WT community, and this catalyzed the participation of experts in endocrinology and preventive medicine in the Task Force work.

The Task Force met twice a month in a restaurant in the community. In the end, the group produced the report entitled *Diabetes in Humboldt Park: A Call to Action* (The Humboldt Park Diabetes Task Force, 2006). The report was prepared in time to coincide with the date of publication of the journal article. Thus, instead of the news being limited to the devastating impact of diabetes in Humboldt Park, equal attention was given to the community's demand for action. Action steps called for in the Task Force report included:

1. Increasing awareness of diabetes and making diabetes a community-wide priority, through: recruitment of an oversight board; engagement of community groups in the design and implementation of efforts to increase awareness of diabetes in the community; conducting a social marketing campaign; and the hiring of outreach workers.
2. Defining the scope of the problem by implementing a community-wide screening campaign for case-finding of persons with diabetes and also for those at risk of developing diabetes, and sharing these findings with the community on a regular basis.

Agenda for the
Chicago City Council Hearings
By the Committees of Health and Human Relations on
Inequities in Health in Chicago's Communities
As presented by the
Sinai Health System's Improving Community Health Survey

Tuesday, March 9, 2004
9:30 – noon
Association House of Chicago, 1116 North Kedzie Avenue

Welcome to Association House:	Harriet Sadauskas, Executive Director, Association House of Chicago (5 mins)
Context for Today's Hearings:	Madeline Roman-Vargas, Dean, Humboldt Park Vocational Center of Wilbur Wright College (10 mins)
Introduction of the Issues:	Benn Greenspan, C.E.O., Sinai Health System (10 mins)
Findings from Two Main Studies:	Steven Whitman, Ph.D., Director Sinai Urban Health Institute (30 mins)
Community Participation:	Cynthia Williams, M.S., Director of Family Education, Sinai Community Institute (10 mins)
Breast Cancer – a Patient's View:	Ms. Darnie Holmes (10 mins)
Mother of Child Who Was Obese:	Ms. Griselda Tejeda (10 mins)
Response:	Susan Scrimshaw, Ph.D., Dean, School of Public Health, UIC (15 mins)
Community Perspective:	Eliud Medina, Executive Director, Near Northwest Neighborhood Network/Humboldt Park Empowerment Partnership (5 mins)
	Miguel Palacio, Assoc. Director, Association House of Chicago (10 mins)

Figure 10-1   Agenda for the Chicago City Council Hearings, March 9, 2004, to present data about health inequities in Chicago's communities

3. Implementing a program of primary prevention to reduce the number of people who develop diabetes. This program would include the creation of a community diabetes education center, an intervention program for children identified as "at risk," and the development of multifaceted interventions aimed at diet, physical activity, and behavior change based in worksites and other settings in the community.

**Humboldt Park Health Summit:
Creating a "Community of Wellness"**

October 25, 2004

Dear Friend and Colleague:

The collaboration of agencies and organizations listed below invites you to a Community Health Summit on Tuesday, November 9, 2004, from 9:00 am to 1:00 pm, to be held at the Association House of Chicago, 1116 North Kedzie Avenue, Chicago, Illinois. The main purpose of the summit is to introduce and discuss the concept of a "Community of Wellness", an integrated social approach to health that concentrates on improving basic health and health awareness and knowledge among Humboldt Park residents by making wellness the business of the entire community.

We look forward to your joining community residents and colleagues in the health and wellness field to review this concept of building a Community of Wellness in Humboldt Park and the new initiatives that the Humboldt Park New Communities Program (NCP) Health Committee and the Puerto Rican Agenda developed in response to the Chicago City Council's public hearings of the Committee on Human Relations, chaired by the Hon. Billy Ocasio (Alderman, 26th Ward) and the Committee on Health, chaired by the Hon. Ed Smith (Alderman, 28th Ward) in Humboldt Park on March 9, 2004.

Through the results of the Mount Sinai Health Study of six Chicago communities, compiled by Dr. Steve Whitman of the Sinai Urban Health Institute, the City Council heard residents of the Humboldt Park community document the devastating impact of specific illnesses on them as specific racial and ethnic groups and as a whole. At the summit, we will have a chance to assess the proposed Community of Wellness as a way to ensure that residents take ownership of our own health and health initiatives proposed to begin to address conditions in Humboldt Park.

We value your opinion and hope you will join us on November 9, 2004. Refreshments will be served and registration will begin at 8:15 am. The summit will start promptly at 9:00 am. To confirm your attendance, or if you have any questions, please call Ms. Sabina Romanowska at (773) 489-8935 or you may e-mail her at: sromanowska@ccc.edu.

Sincerely,

Association House of Chicago
Bickerdike Redevelopment Corp./Humboldt Park New Communities Program (NCP)
Consortium to Lower Obesity in Chicago Children (CLOCC)
Co-Op Humboldt Park – VIDA/SIDA
Humboldt Park Empowerment Partnership (HPEP)
McCormick-Tribune YMCA
Puerto Rican Agenda
Puerto Rico Federal Affairs Administration (PRFAA)
Wright College Humboldt Park Vocational Education Center

Figure 10-2 Invitation letter to the Humboldt Park Health Summit, November 9, 2004, to introduce and discuss the establishment of a "Community of Wellness."

4. Improving medical care for people with diabetes by engaging health-care providers in a collaborative network to improve diabetes care, with continuing medical education and quality improvement projects.
5. Helping people with diabetes take better care of their health through resources such as a "diabetes information clearing house," free diabetes

self-management education programs, and community-based resources to support healthful decision-making regarding nutrition and physical activity for persons with diabetes and their families.

The Press Conference and Summit

On December 6, 2006, both the journal article and the report were released at a press conference held at Association House, a social service agency in the HP/WT community. The press conference was attended by over 300 people, including every elected official from the community—at the city, county, state, and federal level (Figs. 10-3 and 10-4). There was an overwhelming response that ranged from anger about the disparity to urgency about the need to take action. The energy of the attendees drove the next step, a plan to further increase community awareness of diabetes and to get input into how to respond to the findings. At this event it was announced that a Diabetes Summit would be held in the community in March (2007), and volunteers were solicited to join the Task Force and help plan the Summit. The purpose of the Summit would be to exchange ideas and information with the community and to make plans for mitigating the damage being done by diabetes in the community.

In response to this request, many individuals stepped forward and volunteered. These people met twice a month for the next 4 months, this time early on Friday mornings at a different community restaurant over breakfast. The Diabetes Summit was held on March 16, 2007, in a community church (*see* Fig. 10-5 for the brochure publicizing the event). In advance of the event, Univision, the television station with the largest news audience in Illinois (in any language), asked to meet with Task Force members. Upon understanding the situation, they agreed to run a news segment describing the upcoming Summit for all 4 nights of the week leading up to the Friday of the event. Over 600 people attended the day-long Summit and learned about the dimensions of the problem, as described by the epidemiology, how to attempt to manage the disease, and where and when to receive screening and other health information. In one sense the Summit became a rally of the many people in Humboldt Park living with or directly impacted by diabetes. The Summit also provided a structure for broader community reaction and input (interpretation) to the findings and the proposed solutions (Figs. 10-6–10-8).

The reach of the Summit was far greater than even the 600 people who attended. One indication of the diffusion into the community came a few days later when a teacher at a public school in the community found the phone number of one of us (SW) on the Web and called to ask if someone

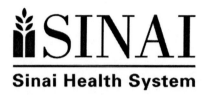

Sinai Health System

Please join
Sinai Urban Health Institute
For a presentation of Sinai Health System's Study on the Extraordinarily High
Prevalence of Diabetes among Puerto Ricans Living In
Humboldt Park and West Town

Wednesday, December 6, 2006
10:00 a.m.
Association House
1116 N. Kedzie Avenue

Sinai Urban Health Institute will release a report on the extraordinarily high prevalence
of diabetes among Puerto Ricans living in Humboldt Park and West Town. The
diabetes prevalence in this community is the highest ever reported for Puerto Ricans
who are already known to have a particularly high prevalence of diabetes nationally.
Diabetes mortality rates were also found to be disproportionately high. The report will
be published in the December 2006 issue of the national <u>Journal of Community Health</u>.

Presented by:
Steve Whitman, Ph.D., Director, Sinai Urban Health Institute
Steve Rothschild, M.D., Chair, Diabetes Task Force, Rush University Medical Center
Jose Lopez, Executive Director, Puerto Rican Cultural Center
Debra Wesley Freeman, CEO, Sinai Community Institute
Elected Officials from Humboldt Park and West Town

Please RSVP to Scofield Communications at (312) 280-7702 or <u>info@scocomm.com</u>

Figure 10-3   Flyer for a meeting at Association House, December 6, 2006, to address
the high prevalence of diabetes among Puerto Ricans living in the Humboldt Park and
West Town Community Areas of Chicago.

would come to talk to her seventh-grade class because her students were asking about the commotion generated by the interest in diabetes. In response,
a presentation was made in front of an assembly of all three seventh-grade
classes in the school. Exactly what was accomplished that day is unclear,
but two observations stood out. First, it appeared that almost everyone in
the community was talking about the problem of diabetes. Second, seventh
graders are very funny and very energetic. Many other presentations and
discussions also took place in the community and the city as a whole in the
months that followed.

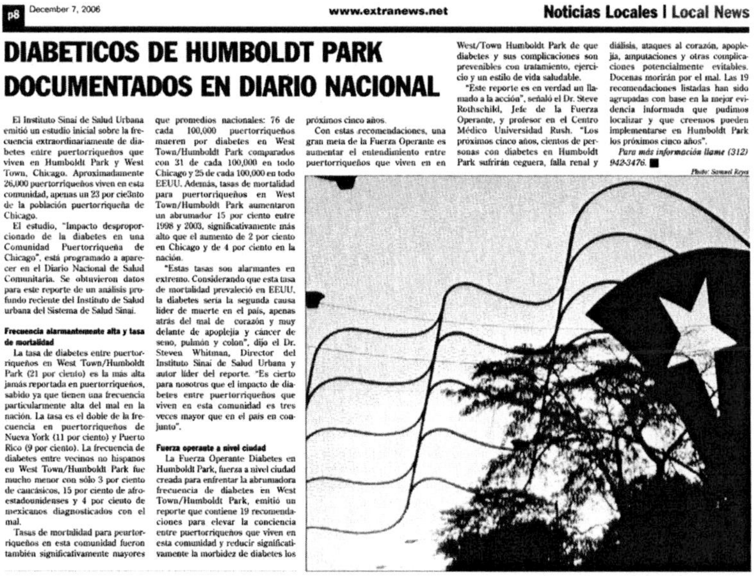

p8 December 7, 2006 www.extranews.net **Noticias Locales | Local News**

DIABETICOS DE HUMBOLDT PARK DOCUMENTADOS EN DIARIO NACIONAL

El Instituto Sinaí de Salud Urbana emitió un estudio inicial sobre la frecuencia extraordinariamente de diabetes entre puertorriqueños que viven en Humboldt Park y West Town, Chicago. Aproximadamente 26,000 puertorriqueños viven en esta comunidad, apenas un 23 por cie3nto de la población puertorriqueña de Chicago.

El estudio, "Impacto desproporcionado de la diabetes en una Comunidad Puertorriqueña de Chicago", está programado a aparecer en el Diario Nacional de Salud Comunitaria. Se obtuvieron datos para este reporte de un análisis profundo reciente del Instituto de Salud urbana del Sistema de Salud Sinaí.

Frecuencia alarmantemente alta y tasa de mortalidad

La tasa de diabetes entre puertorriqueños en West Town/Humboldt Park (21 por ciento) es la más alta jamás reportada en puertorriqueños, sabido ya que tienen una frecuencia particularmente alta del mal en la nación. La tasa es el doble de la frecuencia en puertorriqueños de Nueva York (11 por ciento) y Puerto Rico (9 por ciento). La frecuencia de diabetes entre vecinos no hispanos en West Town/Humboldt Park fue mucho menor con sólo 3 por ciento de caucásicos, 15 por ciento de afroestadounidenses y 4 por ciento de mexicanos diagnosticados con el mal.

Tasas de mortalidad para peurtorriqueños en esta comunidad fueron también significativamente mayores que promedios nacionales: 76 de cada 100,000 puertorriqueños mueren por diabetes en West Town/Humboldt Park comparados con 31 de cada 100,000 en todo Chicago y 25 de cada 100,000 en todo EEUU. Además, tasas de mortalidad para puertorriqueños en West Town/Humboldt Park aumentaron un abrumador 15 por ciento entre 1998 y 2003, significativamente más alto que el aumento de 2 por ciento en Chicago y de 4 por ciento en la nación.

"Estas tasas son alarmantes en extremo. Considerando que esta tasa de mortalidad prevaleció en EEUU, la diabetes sería la segunda causa líder de muerte en el país, apenas atrás del mal de corazón y muy delante de apoplejía y cáncer de seno, pulmón y colon", dijo el Dr. Steven Whitman, Director del Instituto Sinaí de Salud Urbana y autor líder del reporte. "Es cierto para nosotros que el impacto de diabetes entre puertorriqueños que viven en esta comunidad es tres veces mayor que en el país en conjunto".

Fuerza operante a nivel ciudad

La Fuerza Operante Diabetes en Humboldt Park, fuerza a nivel ciudad creada para enfrentar la abrumadora frecuencia de diabetes en West Town/Humboldt Park, emitió un reporte que contiene 19 recomendaciones para elevar la conciencia entre puertorriqueños que viven en esta comunidad y reducir significativamente la morbidez de diabetes los próximos cinco años.

Con estas recomendaciones, una gran meta de la Fuerza Operante es aumentar el entendimiento entre puertorriqueños que viven en en West/Town Humboldt Park de que diabetes y sus complicaciones son prevenibles con tratamiento, ejercicio y un estilo de vida saludable.

"Este reporte es en verdad un llamado a la acción", señaló el Dr. Steve Rothschild, Jefe de la Fuerza Operante, y profesor en el Centro Médico Universidad Rush. "Los próximos cinco años, cientos de personas con diabetes en Humboldt Park sufrirán ceguera, falla renal y diálisis, ataques al corazón, apoplejía, amputaciones y otras complicaciones potencialmente evitables. Docenas morirán por el mal. Las 19 recomendaciones listadas han sido agrupadas con base en la mejor evidencia informada que pudimos localizar y que creemos pueden implementarse en Humboldt Park los próximos cinco años".

Para más información llame (312) 942-3476. ■

Photo: Samuel Reyes

Figure 10-4 Article in "Extra," a Chicago Hispanic newspaper, about the December 6, 2006 meeting at Association House to discuss the high prevalence of diabetes among Puerto Ricans living in Chicago.

Source: *Extra*, December 7, 2006, p. 8

Making Something Happen

The increased community interest and momentum generated by the Summit made it clear to the Task Force that an intervention was needed—sooner rather than later. The ideal intervention was described in the Task Force report. It consisted of selecting a 72-block area of HP/WT and making the reduction of diabetes and its complications the highest possible health priority by implementing measures of primary, secondary, and tertiary prevention. Most importantly, the Task Force included key community leaders and organizations committed to impacting the ideology and culture of the community to help make diabetes a primary concern, thus facilitating "ownership" of the community's health (Ansell, 2010). This is envisioned as an example consistent with Freire's conscientization (Freire, 1972; Elias, 1976). Intervening in the entire HP/WT area was not feasible because it was too large (consisting of 108,000 people). The selected 72-block area contains 37,000 people, 27% Mexican, 33% Puerto Rican, 13% Black, 16% White, and 11% Hispanic people of other origins. The project quickly acquired the community name of the "Block-by-Block Project," and people would routinely ask Task Force members about it as they walked down the street. And they are still talking about it.

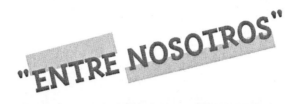

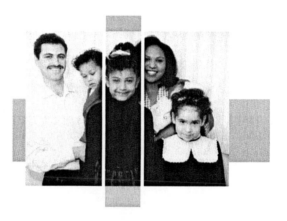

"ENTRE NOSOTROS"

A Summit On **Diabetes**
and Latino Healthcare

Friday, March 16, 2007
PROGRAM

Rebaño Compañerismo Cristiano Church
Chicago, Illinois

diabeteschicago.com

Figure 10-5 Front cover of the Program for the Summit on Diabetes, March 16, 2007, held in response to the "Call to Action" of public health workers, community activists, local politicians and health researchers concerning high diabetes prevalence among Puerto Ricans living in Chicago.

A recent study by the Sinai Urban Health Institute shows that Puerto Ricans in Humboldt Park have one of the highest prevalence rates of Diabetes ever reported among any group of people. Other parts of this community also have rates of the disease. Even more alarming, the Diabetes mortality rate for **Puerto Ricans living in Humboldt Park** is two times that of the city of Chicago and almost **three times that of the rest of the nation.**

Target Audience

- Community residents and people directly or indirectly affected by diabetes and other chronic conditions
- Healthcare and human service providers (e.g., physicians, nurses, health educators/health promoters).
- Community-based leaders and organizations.
- Elected and appointed policy-makers.
- Students/Researchers.

Rebaño Compañerismo Cristiano Church
2435 W. Division Street
Chicago, IL 60622
from 8:00 am – 4:30 pm
For more info (773) 456-7496

Figure 10-6 Poster Advertising "Entre Nosotros," the Summit held on March 16, 2007, in Humboldt Park, to address the problem of alarming rates of diabetes.

Initially one of the district's state legislators and a supporter of these efforts placed funding in the state budget, which was approved. However, the Illinois state budget started running out of money, and thus, although approved, the project was not funded. Toward the end of 2008 the Polk Bros. Foundation of Chicago (http://www.polkbrosfdn.org/) invited members of the Task Force to make a presentation to its Board. This resulted in a 1-year planning grant for the "Block-by-Block Project."

While all of this was going on, the authors, in collaboration with the Humboldt Park COW and the PRCC, submitted a substantial proposal to the U.S. National Institutes of Health for a community-based participatory research project to implement the "Block-by-Block Project." This project was funded for $2,000,000 for 4 years starting in mid-2009. It is worth noting

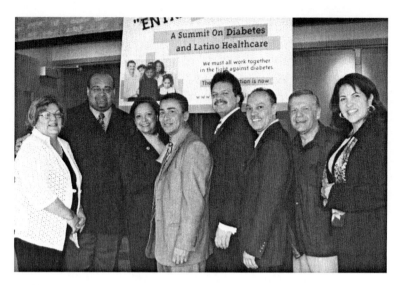

Figure 10-7 Photograph of the speakers at the "Entre Nosotros" event on March 16, 2007, which appeared in *La Raza*, a local Hispanic newspaper.

Source: *La Raza*, April 7, 2007, p. 34.

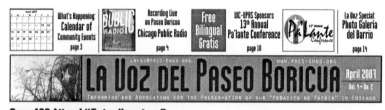

Over 400 Attend "Entre Nosotros"–
Humboldt Park Hosts Historic Diabetes Summit:
Elected Officials, Community Leaders, Health Providers and Residents Unite to Address Puerto Rican Diabetes Crisis

Miguel Angel Morales

Diabetes is a real killer in the Puerto Rican community of East Humboldt Park—three times the national average according to a study released on December 6, 2006. "Disproportionate Impact of Diabetes in a Puerto Rican Community of Chicago." The Sinai Urban Health Institute (SUHI) conducted the study and it asserted that almost 21% of Puerto Ricans in this area were diagnosed with diabetes, compared to whites (3.1%) and African Americans (14.5%) who live in West Town-Humboldt Park.

The Humboldt Park Diabetes Task Force, composed of community based organizations and agencies, research institutes and hospitals,

decided it wasn't enough to merely report the results. They released the SUHI study with a set of recommendations. One of these recommendations, to "Increase awareness of diabetes and make diabetes a community wide priority," was realized just last month

On Friday, March 16, Humboldt Park community organizations and elected officials held a conference entitled "Entre Nosotros" A Summit On Diabetes and Latino Healthcare. Over 400 community residents, public health folks, medical professionals, city officials and elected officials attended the summit held at Rebaño Compañerismo Cristiano Church on Paseo Boricua. State Senator Willie Delgado

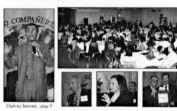

Diabetes Summit... page 9

Figure 10-8 Article and photographs from the "Entre Nosotros" event, March 16, 2007, appearing in *La Voz del Paseo Boricua*, a local newspaper dedicated to "Informing and Advocating for the Preservation of a Little Bit of Our Homeland."

Source: *La Voz Del Paseo Boricua*, April 2007, p. 1.

that the submitted proposal received very good scores. However, there was one substantial concern: that the community support for this project was so strong and well-organized that this project may not be replicable. We will deal with this "dilemma" when we come to it. Meanwhile, we enjoy its success and potential.

Observations and Implications

In a book like this that is so concerned with praxis, it makes sense to reflect on the events described above. The introduction to this book presented what we call the Sinai Model for trying to bring about health equity. Many of the aspects of the work described in this chapter conform to this model:

- Data that turned out to be provocative were gathered at the local level;
- the community (in this case HP/WT) was involved in the mission of the survey and the creation of the questions contained in the survey;
- data and findings were made available to the community as quickly as possible. A common complaint communities have of research studies is the huge time gap between when the data are gathered and when they are put into action. We refused to repeat such an error;
- because the community was so engaged in these efforts (and indeed was leading them), huge community forums were held. These, in turn, brought out all the politicians and the Spanish language media;
- the attention to the problem of diabetes was elevated by a very public dialogue extending even to middle school students. A concept put forward by the community and associated researchers was that an effort was being made to shift the ideology surrounding diabetes. All indications are that this effort is beginning to be successful;
- funders took note at the state level, among foundations and at the NIH; and
- substantial funding was acquired and the intervention has begun.

In all of this work, the power of the people in the community and the community-based organizations cannot be overestimated. In fact, these early successes can also be described by what did not happen rather than by what did. For example, in the 5 years or so described above, never once were there any "turf battles" or any competition among community organizations, politicians, or medical institutions. And, although everyone was disappointed about how slowly this process moved, no one criticized anyone for this. Much of this resulted from the fact that throughout the process the people of the community remained in charge. It was not that researchers, physicians, and medical centers were nice, well-intentioned people (they were) but that the choice was not theirs to make. They could join the community efforts or they could go home. Fortunately, they have chosen to join.

Acknowledgments

This project could not have been done without the support, time, and dedication of the HP/WT community, the community-based organizations that were the engine of the work (and who are named above), members of the Task Force, and researchers at the Sinai Urban Health Institute. Generous funding for this project was provided by the Robert Wood Johnson Foundation (Grant # 043026) and the Chicago Community Trust (Grant # C2003-00844), in addition to the grants from the Polk Bros. Foundation and NIH described in the text.

References

Ansell, Leah. 2010. Community-based interventions: Past, present, and future. In *Urban Health: Combating Disparities with Local Data*, ed. Steven Whitman, Ami M. Shah, and Maureen Benjamins, Chapter 13. New York: Oxford University Press.

Behavioral Risk Factor Surveillance System. Online. Available: http://apps.nccd.cdc.gov/brfss/display.asp?cat=DB&yr=2004&qkey=1363&state=US. Accessed June 21, 2008.

Benjamins, Maureen. 2010. The Jewish Community Health Survey of Chicago: Methodology and key findings. In: *Urban Health: Combating Disparities with Local Data*, ed. Steven Whitman, Ami M. Shah, and Maureen Benjamins, Chapter 4. New York, NY: Oxford University Press.

Black, Sandra A. 2002. Diabetes, diversity, and disparity: What do we do with the evidence? *American Journal of Public Health* 92:543–548.

Centers for Disease Control and Prevention. 1999. *Diabetes Surveillance, 1999*. Atlanta, GA: U.S. Department of Health and Human Services.

Centers for Disease Control and Prevention. 2003a. *National Diabetes Fact Sheet 2003*. Atlanta, GA: U.S. Department of Health and Human Services. Online. Available: http://www.cdc.gov/diabetes/pubs/pdf/ndfs_2003.pdf. Accessed June 21, 2008.

Centers for Disease Control and Prevention. 2003b. Self-reported heart disease and stroke among adults with and without diabetes—United States, 1991-2001. *Morbidity and Mortality Weekly Report* 52:1065–1070.

Centers for Disease Control and Prevention. 2004. Prevalence of diabetes among Hispanics—selected areas, 1998–2002. *Morbidity and Mortality Weekly Report* 53:941–944.

Coffey, Rosanna M., Trudy L. Matthews, and Kelly McDermott. 2004. Diabetes care quality improvement: A resource guide for state action. (Prepared by The Medstat

Group, Inc. and The Council of State Governments under Contract No. 290-00-0004). Rockville, MD: Agency for Healthcare Research and Quality, Department of Health and Human Services, AHRQ Pub. No. 04-0072.

Diabetes Control and Complications Research Group. 1993. The effect of intensive diabetes treatment on the development and progression of long-term complications in insulin-dependent diabetes mellitus: The Diabetes Control and Complications Trial. *New England Journal of Medicine* 329:977–1027.

Elias, John L. 1976. *Conscientization and Deschooling. Freire's and Illich's Proposals for Reshaping Society.* Philadelphia, PA: Westminster Press.

Freire, Paulo. 1972. *Pedagogy of the Oppressed.* London: Penguin.

Harris, Maurren I., Katherine M. Flegal, Catherine C. Cowie, Mark S. Eberhardt, David E. Goldstein, Randie R. Little, et al. 1998. Prevalence of diabetes, impaired fasting glucose, and impaired glucose tolerance in U.S. adults. The Third National Health and Nutrition Examination Survey, 1988–1994. *Diabetes Care* 21:518–524.

Hoyert, Donna L. and Ann R. Lima. 2005. Querying of death certificates in the United States. *Public Health Reports* 120:288–293.

Hu, Frank B., JoAnn E. Manson, Meir J. Stampfer, Graham Colditz, Simin Liu , Caren G. Solomon, et al. 2001. Diet, lifestyle, and the risk of type 2 diabetes mellitus in women. *New England Journal of Medicine* 345:790–797.

Kochanek, Keneth D., Sherry L. Murphy, Robert N. Anderson, and Charles Scott. 2004. Deaths: Final data for 2002. *National Vital Statistics Reports.* Hyattsville, MD: National Center for Health Statistics.

Lethbridge-Cejku, Margaret, Jeannine S. Schiller, and Luther Bernadel. 2004. Summary health statistics for US Adults: National Health Interview Survey, 2002. National Center for Health Statistics. *Vital Health Statistics 10*, 222:1–151.

McGinnis, J. Michael. 2002. Diabetes and physical activity: Translating evidence into action. *American Journal of Preventive Medicine* 22(4S):1–2.

Melnik, Thomas A., Akiko S. Hosler, Jackson Sekhobo, Thomas P. Duffy, Edward F. Tierney, Michael M. Engelgau, et al. 2004. Diabetes prevalence among Puerto Rican adults in New York City, NY 2000. *American Journal of Public Health* 94:434–437.

Mokdad Ali H., Earl S. Ford, Barbara A. Bowman, David E. Nelson, Michael M. Engelgau, Frank Vinicor, et al. 2000. Diabetes trends in the U.S.: 1990–1998. *Diabetes Care* 23:1278–1283.

Nathan, David M. and William H. Herman. 2004. Screening for diabetes: Can we afford not to screen? *Annals of Internal Medicine* 140:756–758.

National Institutes of Health. 1998. Clinical guidelines on the identification, evaluation, and treatment of overweight and obesity in adults: The evidence report. Publication no. 98-4083.

Perez-Cardonna, Cynthia. M. and Rosa Perez-Perdomo. 2001. Prevalence and associated risk factors of diabetes mellitus in Puerto Rican adults: Behavioral Risk Factor Surveillance System, 1999. *Puerto Rico Health Sciences Journal* 20:147–155.

Saydah, Sharon H., Mark S. Eberhardt, Catherine M. Loria, and Frederick L. Brancati. 2002. Age and the burden of death attributable to diabetes in the United States. *American Journal of Epidemiology* 156:714–719.

Schenker, Nathaniel and Jane F. Gentleman. 2001. On judging the significance of differences by examining the overlap between confidence intervals. *The American Statistician* 55:182–186.

Shah, Ami M., and Steven Whitman. 2010. Sinai Health System's Improving Community Health Survey: Methodology and key findings. In *Urban Health: Combating*

Disparities with Local Data, ed. Steven Whitman, Ami M. Shah, and Maureen Benjamins, Chapter 3. New York, NY: Oxford University Press.

Stata Corporation. 2003. STATA Statistical Software, Release 8.0 (Windows). College Station, TX: STATA Corporation.

Task Force on Community Preventive Services. 2002. Recommendations for healthcare system and self-management education interventions to reduce morbidity and mortality from diabetes. *American Journal of Preventive Medicine* 22:10–14.

The Humboldt Park Diabetes Task Force. 2006. *Diabetes in Humboldt Park: A call to action*. Online. Available: http://www.suhichicago.org/files/publications/Q.pdf. Accessed December 21, 2009.

U.S. Department of Health and Human Services. 1991. *Healthy People 2000: National Health Promotion and Disease Prevention Objectives*. Washington, DC: Public Health Service, Publication 91-50212.

U.S. Department of Health and Human Services. 2000. *Healthy People 2010: Understanding and Improving Health*. Washington, DC: Public Health Service.

Whitman, Steve, Abigail Silva, and Ami Shah. 2006. Disproportionate impact of diabetes in a Puerto Rican community of Chicago. *Journal of Community Health* 31(6):521–531.

Whitman, Steve, Cynthia Williams, and Ami Shah. 2004. *Sinai's Improving Community Health Survey: Report 1*. Chicago, IL: Sinai Health System.

11

PEDIATRIC ASTHMA IN BLACK AND LATINO CHICAGO COMMUNITIES: LOCAL LEVEL DATA DRIVES RESPONSE

**Helen Margellos-Anast and
Melissa A. Gutierrez**

Background

Asthma is a chronic respiratory disease characterized by swelling and narrowing of the lung airways. The airways of people with asthma are sensitive and react to different stimuli called triggers. Some examples of triggers for asthma include cigarette smoke, allergens (e.g., pollen, pet hair, etc.), mold, cockroaches, and rodents. Although asthma can be a detrimental disease if not managed properly, it can be controlled via the proper use of medications, trigger avoidance, early recognition of symptoms, and appropriate and timely response to symptoms. When asthma is well-controlled, people with asthma and their families can live healthy and productive lives. This chapter discusses how local-level data pertaining to the prevalence and effects of pediatric asthma in six diverse Chicago communities led to culturally appropriate action to improve asthma outcomes among children living in some of the city's most affected communities.

Epidemiology of Asthma

Asthma is the most common chronic disease of childhood, affecting 14% of U.S. children under age 18 years (10 million) and resulting in more school days missed than any other disease (Centers for Disease Control and Prevention [CDC], 2009a; Akinbami, 2007). In 2003, children missed 12.8 million days of school because of asthma (Akinbami, 2007). Poorly controlled asthma can result in increased utilization of urgent health care and therefore substantial health-care costs. In 2004, children younger than 18 years had 754,000 emergency department (ED) visits (103 per 10,000) and 198,000 hospitalizations (27 per 10,000) for asthma (Moorman et al., 2007). Asthma medical expenditures (hospitalizations, ED visits, physician services, and medications) in the United States were estimated at $14.7 billion in 2007 (National Institutes of Health, National Blood, Lung and Heart Institute, 2007).

Asthma prevalence rates nationally are known to be highest among Puerto Rican children (31%), followed by non-Hispanic Black children (17%); they are lowest among Mexican children (10%) (CDC, 2009a; Lara et al., 2006; Akinbami, 2007). Notably, between 1980 and 2001, the mortality rate resulting from asthma increased among Black children despite significant improvements in medications and knowledge of how to control the disease over the same interval. By 2001, Black children were 5.6 times more likely to die from asthma than non-Hispanic White children (Gupta, Carrión-Carire, and Weiss, 2006). Black children are also over 3.5 times more likely to visit the ED for asthma-related problems than are non-Hispanic White children (263.6 per 10,000 vs. 73.0 per 10,000) (Akinbami, 2007).

Motivation for the Survey

In the time leading up to *Sinai's Improving Community Health Survey* (Sinai Survey), which took place between September 2002 and April 2003 (*see* Chapter 3) (Shah and Whitman, 2010), data had begun to emerge suggesting that Chicago might be among the cities hardest hit by asthma, with higher than national asthma-related mortality and morbidity rates (Weiss and Wagener, 1990; Marder et al., 1992; Targonski et al., 1994; Thomas and Whitman, 1999; Mannino et al., 2002). In 1996, the asthma hospitalization rate for Chicago was 42.8 per 10,000, more than twice the U.S. rates (Thomas and Whitman, 1999). In addition, the 1996 age-adjusted asthma mortality rate in Chicago was 4.7 times higher in non-Hispanic Blacks than in non-Hispanic Whites (Thomas and Whitman, 1999). A study in the nation's largest city, New York City, had demonstrated that hospitalization and mortality rates varied by neighborhood (Carr, Zeiel, and Weiss, 1992). Chicago, the nation's third largest city, has 77 officially designated community areas (Chicago Fact Book Consortium, 1995), many of which are quite segregated. Therefore, one might ask if asthma prevalence and severity rates vary by community area in Chicago.

Sources such as the National Health Interview Survey (NHIS), the Behavioral Risk Factor Surveillance System (BRFSS) Survey, the National

Hospital Ambulatory Medical Care Survey (NHAMCS), and the Illinois Health Care Cost Containment Council (IHCCCC) provide a great deal of information about the prevalence, morbidity, and costs associated with pediatric asthma on the national and state level. Vital statistics data allows for the analysis and display of asthma mortality data by smaller geographical areas such as city, community, and neighborhood, whereas hospitalization rates can be broken down to the zip code level. However, at the time when the Sinai Survey was being conceived, there was little other information available regarding asthma prevalence or severity at the city or community level. It was therefore not known, for example, whether reports of higher asthma morbidity and mortality in certain inner city populations compared with others could be attributed to differences in asthma prevalence or, rather, to differences in the severity and control of the disease. The lack of community-level information pertaining to asthma prevalence, severity, and control was a substantial deficit, and one that needed to be addressed if interventions aimed at preventing the development and exacerbation of the disease were to be appropriately targeted to those most at risk.

Therefore, obtaining data on pediatric asthma that could inform local-level interventions and policy to quell the epidemic was a priority of the Sinai Survey.

This chapter pursues three main purposes:

1. First, local-level data pertaining to the prevalence, morbidity, severity, and control of asthma in children age 12 years and younger living in the six surveyed communities in Chicago are presented. Data are compared with existing city and national estimates whenever possible.
2. Second, the findings of the survey are discussed in the context of the action that resulted from them. Specifically, the survey findings led directly to the development of interventions to address the disproportionate burden of asthma suffered by certain communities and groups of people and offered insight on how to combat the epidemic on the local, city, and state level.
3. Third, the lessons learned along the way and their implications are presented.

The Data

Methods

The survey from which the data were obtained is described in detail in Chapter 3 and the demographics of each surveyed community are presented in Table 3-2 (Shah and Whitman, 2010). In households where a child (12 years and under) resided, the interview included a pediatric component addressed to the primary caregiver of one randomly selected child. The child module of the survey contained 22 questions specific to pediatric asthma. The question of asthma prevalence (i.e., how many children have asthma) was pursued in three ways. First, the lifetime prevalence of asthma was assessed by asking whether the child had ever received a diagnosis of asthma. The question used was: "Have you ever been told by a doctor, nurse, or other health professional that your child had asthma?" and is a slight modification of the question used by the National Health Interview Survey (NHIS). Next, the prevalence of asthma episodes and attacks was assessed by asking the question: "During the last 12 months, has your child had an episode of asthma or an asthma attack?" This question also comes from NHIS and is worded exactly the same. Finally, to approximate the prevalence of undiagnosed pediatric asthma in these communities, questions from the validated Brief Pediatric Asthma Screen (BPAS) were included (Wolf et al., 1999). The BPAS consists of four questions that, when answered in a certain combination, reveal that the child likely has asthma.

A number of questions were intended to determine the burden that pediatric asthma exerts on certain communities. For example, there was a series of questions intended to assess whether children with asthma had their asthma under proper control. The National Heart, Lung, and Blood Institute's (NHLBI) standards for properly controlled asthma were used as the criteria (NHLBI, 1997; 2002). A child was determined to have poorly controlled asthma if any of the following criteria applied:

1. Four or more asthma attacks in the past 12 months;
2. Four or more wheezing episodes in the past 12 months;
3. Five or more nights of disturbed sleep in the past 30 days;
4. Four or more incidents of urgent health resource utilization in the past 12 months (e.g., sum of emergency department/urgent care center visits, hospitalizations, and urgent clinic visits);
5. Having had asthma symptoms severe enough to limit speech to only one or two words at a time between breaths within the past 12 months.

Finally, the data were analyzed considering data from the adult survey about cigarette smoking in the household to determine the proportion of children with asthma who were consistently exposed to the universal trigger of secondhand cigarette smoke (*see* Chapter 7 for more information) (West and Gamboa, 2010).

Data Analysis

All observations were weighted to account for the probability of selection (at the block, household, and respondent levels) and to ensure that the sample accurately reflected the socio-demographic characteristics of the base populations per the 2000 Census. Data were analyzed using SAS version 9 (SAS Institute Inc., 2002–2003), which allows for sampling design effects to be considered.

Results

Prevalence

The prevalence of physician-diagnosed asthma in the six communities ranged from 6% in South Lawndale to 20% in West Town, with four of the six communities exceeding the national rate of 12% during the same time-interval (Centers CDC, 2009b). Caregivers who did not report that their child had ever been diagnosed with asthma were screened via the BPAS (Wolf et al., 1999). Those who screened positive for asthma via the BPAS likely had asthma. Figure 11-1 presents the proportion of children with diagnosed asthma, screened asthma, and the combined total in each community. The prevalence of diagnosed asthma could be seen as the low end of a range, whereas the total of those with a diagnosis and those with screened asthma could be seen as the high end of the range. The combined total will be referred to as *potential asthma* from this point forward. The prevalence of potential asthma exceeded 20% in four of the six communities: Humboldt Park (28%), West Town (28%), North Lawndale (23%), and Roseland (23%).

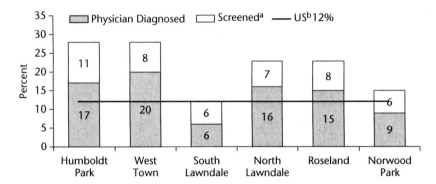

Figure 11-1   Proportion of Children with Physician-Diagnosed and Screened Asthma by Community Area

Source: Sinai's Improving Community Health Survey, 2002–2003.

Notes: [a]Screened positive for asthma via *Brief Pediatric Asthma Screen.*
[b]Comparison data is the prevalence of physician diagnosed asthma, National Health Interview Survey, 2003.

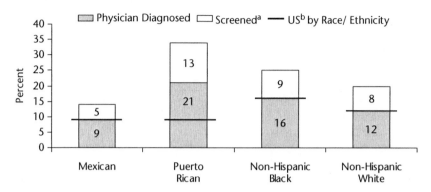

Figure 11-2 Percent of Children with Physician-Diagnosed and Screened Asthma by Race/ Ethnicity

Source: Sinai's Improving Community Health Survey, 2002–2003.

Notes: [a]Screened positive for asthma via *Brief Pediatric Asthma Screen.*
[b]Comparison data is the prevalence of physician diagnosed asthma, National Health Interview Survey, 2003.

In other words, in four of the six surveyed communities, the prevalence of pediatric asthma might be twice as high as it is for the United States as a whole (12%) (CDC, 2009b).

When the data are presented by race and ethnicity (Fig. 11-2), the highest rates of potential asthma are among Puerto Rican (34%) and non-Hispanic Black (25%) children. These trends resemble what is found nationally, with Puerto Rican and non-Hispanic Black children having the highest rates. But, although the trend is similar, the rates are higher among surveyed Chicago children than they are nationally, where 27% of Puerto Rican and 17% of non-Hispanic Black children have physician-diagnosed asthma (Akinbami, 2006; Lara et al., 2006, Akinbami, 2007).

These survey findings were the first to officially document the prevalence of asthma in certain Chicago communities that had long been suspected of suffering an immense asthma burden. Around the same time that the findings of the Sinai Survey were being analyzed and prepared for dissemination, preliminary findings from the Harlem Children's Zone asthma study were highlighted on the front page of *The New York Times* (April 19, 2003). The article reported that "One of every four children in central Harlem has asthma, which is double the rate researchers expect to find and, researchers say, is one of the highest rates ever documented for an American neighborhood." However, the prevalence of asthma was equally high for several of the Chicago neighborhoods surveyed, especially for Black and Puerto Rican children. Thus, what made front-page news in *The New York Times* is an every day reality for children living in certain Chicago communities. Later findings from the Harlem Children's Zone revealed that 30% of screened children had potential asthma (Nicholas et al., 2005). Several other studies that have since been conducted in Chicago (Quinn et al, 2006; Shalowitz et al., 2007; Gupta et al., 2008) and other big cities (Simon et al., 2003; Nicholas et al., 2005) have corroborated that the prevalence of asthma in inner-city, minority, disadvantaged communities approaches, and even exceeds, 25%.

Asthma Burden and Control

In addition to having a higher prevalence of asthma, it has been documented that minority children living in inner-city communities also suffer disproportionately from it, as shown by their morbidity and mortality rates (Weiss and Wagener, 1990; Halfon and Newacheck, 1993; Finkelstein et al., 1995; Lara et al., 2006;). Findings from the Sinai Survey lend further evidence to this assertion. For example, between 26% and 54% of children with diagnosed asthma in five of the communities had asthma that could be considered poorly controlled per the NHLBI's standards, as shown in Table 11-1 (NHLBI, 1997; NHLBI, 2002). This finding is not surprising given that in most surveyed communities, more than 50% of children with an asthma diagnosis were not currently using a controller medication[1] (Table 11-1). In fact, in four of the communities, more than 40% of children with diagnosed asthma did not have access to any medication (Table 11-1). It is extremely dangerous

TABLE 11-1 Asthma Burden and Control for Children with an Asthma Diagnosis by Community Area

Outcome	Humboldt Park (%)	West Town (%)	South Lawndale (%)	North Lawndale (%)	Roseland (%)
Poorly Controlled Asthma[a]	54	26	44	33	39
No Controller Medication	52	76	54	80	78
No Controller or Rescue Medication	16	50	48	38	73
Children with potential asthma[b] who live with a smoker	48	20	12	48	61

Source: Sinai's Improving Community Health Survey, 2002–2003 (Norwood Park was omitted because only five children had an asthma diagnosis).

Notes: [a]As defined by the National Heart Lung and Blood Institute.
[b]Potential Asthma is defined as physician diagnosed plus screened positive per the *Brief Pediatric Asthma Screen*.

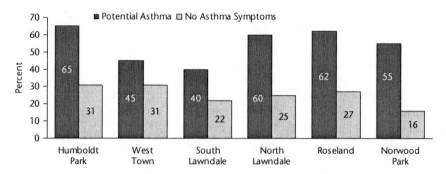

Figure 11-3   Percent of Children with at Least One Emergency Department Visit in the Last 12 Months by Asthma Status

Source: Sinai's Improving Community Health Survey, 2002–2003.

for a child with asthma to not have access to a quick-relief medication,[1] which could save his/her life in case of an attack. In Roseland, a shocking 73% of children with diagnosed asthma did not have access to a single medication.

The Sinai survey data supports findings by other researchers suggesting that children from poor, inner-city, and minority communities with asthma exert a great toll on the emergency health-care system (Halfon and Newacheck, 1993; Singh et al., 1993; Finkelstein et al., 1995; Woodruff et al., 1999; Rand et al., 2000). Figure 11-3 shows the proportion of children who went to the ED at least once in the past year, dividing the children into those with potential asthma and those without any symptoms of asthma. Note that in four of the six surveyed communities, more than 50% of children with potential asthma indicated having used the ED in the past year. In all cases, ED use by children with potential asthma exceeded ED use among children with no asthma symptoms, and in many instances children with potential asthma were two to three times more likely to use the ED than children with no symptoms (Fig. 11-3).

The detrimental effects of tobacco smoke on children who have asthma have been well-established (Chiomonczyk et al., 1993). In fact, exposure to cigarette smoke, whether primary or secondary, is recognized as the one universal trigger of asthma. Nonetheless, the survey revealed that in three of the surveyed communities, the proportion of children with potential asthma living with a smoker approached or exceeded 50% (Table 11-1). Given the high smoking rates in several of these communities (*see* Chapter 7) (West and Gamboa, 2010), children with asthma are likely to be frequently exposed to secondhand smoke, further exacerbating the burden asthma exerts on their lives.

Implications

It has been well-established that Chicago is one of the cities hardest hit by the surging asthma epidemic (Weiss and Wagener, 1990; Marder et al., 1992;

Targonski et al., 1994; Thomas and Whitman, 1999; Naureckas and Thomas, 2007). However, prior to the Sinai Survey, there was no hard evidence to back up the prevalent suspicion that children living in Chicago's most disadvantaged, minority communities might bear the greatest burden. The Sinai Survey provided that evidence when it revealed that one of every four children in four of the surveyed Chicago communities likely had asthma. Furthermore, children in poorer and minority communities surveyed tended to have asthma that was poorly controlled, meaning they often suffered needlessly as a result of the disease.

Although asthma is a chronic disease and cannot be cured, it can be controlled with proper medications, symptom monitoring, and trigger avoidance. When asthma is well-controlled, children can live normal and productive lives, reaching their full potential. However, when it is not, the effects stem far beyond the immediate to potentially compromise a child's long-term health and quality of life. For example, some of the potential short-term effects of poorly controlled asthma might be that the child does not sleep well at night and therefore is not fully alert when at school, he/she may miss school frequently (which often results in the parent missing work), and he/she may not be able to play fully nor participate in structured activities or sports. The short-term consequences have potential long-term effects, including remodeling of the lungs, resulting in a greater risk for future lung disease; compromising the quality of education that the child receives, thereby affecting his/her future career prospects; and impairing social skills and self-confidence.

Although no one familiar with asthma in Chicago was surprised by the immense burden revealed by the Sinai Survey, those outside the asthma community were now mobilized to provide the resources necessary to address the situation. Several additional studies followed that substantiated the survey data discussed herein and definitively proved that children in poor, minority, urban communities are at an increased risk of having asthma and of suffering needlessly from poorly controlled asthma (Nicholas et al., 2005; Quinn et al., 2006; Shalowitz et al, 2007; Gupta et al., 2008).

Local-level data reveal disparities in asthma prevalence, severity, and management, which are likely attributable to a combination of personal, social, and environmental factors. Furthermore, national and city-wide data may seriously underestimate the prevalence of pediatric asthma in urban communities. Poorly controlled asthma in childhood has grave economic and social ramifications, not only for the individual child but also for their families and the community. Interventions and policies are most effective when they target communities most in need and when they consider the social and environmental context of the problem. Armed with local-level data, community leaders and policymakers may foster effective health planning and bring greater resources to these marginalized communities.

The Response: Data Drives Change

The Sinai Survey took place in 2002 to 2003, with the first report documenting key findings from the survey published in 2004 (Whitman, Williams,
and Shah, 2004). The report was quickly disseminated to those with a vested
interest in the findings, particularly to community partners, researchers,
funders, and policymakers. The months immediately following the survey
were devoted to making numerous presentations on the key findings of the
survey and discussing those findings with stakeholders. Chapter 3 presents
more details on these activities. Briefly, the pediatric asthma findings generated substantial buzz among all audiences to which they were presented,
both community and professional. The perceived importance of the findings
to the local, asthma professional community is evident in the fact that the
data were presented at the unveiling of the Chicago Asthma Action Plan on
World Asthma Day (May 1, 2004). Significant media attention followed the
release of the data (Fig. 11-4) and the Chicago Asthma Action Plan. Some
of the specific headlines included: "City 'sick with asthma,' but experts have

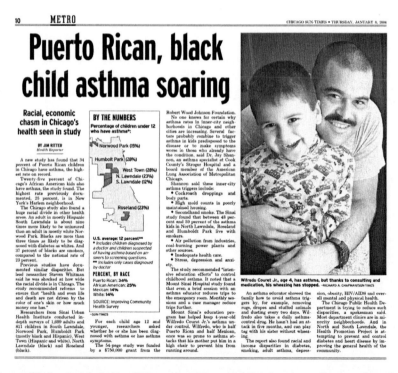

Figure 11-4   Article in the *Chicago Sun-Times* highlighting the pediatric asthma findings of *Sinai's Improving Community Health Survey*

Source: Jim Ritter, "Puerto Rican, black child asthma soaring: Racial, economic chasm in
Chicago's health seen in study," *Chicago Sun-Times,* January 8th, 2004, Metro Section.

plan to get well" (*Chicago Sun Times*, May 4, 2004) and "Chicago told it has an asthma epidemic" (*Chicago Tribune*, May 5, 2004). The survey findings, their implications, the work of other Chicago-area researchers, and efforts to reduce asthma disparities were also highlighted in a special feature entitled "Waiting to Inhale," published by *Chicago Reporter* in September 2004 (vol. 33, no. 7). The survey findings also generated an interest in conducting future research to substantiate its findings. Finally, the survey findings mobilized researchers and communities toward action to address the problem. A multitude of interventions followed. Those instigated by the Sinai Urban Health Institute (SUHI) and Sinai Children's Hospital (SCH) are discussed in greater detail below.

Sinai Urban Health Institute Pediatric Asthma Interventions

SUHI and SCH have been working together since July 2000 to address the unacceptable burden poorly controlled asthma has on the communities served by the Sinai Health System. The Sinai Health System is located in the poor, predominately Black community of North Lawndale, where the survey revealed that nearly one of every four children likely has asthma. Not only are children in North Lawndale more likely to have asthma than many of their counterparts in other Chicago communities, but the survey also revealed that only 15% of children in North Lawndale with diagnosed symptomatic asthma are on proper medications and that nearly half are exposed to tobacco smoke on a daily basis.

Although the survey data would not become available until 2004, the high volume of children coming through Sinai's Emergency Department for asthma, combined with the experiences of area physicians with many poorly controlled asthma patients, led to the establishment of the first Pediatric Asthma Initiative (PAI-1) in 2000. A series of four comprehensive asthma interventions, each building on the successes and shortcomings of its predecessors, have followed and have resulted in substantial knowledge about how best to address the suffering resulting from asthma in poor, minority, urban communities. A description of each of these efforts and their outcomes follows, highlighting the improvement that these programs have made in the lives of several hundred children, their families, and the community.

The Community Health Worker (CHW) Model is an integral part of each of the interventions. CHWs are laypeople who live in the community that the project serves. They share a cultural and communal connection with those targeted by the intervention. As a result, they are often better able to establish the relationship of trust needed to successfully identify and address barriers to proper disease management. CHWs do not need to have any prior experience in the field, as they are trained by the program to teach children and their families how to more effectively manage asthma. Other synonymous terms include community health educator, peer educator, lay health educator, *promotora de salud,* and outreach educator, among others. Several published literature reviews have summarized the findings from studies assessing the effectiveness of CHWs in preventing (primary prevention), identifying (secondary prevention), and managing (tertiary prevention) various chronic diseases (Swider, 2002; Nemcek and Sabatier, 2003; Persily, 2003; Andrews et al., 2004; Brownstein et al., 2005; Lewin et al., 2005; Norris et al., 2006).

Each of the interventions described on the following pages has included a sound evaluation component, with findings documenting significant improvements in asthma control as indicated by decreased asthma morbidity (e.g., urgent health resource utilization, ED visits, and symptoms). Subsequently, several of the interventions also were associated with increases in quality of life, self-efficacy, and asthma knowledge. In short, the lives of the families served by the projects have dramatically improved. A brief synopsis of each project follows in chronological order, ending with the most comprehensive intervention to date, *Healthy Home, Healthy Child: The Westside Children's Asthma Partnership.* Table 11-2 provides demographic and baseline characteristics of the participants of each of these programs.

Pediatric Asthma Intervention-1 (PAI-1)

SUHI and SCH first responded to the pediatric asthma problem plaguing the Westside of Chicago in July 2000 with the launch of the original Sinai PAI-1 (Karnick et al., 2005). The central hypothesis of this sequential randomized clinical trial was that the most economic and effective path to maximizing the health status of inner-city children with asthma is through a process of case-specific, one-on-one reinforced health education combined with case management services. Study participants included children (1–16 years) with asthma who were randomized into three groups: Group One (G1) received a single, one-on-one asthma education session with a trained CHW; Group Two (G2) received the same initial asthma education session, but that education was reinforced on a monthly basis via phone calls; and Group Three (G3) received reinforced asthma education with the addition of case management. All participants in each group received an evaluation by a pediatric pulmonologist at their initial visit to ensure proper medical management. The initial education session occurred during this visit and, therefore, in a clinic setting.

Two hundred twelve children were enrolled in the project, of which 165 (78%) completed the 9 months of follow-up. Table 11-2 summarizes participant characteristics and demographics. Participants were generally high utilizers of urgent health-care services, with the average child having two ED visits and one hospitalization for asthma in the year prior to enrollment.

TABLE 11-2 Sinai Urban Health Institute Pediatric Asthma Intervention Characteristics, Participant Demographics, and Baseline Data

	PAI-1[a]	PAI-2[b]	CPATC[c] (Chicago Sample)
Funding Period	7/01/2000–5/31/2002	11/01/2004–8/31/2006	4/01/2006–12/31/2008
Funder	Michael Reese Health Trust and Crown Foundation	Illinois Department of Public Health	Illinois Department of Public Health
Participant Recruitment	Sinai Patients	African American Children living on the Westside of Chicago	Children living on the Westside and Southside of Chicago
Location of Visits	Clinic	Participant's Home	Participant's Home
Race/Ethnicity	66% Non-Hispanic Black 34% Hispanic	100% Non-Hispanic Black	61% Non-Hispanic Black 30% Hispanic 7% Hispanic Black 2% Mixed
Age (mean)	6 years	7 years	7 years
Gender (% male)	59.9%	57.1%	55.1%
% Medicaid/All Kids[d] Insured	89.0%	95.7%	74.8%
Total Enrolled in Study	212	70	334
Number Completing Follow-up period	165	50	234
Nighttime Symptoms in the past 2-weeks at baseline (mean)	—	4.0	3.5
Emergency Department Visits in the year prior to baseline (mean)	1.9	3.1	2.4
Sum Urgent Health Resource Utilization[e] in the year prior to baseline (mean)	5.7	6.5	5.3

Notes: [a]Pediatric Asthma Intervention-1.
[b]Pediatric Asthma Intervention-2.
[c]Controlling Pediatric Asthma Through Collaboration and Education.
[d]All Kids is a state run health insurance program available to all children in the state of Illinois.
[e]Sum of urgent health resource utilization variables (hospitalizations, ED visits, and urgent clinic visits).

TABLE 11-3   Outcome Data for Sinai Urban Health Institute Pediatric Asthma
Interventions - PAI-1, PAI-2, and CPATCE

Outcome	PAI-1(n = 165)[a]	PAI-2 (n = 50)[b]	CPATCE—Chicago Sample (n = 234)[c]
Asthma ED[d] Visits	64.0% decline*	73.5% decline*	49.5% decline*
Asthma Hospitalizations	81.0% decline*	71.4% decline*	60.6% decline*
Urgent Health Resource Utilization	67.6% decline*	69.3% decline*	53.9% decline*
Nighttime Asthma Symptoms	—	51.6% decline*	57.7% decline*
Quality of Life[e]	—	Increased by 0.8*[e]	Increased by 0.54*[e]

*Statistically significant $p < 0.05$ per Wilcoxon signed rank sum test for non-parametric data

Notes: [a]Pediatric Asthma Intervention-1 (PAI-1). Percentages are based on the difference between means at baseline and data collected through nine months of follow-up and extrapolated out to represent one year post-baseline.
[b]Pediatric Asthma Intervention-2 (PAI-2). Percentages are based on the difference between means at baseline and data collected through one year post baseline.
[c]Controlling Pediatric Asthma Through Collaboration and Education (CPATCE). Percentages are based on the difference between means at baseline and data collected through 6 months of follow-up and extrapolated out to represent one year post-baseline.
[d]ED = Emergency Department.
[e]An increase of 0.5 is clinically significant.

Participants in all three groups utilized significantly fewer urgent health-care services in the follow-up year. Averaged across all three groups, the magnitude of the decline in utilization was substantial: about 81% for hospitalizations, 69% for hospital days, 64% for ED visits, and 58% for urgent clinic visits (Table 11-3). Although there were no statistically significant differences between study groups for four of the five main outcome measures, G3 participants consistently improved to a greater degree than G1 or G2. Furthermore, the PAI-1 project also proved to be cost-effective. In fact, the G3 intervention resulted in an estimated $4,778 saved per patient/year over costs incurred during the baseline year. This translates to $13.29 saved per dollar spent on the intervention. The findings of PAI-1 were published in the *Journal of Asthma* (Karnick et al., 2005).

The findings of PAI-1 clearly support the utility and cost–benefit associated with the combined provision of health education utilizing a CHW and case management services for pediatric patients who are high utilizers of urgent health-care services. Other studies have also supported the utility of individualized, case-specific asthma education and case management provided by health professionals (e.g., nurses, social workers, CHWs, and others in improving asthma outcomes) (Butz et al., 1994; Evans et al., 1999;

Greineder, Loane, and Parks, 1995; Greineder, Loane, and Parks, 1999; Hughes et al., 1991; Kelly et al., 2002; Stout, White, and Rogers, 1998).

Lessons Learned and Challenges   Several important lessons learned via PAI-1 have proved instrumental in the development of subsequent Sinai interventions. First, because PAI-1 preceded the Sinai Survey, the baseline data provided a first glimpse into how asthma impacted the lives of children living in the communities served by the Sinai Health System. PAI-1's eligibility criteria did not require that a child have poorly controlled asthma, yet the average participant had been to the ED nearly twice in the year prior to enrolling and had utilized urgent health-care services of some sort (e.g., ED, hospitalizations, and urgent clinic visit) nearly six times. This information strengthened the desire for asthma-specific data from these communities that could be used as a benchmark for the evaluation of future interventions.

Second, PAI-1 suggested that even a one-time, individualized asthma education session with a CHW could result in improved asthma control. Whereas G3 participants consistently improved to the greatest degree, the basic intervention provided to G1 participants was also associated with improved outcomes. Therefore, it is important to target the approach to the needs of the person being served, but some intervention is better than nothing at all. It should be noted, however, that the interpretation of the results is complicated by the fact that all study participants saw a pulmonologist upon enrollment, making it difficult to separate out how much of the noted improvement among participants resulted from health education/case management and how much resulted from changes in medical management. However, evidence has consistently pointed to the need for education in addition to the proper prescribing of medications in properly managing asthma. Both the NHLBI guidelines (NHLBI, 1997; 2002) and an expert panel report of policy recommendations (Lara et al., 2002) have emphasized the importance of health education/case management in addition to better prescribing in maximizing asthma control. Therefore, it is unlikely that the dramatic improvements noted would have been observed with medication changes alone.

Third, primary care providers face many obstacles to applying the NHLBI asthma treatment guidelines to patient care, particularly in the inner city, where reimbursement for services often is at or below the cost of delivering quality care. Realistic mechanisms and incentives are needed to ensure that patients receive care consistent with the NHLBI standards. Medicaid funding support for health education, with or without case management, is a realistic program for improving quality of life and asthma care in the inner city while reducing public expenditures.

There were certain methodological challenges associated with PAI-1 that should be mentioned. For one, funding constraints limited the follow-up period to 9 months. As such, 9 months of follow-up data was extrapolated to 12 months to make comparisons with the baseline year. Although seasonal trends in asthma symptoms, severity, and health resource utilization have been documented in the literature (Thomas and Whitman, 1999; Weiss, 1990) an analysis of PAI-1 data by season showed no trend, making it unlikely this limitation affected the results. Second, the study is limited by the fact that the baseline data was collected retrospectively and that all data was collected via participant recall. Therefore, the ability of the caregivers to accurately remember information may have affected findings (i.e., recall bias). Social desirability bias may also have been a factor given that the CHW was responsible for some of the data collection and respondents may have wanted to answer favorably to please the CHW. However, given the main outcomes assessed (e.g., ED visits, hospitalizations, etc.) are generally memorable, and given the extent of improvement between the baseline and follow-up year, it is unlikely that the overall conclusion of the evaluation was impeded upon by these limitations.

A final notable challenge involves the fact that the intervention occurred in the clinic and over the phone. Given asthma is a condition that can be affected immensely by the home environment, it was difficult to fully and completely educate the family on environmental triggers that might be aggravating the child's asthma without going into the home. Also, it was possible that by conducting the intervention in a clinic setting, some of the most vulnerable children were being missed because of the fact that they were unlikely to be seen in the clinic and might be relying predominantly on the ED for asthma care.

Pediatric Asthma Intervention-2 (PAI-2)

In 2004, with pilot funding from the Illinois Department of Public Health (IDPH)[2], SUHI and SCH were able to implement a project to assess the feasibility and effectiveness of an approach utilizing CHWs making home visits in improving asthma management among Black children with severe asthma living in inner-city neighborhoods. This pilot funding was stimulated directly by the pediatric asthma findings of the Sinai Survey (Figs. 11-1, 11-2, 11-3; Table 11-1). The developed approach built on the successes and limitations of PAI-1, while also considering the existing literature pertaining to effective asthma interventions with inner-city children (Butz et al., 1994; Garret et al., 1994; Stout, White, and Rogers, 1998; Kelly et al., 2002; Kinney et al., 2002; Morgan et al., 2004). It was also felt to be imperative that this next intervention should occur primarily in the family's home.

The pilot project, PAI-2, utilized CHWs recruited from the same inner-city, predominantly Black communities served by the project and trained to serve as asthma educators. The CHWs sought to teach and empower children and their families to more effectively manage asthma. The education provided to the family was individualized and was provided in the family's home whenever possible. The CHW also aimed to facilitate the establishment of a relationship with a primary care provider. The CHWs did not need to have any prior experience with asthma. Rather, the intent was to locate individuals with a cultural connection to the target communities and a passion for positively impacting the lives of the people living within those communities. Once the CHWs were identified, they participated in a 5-day intensive asthma training class conducted by a certified asthma educator who specializes in training asthma CHWs. In addition to the formal training sessions, the selected CHWs received further training by working closely with their supervisor, who was also the Pediatric Asthma Educator for SCH.

Methods   Participants were recruited primarily from the ED and inpatient units of SCH and also via referrals from community physicians. Eligible children had severe, poorly controlled asthma, were between the ages of 2 and 16 years, and were Black (because of funding requirements). The CHWs conducted three to four home visits over a 6-month period with each participating family. The CHW also served as a liaison between the family and the medical system, helping to bridge the gap between parents and medical providers—particularly primary care providers. When necessary, the CHW, in consultation with her supervisor and appropriate Sinai staff, also provided basic case management services.

The success of PAI-2 in meeting its goals was evaluated using a pre–post test methodology with each child serving as his/her own historical control. Participants were followed for 1 year post-baseline for evaluation purposes. The main outcomes assessed included asthma symptom severity (in the past 2 weeks), frequency of asthma-related emergency health resource utilization, caregiver quality of life (Juniper et al., 1996), asthma-related knowledge of the caregiver, and the belief (self-efficacy) of the caregiver that he/she is able to manage the child's asthma (Telleen, 2000). Other outcomes of interest included whether the intervention was effective in decreasing the number of triggers to which the child is exposed and whether medications were being used correctly. Another project goal involved ensuring that each participating child had an Asthma Action Plan (AAP) signed by his/her physician. An AAP is a set of individualized instructions that detail how a person with asthma should manage the condition at various stages. The CHW would not only ensure that the family had an AAP but that the caregiver and child (given that the child exhibits a certain level of comprehension) understood how to implement the AAP.

Results   Between November 15, 2004 and July 15, 2005, 70 children were enrolled into PAI-2. Table 11-2 displays the baseline characteristics and demographics of enrolled participants. Participants were often high utilizers of emergency health services, as evidenced by the fact that the average participant had visited an ED, been hospitalized, or visited a physician for worsening asthma 6.5 times in the year prior to participation. Fifty-four percent of enrolled children lived with a smoker. Fifty-eight (83%) completed the 6-month intervention phase. The outcome analysis was limited to the 50 (71%) children who completed the entire 12-month evaluation phase.

The findings strongly suggest that the primary goal of improving asthma control and thus decreasing asthma-related morbidity and improving quality of life was met. With regard to asthma-related morbidity, the specific outcomes examined included four symptom-related variables, asthma exacerbations, wheezing episodes, and urgent health resource utilization. Statistically significant improvements were noted for the majority of examined outcomes. For example, the frequency of nighttime asthma symptoms decreased from 3.1 nights of disturbed sleep in the 2 weeks preceding the baseline visit to an average of 1.5 nights of disturbed sleep per 2-week interval over the course of the 12-month follow-up. This is a 52% decrease in nighttime symptom frequency (Table 11-3). Daytime symptom frequency decreased by a similar magnitude. Urgent health resource utilization also decreased significantly over the follow-up period. For example, ED visits decreased from 3.4 times in the year prior to the study to 0.9 in the year following, a 74% decrease ($p < 0.05$; Table 11-3).

The study's second primary goal was to improve the family's quality of life. A validated tool, the *Pediatric Asthma Caregiver's Quality of Life Questionnaire* was used to assess progress toward this goal (Juniper et al., 1996). The caregiver's quality of life is an indicator of the impact of improved asthma control on the family's overall well-being. Caregiver Quality of Life scores increased significantly from 5.2 (out of a maximum of 7) at the time of enrollment in the intervention to 6.0 ($p < 0.05$) by month 12. Other studies have suggested that changes of this magnitude are associated with clinically significant improvements in asthma outcomes (Juniper et al., 1994).

The project also had four secondary goals (variables on the pathway to successfully meeting the primary goals). Over the follow-up period, improvements were noted for the majority of outcomes utilized in measuring the intervention's progress in meeting these secondary goals. Specifically, asthma-related knowledge improved significantly, exposure to asthma triggers in the home decreased (most notably, exposure to secondhand cigarette smoke), medication use improved, and there was a notable increase in the obtainment of AAPs.

The PAI-2 project was also associated with substantial cost savings. In fact, the intervention was associated with an estimated $2,561.60 saved per participant per year. This translates to $5.58 saved per dollar spent on the intervention.

Lessons Learned and Challenges   Several important lessons were learned through the process of this pilot intervention. First, having a CHW from the target community who shares a cultural connection with participants is vital in establishing the relationship of trust needed to ensure the acceptability of the intervention and its success. Second, when hiring a CHW, one should look for an individual who possesses a true passion for giving back to the community, is willing to take initiative and go the extra mile in ensuring that families have the information and resources they need, and is able to think critically and problem-solve. It is important to devote time upfront in properly training CHWs and to also make a commitment to ongoing continuing education. Third, home visits help ensure that the most vulnerable of families, and therefore those most in need of intervention, are reached. Fourth, many children have multiple caregivers, and the intervention will be most effective when as many of the people as possible who are involved in the child's daily care are educated.

The project experienced certain challenges worth mentioning. One substantial challenge involved the transient nature of the target population and the instability of their lives. Many of the caregivers who participated lived with another family member or friend and, therefore, did not have total control over the environment in which they lived. Many families were seeing multiple physicians (i.e., seeing whichever physician was convenient at the time), and as a result most children did not have an established relationship with one doctor who was managing their asthma. Finally, the level of cigarette smoke exposure to which participating children were subjected on a daily basis was extraordinarily high, with 31% of caregivers reporting their child was exposed to cigarette smoke at least once a day and 54% of children living with a smoker. Evaluation findings suggested that cigarette smoke exposure significantly decreased between baseline and the 12-month follow-up, with 17% of caregivers reporting their child was exposed to cigarette smoke at least once daily ($p < 0.0001$) and 46% of children living with a smoker ($p = 0.0215$). It is difficult to conclude whether these were true changes or were the results of social desirability bias.

Conclusion   The findings suggest that individualized, one-on-one asthma education provided by a trained, culturally competent CHW in the home environment is an effective means of improving asthma management among inner-city Black children with poorly controlled asthma. The pilot study provided evidence of improved asthma outcomes, quality of life and asthma-related knowledge, and decreased exposure to triggers among families participating in the intervention. Given the degree of improvement in urgent health resource utilization combined with the relative low cost of the intervention, the PAI-2 model is also cost-effective. Nonetheless, further studies are needed to affirm the results and assess whether the model can be translated to other high-risk populations.

Controlling Pediatric Asthma Through Collaboration and Education (CPATCE): a Statewide Initiative

Introduction   The promising results of PAI-2 led the IDPH[2] to incorporate the PAI-2 Community Health Educator model as a key component of a larger state-wide initiative, *Controlling Pediatric Asthma through Collaboration and Education (CPATCE)*. CPATCE sought to improve asthma management among high-risk children in Illinois, thereby reducing asthma-related health-care expenditure and asthma-related morbidity and mortality. The CPATCE initiative was launched in the spring of 2006. SUHI and SCH were funded to serve as the coordinating, training, and evaluation entity for the initiative.

CPATCE expanded the PAI-2 CHW model to six additional areas targeted by IDPH because of disproportionately high asthma hospitalization rates (above the State average). Each target area also had an established asthma consortium within it that was funded to implement the Sinai CHW model in that area. The six areas selected to participate are diverse in terms of urbanicity, race/ethnicity, and socio-economic status. Table 11-4 shows the program delivery areas and their corresponding asthma consortia.

Methods   SUHI and SCH undertook three specific activities as part of this expansion. First, the PAI-2 CHW model was expanded locally to continue addressing the unique needs of disadvantaged, minority children with asthma

TABLE 11-4   Controlling Pediatric Asthma through Collaboration and Education Site Areas and Asthma Consortia

Site Name	City/County	Area Type
Sinai Urban Health Institute & Sinai Children's Hospital	Chicago, Cook Co., IL	Metropolitan
Chicago Asthma Consortium/Respiratory Health Association	Chicago, Cook Co., IL	Metropolitan
Decatur Area Asthma Collation	Decatur, Macon Co., IL	Small Metropolitan
Bureau/Putnam Asthma Team	Bureau Co., Putnam Co., IL	Rural
Rockford Asthma Coalition	Rockford, Winnebago Co., IL	Small Metropolitan
Northwestern Asthma Consortium	Knox Co., Henry Co., Stark Co., IL	Rural
Washington County	Washington Co., IL	Rural

living in Chicago. The expansion resulted in the program being offered to all children with poorly controlled asthma living in targeted neighborhoods as opposed to only Black children (as in PAI-2). More CHWs were hired, including a CHW fluent in Spanish. Also, SUHI/SCH worked closely with another CPATCE-funded Chicago site, the Chicago Asthma Consortium/ Respiratory Health Association of Metropolitan Chicago (CAC), to more completely cover the "hotspots" of asthma in Chicago. Second, SUHI/SCH established the Sinai Asthma Education Training Institute (SAETI) to coordinate the training of CHWs at the six new sites, and the implementation of the Sinai CHW model on a wider scale. An asthma training curriculum was developed and adapted to meet the needs of the different sites. The intervention process was standardized, and a formal education guide was assembled. This education guide was to be used by CHWs in conducting their home visits. Third, SUHI served as the primary evaluator of the initiative's success for each participating site. Results were carefully monitored at all sites to ensure that the program met its goals, efforts were effective, and findings would guide future work.

CPATCE utilized CHWs from the communities targeted by the intervention to deliver case-specific asthma education in the home environment. Once identified, the CHWs participated in an 18-hour train-the-trainer asthma workshop hosted by SAETI. Each site then began recruiting for their respective program. Recruitment sources utilized by different sites included EDs, inpatient units, physician referrals, Women Infant and Children (WIC) programs, daycares, pharmacies, and schools, among others. Eligible children were between the ages of 2 and 16 years, had a prior diagnosis of asthma, and had severe, uncontrolled asthma as defined by NHLBI guidelines (NHLBI, 2002).

The CHWs met with families three times over a 6-month period. The education was tailored to the family's unique needs and was provided in the family's home whenever possible. Each session lasted between 60 and 90 minutes. Although the primary caregiver was the main focus of the education, the asthmatic child was also included in an age-appropriate manner whenever possible. Other caregivers of the child were also frequently present and included in the educational session. The CHW also served as a liaison between the family and the medical system, encouraging caregivers to see their child's primary care physician (PCP) regularly, providing referrals to those without a PCP, and working with PCPs in the development and teaching of an AAP.

The project's goals were evaluated using a pre–post test methodology with each child serving as his/her own historical control. Data collection timepoints and methodology differ slightly between SUHI/SCH and the other sites. At SUHI/SCH, data was collected at baseline, every month following, and at the two subsequent home visits. At each of the other sites, data was collected at baseline, the 2-month home visit, via phone at 4 months post-enrollment, and at the 6-month home visit. SUHI/SCH also collected data for 1 year following the baseline visit; however, for the sake of clarity, this chapter presents data through 6 months of follow-up for all sites.

Because CPATCE's goals were similar to its predecessor, PAI-2, the outcomes assessed were the same, including asthma symptom severity, asthma-related emergency health resource utilization, caregiver quality of life, asthma-related knowledge of the caregiver, and the belief (self-efficacy) of the caregiver that he/she is able to manage the child's asthma. Because of advances in scale development, a new self-efficacy tool was used in the CPATCE study (Bursch et al., 1999).

Results   Five of the six new sites implemented the intervention to some degree. One of the asthma coalition was unable to successfully implement the CHW model in their small rural community. Washington County is a rural county and had the smallest population of all selected target areas (15,124 per 2005 Census estimates), with are only about 3,800 children in the entire county. The local health department is small and was already overcommitted. It also proved difficult to establish buy-in for the program from both local professionals and community members. In fact, all of the rural counties struggled to implement the intervention to the full degree. This is discussed further in the "Lessons Learned and Challenges" Section below.

Four hundred fifty-five children were enrolled into CPATCE statewide between October 2006 and June 2008, of which 326 (72%) completed the entire 6-month intervention and data collection follow-up. Two hundred thirty-six of the enrolled children were from Sinai, whereas 98 were from CAC. These two sites combined created a larger Chicago sample ($n = 334$). Table 11-5 presents the demographic characteristics of study participants from the three sites with large enough sample sizes to protect personal information and annonymity. Table 11-2 provides the demographic characteristics of the combined Chicago sample. Two hundred and thirty-four (70%) of Chicago participants completed the entire 6-month intervention phase.

The findings described herein are for the pooled Chicago sample of Sinai and CAC participants, a sample representing many of the asthma "hotspots" in the city. The Decatur Area Asthma Coalition had similar findings to those of the Chicago sites, but these are not presented in this chapter. The remaining three sites did not have a large enough enrollment to analyze data through 6 months.

Findings indicate that Chicago-area CPATCE participants improved significantly with regard to urgent health resource utilization between the year

TABLE 11-5   CPATCE Participant Demographics and Baseline Characteristics by Site

	CAC[a] (n = 98)	Decatur (n = 84)	Sinai (n = 236)
Race/Ethnicity			
non-Hispanic Black	90%	65%	49%
Hispanic Black	4%	0%	8%
Hispanic	3%	0%	41%
non-Hispanic White	0%	20%	0%
Mixed race/ethnicity	3%	15%	2%
Age (mean)	8 years	7 years	7 years
Gender—% male	44%	55%	59%
Insurance			
Medicaid/All Kids[b]	64%	97%	79%
Education of Caregiver			
High School Grad. or less	39%	67%	60%
Nighttime Symptoms in the past 2-weeks at baseline (mean)	3.4	3.7	3.6
Emergency Department Visits in the year prior to baseline (mean)	2.2	2.1	2.5
Sum Urgent Health Resource Utilization[c] in the year prior to baseline (mean)	4.4	5.7	5.7

Notes: [a]*Chicago Asthma Consortium.*
[b]All Kids is a state run health insurance program available to all children in the state of Illinois.
[c]Sum of urgent health resource utilization variables (hospitalizations, ED visits, and urgent clinic visits).

prior to and the year following the intervention (Table 11-3). For example, Chicago participants experienced a 50% decrease in ED visits and a 61% decrease in hospitalizations. On average, participants also experienced statistically and clinically significant increases in quality of life and asthma knowledge and significant reductions in the presence of asthma triggers. One key component of the model is to improve the relationship between the client and a primary care provider. It is therefore interesting to note that the data show a significant increase in regular asthma clinic visits. These increases lend power to the notion that the Sinai CHW model bridges the gap between the patient and the primary care provider.

Lessons Learned and Challenges   A large state-wide initiative of this nature provides a wealth of information on successes and challenges. Several key lessons were learned through the process of implementing and evaluating CPATCE. First, a coordinating site is vital to the success of a multisite project such as this. SUHI's role as the coordinating, training, and evaluation site for the project was crucial to the successful roll out of the project. Second, sufficient time and resources need to be allocated specifically to establishing relationships within the community, publicizing the program, securing buy-in, and identifying viable recruitment sources. When adequate time and resources are not allocated to these activities, recruitment and retention suffer. It is also virtually impossible to successfully implement a community-based intervention without support and buy-in from community leaders. To ensure success, the entire community must be saturated with information about the program, and activities must coordinate with existing programs and services. The most important method to improving retention is for the CHW to simply establish a good relationship with the family and to gain the family's trust.

Although the intervention was a great success in three of the seven sites, the more rural communities faced some problems in implementing the model that are worth noting. Specifically, the implementation of the CHW model within rural Illinois communities proved to be particularly challenging. Although CHW models have been utilized effectively in other rural communities both in the United States and other countries, it does not seem that Illinois rural communities are ready to embrace this approach. Given a CHW model may be ideal in supplementing coverage within medically underserved rural communities, hopefully this mindset will change over time. However, considerable resources would need to be devoted to overcoming barriers and establishing support for a CHW model in rural Illinois communities.

Conclusions   The results of CPATCE show that the SUHI CHW model translates well to other urban and metropolitan environments. Although this particular project had difficulty in rural communities, there is no reason to believe that CHW models cannot and do not work in rural environments. CHW models have been used extensively in both rural and urban communities (Butz et al., 1994; Kelly et al. 2002; Kinney et al., 2002; Krieger et al., 2004; Morgan et al., 2004; Butz et al., 2005; Krieger et al., 2005; Martin et al., 2006). Unfortunately, CHW interventions are not often vigorously evaluated. It is vital that more resources be devoted to both the implementation and evaluation of CHW models in both rural and urban environments so that findings can impact policy, resulting in sustainable programs. Despite the fact that only three of the six sites were able to implement the model with enough participants to allow for evaluation, the consistency of findings between PAI-2 and CPATCE sites strongly suggest that culturally appropriate CHWs are an effective means of improving asthma management in urban and smaller metropolitan areas.

Healthy Home, Healthy Child: The Westside Children's
Asthma Partnership (HHHC)

Background   Nine years of experience by SUHI/SCH aimed at improving asthma management among children living in disadvantaged communities has led to two important conclusions: *(1)* CHWs are effective in establishing relationships of trust with the families they serve and consequently are in a position to comprehensively address the barriers families face in properly managing a child's asthma; and *(2)* the social and economic issues that impede a family's ability to manage asthma are complex and often require expertise that goes beyond that of a medical professional or CHW. Therefore, in September 2008, with funding from the CDC[3], SUHI/SCH initiated its most comprehensive initiative to date: *Healthy Home, Healthy Child: The Westside Children's Asthma Partnership (HHHC).*

HHHC aims to translate the Seattle-King County Healthy Homes (SKCHH) Phase I (Krieger et al., 2004; Krieger et al., 2005) environmental intervention model into one that is culturally appropriate and effective for children with poorly controlled asthma living on Chicago's Westside. The SKCHH project (Phase I) sought to reduce asthma-related morbidity by reducing exposure to indoor asthma triggers among low-income children with asthma living in urban households. The approach utilized CHWs who were trained to serve as Community Home Environmental Specialists. A total of 274 low-income households with a child 4 to 12 years who had persistent asthma were enrolled and randomized into either a high- or low-intensity intervention. The high-intensity group received seven home visits over the course of a year. The home visits entailed structured home environmental assessments, preparation and teaching of an AAP, social support, and a full set of resources to reduce exposures (e.g., allergy-control pillow and mattress encasements, smoking cessation counseling, etc.). Those in the low-intensity group received a single CHW visit and some supplemental materials. Evaluation findings suggested that those in the high-intensity group improved to a significantly greater degree with regard to caregiver quality of life, urgent health resource utilization, and actions to reduce dust in the home. The methods and findings of the SKCHH have been published (Krieger et al., 2004; Krieger et al., 2005). Two other significant initiatives have included components of the SKCHH approach within an intervention utilizing CHWs making home visits and have also yielded significant improvements in outcomes (Spielman et al., 2006; Parker et al., 2008).

Although the SKCHH project has demonstrated considerable success in the Seattle-King County Community among diverse minority, lower-income populations, the communities on Chicago's Westside offer a different climate in which to implement the intervention, evaluate its effectiveness, and document the process and feasibility of translating the model to other populations. HHHC is utilizing a collaborative approach drawing on the strengths of several partners and incorporating full and meaningful participation by the community.

Intervention   The HHHC intervention works with children between the ages of 2 and 14 years with poorly controlled asthma as well as their caregivers. Children must live in one of Chicago's Westside, predominantly Black communities to participate in the program. HHHC seeks to empower families to make the changes necessary to improve their child's asthma management and, thereby, the family's quality of life. The Sinai CHW home visit model remains at the heart of the approach. The home visits focus on both improving asthma management by educating caregivers and children to better manage asthma medically while also addressing the disproportionate presence of asthma triggers in the home environment. CHWs work with families to set achievable goals that will move them toward optimal health. Figure 11-5 presents the intervention model in more detail.

Partners in this endeavor include the Chicago Asthma Consortium (CAC), Health & Disability Advocates (HDA), the Metropolitan Tenant's Organization

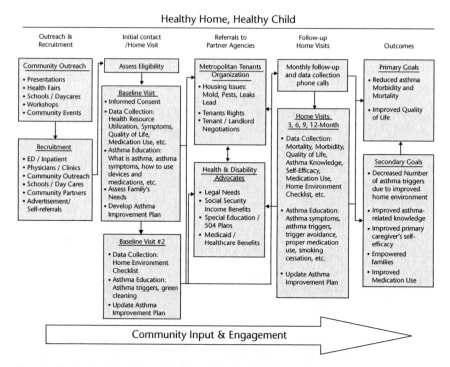

Figure 11-5   Healthy Home, Healthy Child Intervention Model

(MTO), and the Sinai Community Institute (SCI). The CAC, established in 1996, is a coalition of medical and public health professionals, business leaders, government agencies, community-based organizations, and individuals dedicated to improving the quality of life for people with asthma through networking, information sharing, and collaboration. HDA, a nonprofit legal and policy organization based in Chicago, Illinois, protects and promotes healthcare access, healthy housing, and income security for low-income populations, including children and their families, people with disabilities, and older adults. For more than 20 years, the MTO, a nonprofit organization, has educated, organized, and empowered tenants to have a voice in the decisions that affect the availability and affordability of safe and decent housing. MTO is the largest organizer of tenants in Chicago and serves more than 15,000 tenants annually. The SCI, located in North Lawndale, is committed to improving the overall health of Chicago residents by implementing a comprehensive array of health improvement and social service programs. All SCI programs address social, economic, and environmental factors that influence the health of residents of Chicago's Westside communities.

Each of these partners brings unique strengths to the project. MTO provides support in training CHWs to conduct a thorough environmental assessment and to work with families in modifying the home environment and behaviors to reduce exposure to asthma triggers. A MTO Housing Advocate handles environmental situations beyond the expertise of the CHW. Attorneys working for HDA provide *pro bono* assistance in resolving housing and other issues requiring legal intervention. A Community Advisory Board comprised of community leaders, representatives, and residents has been assembled by SCI and CAC to inform the project and its approach.

The program objective is to significantly impact asthma-related measures of morbidity, urgent health resource utilization, and quality of life. Therefore, progress is being monitored toward two primary goals (to decrease asthma-related morbidity and to improve quality of life) and three intermediate goals (to decrease the number of asthma triggers in the home environment, to improve asthma-related knowledge of the child's primary caregiver, and to improve the caregivers' confidence in their ability to properly manage asthma).

To introduce the HHHC program to the community, a launch event was held in the North Lawndale community on May 5, 2009. The HHHC Launch Event garnered much media attention. Several stories appeared on local television and radio stations, including WBBM-TV CBS 2 Chicago and WBEZ-Chicago Public Radio. A news article by Agnes Jasinski appeared in the *Chicago Tribune* on May 15, 2009, entitled, "Program makes asthma a little easier to live with: Health educators visit homes to help families eliminate asthma triggers." Figure 11-6 presents another article that appeared in the local communtiy newspaper, the *North Lawndale Community News.*

Enrollment began February 2009 and will continue for 17 months, ending on June 30, 2010. HHHC hopes to help 300 families living on Chicago's Westside to better manage their child's asthma by improving medical management while also reducing the presence of triggers in the home. By building on the strengths and expertise of several partners, HHHC is now poised to address many of the barriers that limit a family's ability to properly manage asthma and is therefore optimally positioned to make an impact on the lives of children with poorly controlled asthma living on Chicago's resource poor Westside.

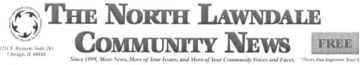

SINAI URBAN HEALTH INSTITUTE KICKS OFF FREE ASTHMA CARE IN NORTH LAWNDALE

"Healthy Home, Healthy Child" is a New Coalition Fighting Asthma in West Side Children
Krista Christophe

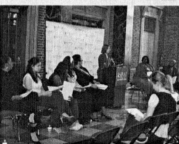

Mt. Sinai health administrators and asthma health advocates launch "Healthy Home, Healty Child program at Douglas Park Cultural Center.

On May 4, Sinai Urban Health Institute launched the asthma care program "Healthy Home, Healthy Child" which offers comprehensive care for 2-14 year olds with asthma in the North Lawndale area. The program's launch took place at the Douglas Park Cultural and Community Center. A number of community members, Mt. Sinai health administrators, and asthma health advocates spoke on the importance of asthma care for children in North Lawndale.

"Healthy Home Healthy Child" provides in-home visits to its participants. During these in-home visits community health educators help identify and eliminate the triggers of asthma in the home of program participants. They also review the use of the medications and equipment involved in asthma care to make sure that the asthmatic child in question is benefiting as much as possible from their prescribed treatment.

The program puts great emphasis on comprehensive care. Dr. Steve Whitman, Director of the Sinai Urban Health Institute stated, "When [Ida B. Wells] was asked what she wanted, she said, 'Well, everything, of course.' I just mentioned that because surely we want that for our children."

In addition to physical care, "Healthy Home, Healthy Child" addresses asthma triggers in the home. Mold, household pets, cockroaches and mice, cigarette smoke, and cleaning products are all household triggers. Sinai Urban Health Institute has partnered with the Metropolitan Tenants Organization and the Chicago Medical-Legal Partnership for Children to ensure that their participants live in an environment that is not hazardous to their health. Other participants include the Chicago Asthma Consortium (CAC) and Breathing Freedom, a community based smoking cessation program.

Asthma is a chronic disorder characterized by restriction, inflammation, and blockage in lungs' airways. Symptoms of an asthma attack include wheezing, shortness of breath, gasping, coughing, and pain or tightness in the chest. Asthma is life threatening and greatly effects the quality of life of those that live with the lung disease.

According to statistics from the Illinois Hospital Association, North Lawndale has one of the highest asthma rates in the city. Children in the neighborhood are 1.5 times more likely to be hospitalized with asthma problems than their peers in other parts of Chicago. If treated early, complications with asthma are better managed later in life. The "Healthy Home, Healthy Child" exists to fight asthma among juveniles in North Lawndale. It is funded by a $1.3 million/ three year grant from the U.S. Centers for Disease Control and Prevention.

Participants in the program
See Asthma - page 5

Figure 11-6   Article in the *North Lawndale Community News,* a local community newspaper, published following *Healthy Home, Healthy Child's* launch event

Source: Krista Christophe, "Sinai Urban Health Institute Kicks off Free Asthma Care in North Lawndale," *North Lawndale Community News*, May 14th–20th, 2009, Volume 11, Issue 20.

Conclusions: Implications and Next Steps

The United States has long recognized the presence of health disparities (U.S. Department of Health and Human Services, 1990; U.S. Department of Health and Human Services, 2000; Keppel, Pearcy, and Wagener, 2002; Agency for Healthcare Research and Quality, 2006; Keppel, 2007) and has even made a commitment to eliminating such disparities (U.S. Department of Health and Human Services, 2000). In Chicago's minority and poor neighborhoods, these disparities and the injustices they represent persist (Silva et al., 2001; Margellos, Silva, and Whitman, 2004; Orsi, Margellos-Anast, and Whitman, 2010). Asthma is one condition that disproportionately affects poor and minority children living in inner-city neighborhoods. Although the prevalence of pediatric asthma nationally increased by 4% per year between 1980 and 1996, it has since stabilized, with approximately 12% of U.S. children suffering from physician-diagnosed asthma (CDC, 2009a). Meanwhile, children in four of the six Chicago communities included in the Sinai Survey were twice as likely to have asthma as children nationally (CDC, 2009a) or in Chicago as a whole (Gupta, Carrión-Carire, and Weiss, 2006). Not only are they more likely to have asthma— they are also more likely to have asthma that is poorly controlled and to suffer needlessly from a condition that can be managed. These findings are consistent with other studies documenting disparities in prevalence and control of asthma by race/ethnicity and suggest that rates and effects are highest in disadvantaged, urban communities (Weiss and Wagener, 1990; Marder et al., 1992; Targonski et al., 1994; Thomas and Whitman, 1999; Simon et al., 2003; Nicholas et al., 2005; Akinbami, 2006; Gupta, Carrión-Carire, and Weiss, 2006; Lara et al., 2006; Quinn et al, 2006; Akinbami, 2007; Naureckas and Thomas, 2007; Shalowitz et al, 2007; Gupta et al., 2008). These survey findings support the need for local-level data by documenting that national- and city-level estimates often mask disparities on the local level. It is difficult to develop and appropriately target interventions and policies without specific information on the communities most in need of them.

Among the factors postulated as contributing to the disproportionate asthma burden experienced by inner-city, minority populations are genetics (Lester et al., 2001), environmental exposures (Infante-Rivard, 1993; Huss et al., 1994; Eggleston, 1998; Eggleston, 2000; Lanphear et al., 2001; Gruchalla et al., 2005; Eggleston, 2007), prenatal exposures (Di Franza, Aligne, and Weitzman, 2004), and access to and quality of care (Crain et al., 1998; Shields, Comstock, and Weiss, 2004; Greek et al., 2006). Although genetics may play a role in the increased burden of asthma experienced by certain populations, the evidence suggests a genetic predisposition combined with early environmental exposure as the pathway to asthma symptoms (Eggleston, 2000; Chan-Yeung et al., 2005). Children living in poor, inner-city neighborhoods often reside in substandard housing, resulting in increased exposure to asthma triggers and allergen sensitization (Gelber et al., 1993; Infante-Rivard, 1993; Willies-Jacobo et al., 1993; Sarpong et al., 1996; Eggleston, 2000; Ashley et al., 2006; Krieger, Takaro, and Rabkin, 2007). Furthermore, the detrimental effects of tobacco smoke on children who have asthma have been well-established (Chiomonczyk et al., 1993). The Sinai Survey data shed light on some of these potential contributing factors, allowing for a more appropriate response.

A recent Cochrane Review of 38 asthma interventions targeting 7,843 children who were enrolled into an educational intervention following a visit to an ED concluded that subsequent ED visits and hospitalizations were significantly reduced among intervention participants as compared to controls (Boyd et al., 2009). However, the studies examined varied widely with regard to the intensity of the intervention, the person providing the education (lay person, nurse, social worker, etc.), the location of the education, and the degree of focus on different aspects of asthma management. No definitive conclusions could be drawn about the specific characteristics of a successful program. This is hardly surprising given that the review included studies conducted in several different countries and in a wide array of communities. What might be appropriate and effective in one community cannot necessarily be translated to another, and local level data pertaining to both the presence of health conditions and their contributing factors are vital to ensuring the most appropriate approach is utilized.

In recent years, the use of CHW (a.k.a. community health educators, lay health educator, peer educator, *promotoral de salud,* etc.) to improve access to health-care services, health knowledge, health outcomes, and health behaviors has become a frequently utilized model among underserved populations. Employing community members as CHWs is a novel way to ensure that the approach is culturally appropriate while also helping to empower disadvantaged communities by building them up from within. As documented above, SUHI has implemented and evaluated a series of pediatric asthma interventions utilizing CHWs and has found the model to be effective and well-accepted by urban communities.

Asthma expenditures were estimated at $14.7 billion in 2007 in the United States (National Institutes of Health, NHBLI, 2007). Although this amount includes costs for care provided in hospitals, ED, physician services, and medications, the greatest portion is associated with urgent health resource utilization that could be avoided if asthma were properly controlled. The CHW model has been demonstrated to effectively improve asthma management and decrease urgent health resource utilization among children with poorly controlled asthma living in urban communities. Given the potential cost savings associated with implementing the model, it should be reimbursed via Medicaid and other insurers, allowing for wider implementation and sustainability.

CHWs have the potential of reducing health-care costs while also making a greater positive impact on the communities in which they live and serve. Furthermore, they empower communities to take control of their own health and inspire a sense of community by building the community from within. Ultimately, CHW programs encourage children with asthma to live healthy and productive lives so that they may grow to be productive and active members of their community and society overall.

One novel aspect of the Sinai Survey is that community members were included in each and every phase of the process, beginning with the selection of survey topics and questions and continuing to the interpretation of findings and the inception of approaches to improve community health based on the findings (Shah and Whitman, 2010). Although SUHI's pediatric asthma work initially began prior to the survey being completed, it has been greatly strengthened over the years as it has continued to evolve into a true partnership with the community.

Unfortunately, health disparities continue to persist in the United States, with certain communities experiencing a disproportionate and unjust prevalence of disease and poor health. Within these communities live real people and children who may be suffering simply because of where they live or the material resources that they have (or don't have). As demonstrated in this chapter, asthma is a condition that exerts an excessive burden on children living in certain communities. Although we do not know how to prevent children from acquiring asthma, we do know how to help them control their disease so that they can live full and productive lives. Findings from the Sinai Survey and the ensuing attention to pediatric asthma, along with the development of culturally appropriate interventions, have made the promise of improved health a reality for children with asthma living in burdened communities in Chicago and Illinois. It is the hope and expectation of the SUHI that the Sinai Model of identifying a health disparity and working with communities to best address it will result in the development of successful interventions (such as the ones described in this chapter), proliferating to other communities across the United States.

Acknowledgments

This work could not have been done without the dedication and time of staff members of the Sinai Urban Health Institute and Sinai Children's Hospital, especially Gloria Seals, who has been instrumental in Sinai's asthma work from the very beginning. Dr. Steve Whitman, Director, Sinai Urban Health Institute, and Dr. Dennis Vickers, Chairman, Sinai Department of Pediatrics, have provided invaluable, continual support and guidance to the projects described herein. Generous funding for the interventions was provided by The Michael Reese Health Trust, The Illinois Department of Public Health, and The Centers for Disease Control and Prevention. The support of partner agencies (who are named above) has been crucial in making each of these interventions a success especially that of the Chicago Asthma Consortium, the Respiratory Health Association of Metropolitan Chicago and the Sinai Community Institute. Finally, we would like to thank all participating families whose invaluable feedback helped shape and inform our interventions, enabling us to better serve the community.

Notes

1. Controller medications (also called preventive or maintenance medications) are generally taken once or twice a day every day (as prescribed) to control and prevent asthma symptoms. Most work by reducing inflammation and sensitivity inside the airways. Controller medications do not work quickly and do not provide immediate relief of asthma symptoms. Controller medications come in a variety of formats, but inhaled steroids are the most common type. Other types include: Leukotrien modifiers, long-acting beta agonists, and immunomodulators. Quick Relief medications (also called reliever medications, rescue medications, short-term medication, and bronchodilators) act quickly to relief asthma symptoms that have already started. These medications work to expand and relax the bronchial airways. They usually work within minutes to provide immediate relief of asthma symptoms such as coughing, chest tightness, shortness of breath and wheezing.
2. This research was supported in part by grants from the Illinois Department of Public Health (Grant Numbers 001-48230-440-0105 & 733-48230-4900-0000). The views expressed are those of the authors and do not necessarily represent the views of the funding agencies.
3. This research was supported in part by grants from the Centers for Disease Control and Prevention (Grant Number 5R18EH000355-02). The views expressed are those of the authors and do not necessarily represent the views of the funding agencies.

References

Agency for Healthcare Research and Quality. 2006 National healthcare disparities report. Rockville, MD: U.S. Department of Health and Human Services, Agency for Healthcare Research and Quality; December 2006. AHRQ Pub. No. 07-0012.

Akinbami, Lara J. 2006. The state of childhood asthma, United States, 1980–2005. Advanced Data from vital and health statistics; no 381, Hyattsville, MD: National Center for Health Statistics.

Akinbami, Lara J. 2007. Asthma prevalence, health care use and mortality: United States, 2003–05. National Center for Health Statistics.

Andrews, Jeanette O., Gwen Felton, Mary Ellen Wewers, and Janie Heath. 2004. Use of community health workers in research with ethnic minority women. *Journal of Nursing Scholarship* 36(4):358–365.

Ashley, Peter, John R. Menkedick, Maureen A. Wooton, Jennifer A. Zewatsky, Steve Weitz, Joanna Gaitens, et al. 2006. Healthy Homes Issue: Asthma. U.S. Department of Housing and Urban Development. Version 3.

Boyd, Michelle, Toby J. Lasserson, Michael C. McKean, Peter G. Gibson, Francine M. Ducharme, and Michelle Haby. 2009. Interventions for educating children who are at risk of asthma-related emergency department attendance. *Cochrane Database of Systematic Reviews,* Issue 2. Art. No.: CD001290. DOI: 10.1002/14651858.CD001290.pub2.

Brownstein, J. Nell, Lee R. Bone, Cheryl R. Dennison, Martha Hill, Myong T. Kim, and David Levine. 2005. Community health workers as interventionists in the prevention and control of heart disease and stroke. *American Journal of Preventive Medicine* 29(5 Suppl 1):128–133.

Bursch, Brenda, Lenore Schwankovsky, Jean Gilbert, and Robert Zeiger. 1999. Construction and validation of four childhood asthma self-management scales: Parent barriers, child and parent self-efficacy, and parent belief in treatment efficacy. *Journal of Asthma* 36(1):115–128.

Butz, Aelene, Luu Pham, LaPricia Lewis, Cassis Lewis, Kim Hill, Jennifer Walker, and Marilyn Winkelstein. 2005. Rural children with Asthma: impact of a parent and child asthma education program. *Journal of Asthma* 42:813–821.

Butz, Arlene M., Floyd J. Malveaux, Peyton Eggleston, Lera Thompson, Susan Schneider, Kathy Weeks, et al. 1994. Use of community health workers with inner-city children who have asthma. *Clinical Pediatrics* 33:135–141.

Carr, Willine, Lisa Zeitel, and Kevin Weiss. 1992. Variations in asthma hospitalizations and deaths in New York City. *American Journal of Public Health* 82:59–65.

Centers for Disease Control and Prevention. 2009a. *Lifetime asthma prevalence percents by age, United States: National Health Interview Survey, 2006.* Online. April 27, 2009. Available: http://www.cdc.gov/asthma/nhis/06/table2-1.htm. Accessed December 18, 2009.

Centers for Disease Control and Prevention. 2009b. *Table 2-1, Lifetime asthma prevalence percents by age, United States: National Health Interview Survey, 2004.* Online. April 27, 2009. Available: http://www.cdc.gov/ASTHMA/nhis/04/table2-1. htm. Accessed December 18, 2009.

Chan-Yeung, M., A. Ferguson, W. Watson, H. Dimich-Ward, R. Rousseau, M. Lilley, et al. 2005. The Canadian childhood asthma primary prevention study: Outcomes at 7 years of age. *Journal of Allergy and Clinical Immunology* 116:49–55.

Chicago Fact Book Consortium. 1995. *Local Community Fact Book: Chicago Metropolitan Area, 1990.* Chicago, IL: Academy Chicago Publishers.

Chiomonczyk, Barbara A., Luis M. Salmun, Keith N. Metathlin, Louis M. Neveux, Glenn E. Palomaki, George J. Knight, et al. 1993. Associations between exposure to environmental tobacco smoke and exacerbations of asthma in children. *The New England Journal of Medicine* 328:1665–1669.

Crain, Ellen F., Carolyn Kercsmar, Kevin B. Weiss, Herman Mitchell and Henry Lynn. 1998. Reported difficulties in access to quality care for children with asthma in the inner city. *Archives of Pediatrics and Adolescent Medicine* 152(4):333–339.

Di Franza, Joseph R., C. Andrew Aligne, and Michael Weitzman. 2004. Prenatal and postnatal environmental tobacco smoke exposure and children's health. *Pediatrics.* 113(4):1007–1015.

Eggleston, Peyton A. 1998. Urban children and asthma: Morbidity and mortality. *Immunology and Allergy Clinics of North America* 18:75–84.

Eggleston, Peyton A. 2000. Environmental causes of asthma in inner city children. The National Cooperative Inner City Asthma Study. *Clinical Reviews in Allergy and Immunology* 18:311–324.

Eggleston, Peyton A. 2007. The environment and asthma in U.S. inner cities. *Chest* 132(5 suppl.):782S–788S.

Evans, R. III, P. J. Gergen, H. Mitchell, M. Kattan, C. Kercsmar, E. Crain, et al. 1999. A randomized clinical trial to reduce asthma morbidity among inner-city children: Results of the National Cooperative Inner-City Asthma Study. *Journal of Pediatrics* 135:332–338.

Finkelstein, Jonathon A., Randall W. Brown, Lynda C. Schneider, Jose M. Quintana, Donald A. Goldmann, and Charles J. Homer. 1995. Quality of care for preschool children with asthma: The role of social factors and practice setting. *Pediatrics* 95:389–394.

Garret, J., J. M. Fenwick, G. Taylor, E. Mitchell, J. Stewart, and H. Rea. 1994. Prospective controlled evaluation of the effect of a community based asthma education center in a multiracial working class neighborhood. *Thorax* 49:976–983.

Gelber, Lawrence E., L. H. Seltzer, James K. Bouzoukis, Susan M. Pollart, Martin D. Chapman, and Thomas A. Platts-Mills. 1993. Sensitization and exposure to indoor allergens as risk factors for asthma among patients presenting to hospital. *American Review of Respiratory Disease* 147(3):573–578.

Greek, April A., Gail M. Kieckhefer, Hyoshin Kim, Jutta M. Joesch, and Nazil Baydar. 2006. Family perception of the usual source of care among children by race/ethnicity, language, and family income. *Journal of Asthma* 43:61–69.

Greineder, Dirk K. Kathleen C. Loane, and Paula Parks. 1995. Reduction in resource utilization by an asthma outreach program. *Archives of Pediatric Adolescent Medicine* 149:415–420.

Greineder, Dirk K., Kathleen C. Loane, and Paula Parks. 1999. A randomized controlled trial of a pediatric outreach program. *Journal of Allergy and Clinical Immunology* 103:436–440.

Gruchalla, Rebecca, Jacqueline Pongracic, Marshall Plaut, Richard Evans III, Cynthia M. Visness, Michelle Walter, et al. 2005. Inner city asthma study: Relationship among sensitivity, allergen exposure, and asthma morbidity. *Journal of Allergy and Clinical Immunology* 115:478–485.

Gupta, Ruchi S., Violeta Carrión-Carire, and Kevin Weiss. 2006. The widening black/white gap in asthma hospitalizations and mortality. *Journal of Allergy and Clinical Immunology* 117:351–358.

Gupta, Ruchi S., Xingyou Zhang, Lisa K. Sharp, John J. Shannon, and Kevin B. Weiss. 2008. Geographic variability in childhood asthma prevalence in Chicago. *Journal of Allergy and Clinical Immunology* 121(3):639–645.

Halfon, Neal and Paul W. Newacheck. 1993. Childhood asthma and poverty: Differential impacts and utilization of health services. *Pediatrics* 91:56–61.

Hughes, Daniel M., Marjorie McLeod, Barry Garner, and Richard Goldbloom. 1991. Controlled trial of a home and ambulatory program for asthmatic children. *Pediatrics* 87:54–61.

Huss, Karen, Cynthia. S. Rand, Arlene M. Butz, Peyton A. Eggleston, Charles Murigande, Lera C. Thompson, et al. 1994. Home environmental risk factors in urban minority asthmatic children. *Annals of Allergy* 72:173–177.

Infante-Rivard, Claire. 1993. Childhood asthma and indoor environmental risk factors. *American Journal of Epidemiology* 137:834–844.

Juniper, Elizabeth F., Gordon H. Guyatt, David H. Feeny, Penelope J. Ferrie, Lauren E. Griffith, and Marie Townsend. 1996. Measuring quality of life in parents of children with asthma. *Quality of Life Research* 5:27–34.

Juniper, Elizabeth J., Gordon H. Guyatt, Andrew Willan, and Lauren E. Griffith. 1994. Determining a minimal important change in a disease-specific Quality of Life Questionnaire. *Journal of Clinical Epidemiology* 47:81–87.

Karnick, Paula, Helen Margellos-Anast, Gloria Seals, Steve Whitman, Gabriel Aljadeff, and Daniel Johnson. 2007. The Pediatric Asthma Intervention: A comprehensive cost-effective approach to asthma management in a disadvantaged inner-city community. *Journal of Asthma* 44:39–44.

Kelly, Cynthia Szelc, Ardythe L. Morrow, Justine Shults, Nermina Nakas, Gerald L. Strope, and Raymond D. Adelman. 2002. Outcomes evaluation of a comprehensive intervention program for asthmatic children enrolled in Medicaid. *Pediatrics* 105:1029–1035.

Keppel, Kenneth G. 2007. Ten largest racial and ethnic health disparities in the United States based on Healthy People 2010 Objectives. *American Journal of Epidemiology* 166(1):97–103.

Keppel, Kenneth G., Jeffrey N. Pearcy, and Diane K. Wagener. 2002. Trends in racial and ethnic-specific rates for Health Status Indicators: United States, 1990-1998. In: *Healthy People Statistical Notes* No: 23. Hyattsville, MD: National Center for Health Statistics.

Kinney, Patrick L., Mary E. Northridge, Ginger L. Chew, Erik Gronning, Evelyn Joseph, Juan C. Correa, et al. 2002. On the front lines: An environmental asthma intervention in New York City. *American Journal of Public Health* 92:24–26.

Krieger, James W., Tim K. Takaro, Carol Allen, Lin Song, Marcia Weaver, Sanders Chai, and Philip Dickey. 2002. The Seattle-King County Healthy Homes Project: Implementation of a comprehensive approach to improving indoor environmental quality for low-income children with asthma. *Environmental Health Perspectives* 110(Suppl 2):311–322.

Krieger, James W., Tim K. Takaro, and Janice C. Rabkin. 2007. Breathe easy in Seattle: Addressing asthma disparities through healthier housing. In: *Eliminating Healthcare Disparities in America*, ed. Richard A. Williams. Totowa, NJ: Humana Press, pp. 313–339.

Krieger, James W., Tim K. Takaro, Lin Song, and Marcia Weaver. 2005. The Seattle-King County Healthy Homes Project: A randomized, control trial of a community health workers intervenient to decrease exposure to indoor asthma triggers. *American Journal of Public Health* 95:652–659.

Lanphear, Bruce P., C. Andrew Aligne, Peggy Auinger, Michael Weitzman, and Robert S. Byrd. 2001. Residential exposures associated with asthma in US children. *Pediatrics* 107(3):505–511.

Lara, Marielena, Lara Akinbami, Glenn Flores, and Hal Morgenstern. 2006. Heterogeneity of childhood asthma among Hispanic children: Puerto Rican children bear a disproportionate burden. *Pediatrics* 117:43–53.

Lara, Marielena, Sara Rosenbaum, Gary Rachelefsky, Will Nicholas, Sally C. Morton, Seth Emont, et al. 2002. Improving childhood asthma outcomes in the United States: A blueprint for policy action. *Pediatrics* 109:919–930.

Lester, Lucille A., Stephen S. Rich, Malcolm N. Blumenthal, Alkis Togias, Shirley Murphy, Floyd Malveaux, et al. 2001. Ethnic difference in asthma and associated phenotypes: Collaborative study on the genetics of asthma. *Journal Allergy and Clinical Immunology* 108:357–362.

Lewin, Simon, Judy Dick, Philip Pond, Merrick Zwarenstein, Godwin N. Aja, Brian E. VanWyk, et al. 2005. Lay health workers in primary and community health care. *Cochrane Database of Systematic Reviews* (1):CD004015.

Mannino David M., David M. Homa, Lara J. Akinbami, Jeanne E. Moorman, Charon Gwynn, and Stephen C. Reed. 2002. Surveillance for asthma—United States, 1980–1999. *Morbidity and Mortality Weekly Report* 51(SS01):1–13.

Marder, David, Paul Targonski, Peter Orris, and Whitney Addington. 1992. Effect of racial and socioeconomic factors on asthma mortality in Chicago. *Chest* 101(Suppl 1):426S–429S.

Margellos Helen, Abigail Silva, and Steve Whitman. 2004. Comparison of health status indicators in Chicago: Are Black-White disparities worsening? *American Journal of Public Health* 94(1):116–121.

Martin, Molly A., Olivia Hernandez, Edward Naureckas, and John Lantos. 2006. Reducing home triggers for asthma: The Latino community health worker approach. *Journal of Asthma* 43:369–374.

Moorman, Jeanne E., Rose Anne Rudd, Carol A. Johnson, Michael King, Patrick Minor, Cathy Bailey, et al. 2007. National surveillance for asthma—United States, 1980–2004. *Morbidity and Mortality Weekly Report Surveillance Summary* 56(8):1–54.

Morgan, Wayne J., Ellen F. Crain, Rebecca S. Gruchalla, George T. O'Connor, Meyer Kattan, Richard Evans, et al. 2004. Results of a home-based environmental intervention among urban children with asthma. *New England Journal of Medicine* 351:1068–1080.

National Heart, Lung, and Blood Institute, National Asthma Education and Prevention Program. 1997. Expert Panel Report 2: Bethesda, MD: US Dept. of Health and Human Services, National Institutes of Health, publication no. 97-4051.

National Heart, Lung, and Blood Institute, National Asthma Education and Prevention Program. 2002. Expert Panel Report 2: Bethesda, MD: US Dept. of Health and Human Services, National Institutes of Health, publication no. 02-5074.

National Institutes of Health, National Blood, Lung and Heart Institute. 2007. *Morbidity and Mortality: 2007 Chartbook on Cardiovascular, Lung and Heart Diseases.* June 2007. Online. Available: http://www.nhlbi.nih.gov/resources/docs/07-chtbk.pdf. Accessed December 18, 2009.

Naureckas, Edawrd T. and Sandra Thomas. 2007. Are we closing the disparities gap? Small-area analysis of asthma in Chicago. *Chest* 132(5 Suppl):858S–865S.

Nemcek, Mary Ann and Rosemary Sabatier. 2003. State of evaluation: community health workers. *Public Health Nursing* 20(4):260–270.

Nicholas, Stephen W., Betina Jean-Louis, Benjamin Ortiz, Mary Northridge, Katherine Shoemaker, Roger Vaughan, et al. 2005. Addressing the childhood asthma crisis in Harlem: The Harlem Children's Zone Asthma Initiative. *American Journal of Public Health* 95:245–249.

Norris, Susan L., Farah M. Chowdhury, K. Van Le, Tonya Horsley, J. Nell Brownstein, Zhang Xuanping, Leonard Jack Jr., and Dawn W. Satterfield. 2006. Effectiveness of community health workers in the care of persons with diabetes. *Diabetic Medicine* 23(5):544–556.

Parker, Edith A., Barbra A. Israel, Thomas G. Robins, Graciela Mentz, Xihong Lin, Wilma Brakefield-Caldwell, et al. 2008. Evaluation of community action against asthma: A community health worker intervention to improve children's asthma-related health by reducing household environmental triggers of asthma. *Health Education and Behavior* 35(3):376–395.

Persily, Cynthia Armstrong. 2003. Lay home visiting may improve pregnancy outcomes. *Holistic Nursing Practice* 17(5):231–238.

Orsi Jennifer M., Helen Margellos-Anast, and Steve Whitman. 2010. Black-White health disparities in the United States and Chicago: A 15-year progress analysis. *American Journal of Public Health* 100:349–356.

Quinn, Kelly, Madeleine U. Shalowitz, Carolyn A. Berry, Tod Mijanovich, and Raoul L. Wolf. 2006. Racial and ethnic disparities in diagnosed and possible undiagnosed asthma among public-school children in Chicago. *American Journal of Public Health* 96:1599–1603.

Rand, Cynthia S., Arlene M. Butz, Ken Kolodner, Karen Huss, Peyton Eggleston, and Floyd Malveaux. 2000. Emergency department visits by urban African America children with asthma. *Journal of Allergy and Clinical Immunology* 105:83–90.

Sarpong, Sampson B., Robert G. Hamilton, Peyton A. Eggleston, and N. Franklin Adkinson Jr. 1996. Socioeconomic status and race as risk factors for cockroach allergen exposure and sensitization in children with asthma. *Journal of Allergy and Clinical Immunology* 97(6):1393–1401.

SAS Institute Inc. 2002-2003. SAS statistical software, version 9.1.3 for Windows@. Cary, NC: SAS Institute.

Shah, Ami and Steve Whitman. 2010. Sinai's Improving Community Health Survey: Methodology and key findings. In *Urban Health: Combating Disparities with Local Data*, eds. Steven Whitman, Ami M. Shah, and Maureen R. Benjamins. New York: Oxford University Press.

Shalowitz, Madeleine U., Laura M. Sadowski, Rajesh Kumar, Kevin B. Weiss, and John J. Shannon. 2007. Asthma burden in a citywide, diverse sample of elementary school children in Chicago. *Ambulatory Pediatrics* 7:271–277.

Shields, Alexandra E., Catherine Comstock, and Kevin B. Weiss. 2004. Variations in asthma care by race/ethnicity among children enrolled in a state Medicaid program. *Pediatrics* 113:496–504.

Silva, Abigail, Steve Whitman, Helen Margellos, and David Ansell. 2001. Evaluation Chicago's success in reaching the Healthy People 2000 goal of reducing health disparities. *Public Health Reports* 116(5):484–494.

Simon, Paul A., Zhiwei Zeng, Cheryl M. Wold, William Haddock, and Jonathan E. Fielding. 2003. Prevalence of childhood asthma and associated morbidity in Los Angeles County: Impacts of race/ethnicity and income. *Journal of Asthma* 40:535–543.

Singh, Anita K., Prescott G. Woodruff, Ray H. Ritz, Diane Mitchell, and Carlos Camargo Jr. 1999. Inhaled corticosteroids for asthma: Are ED visits a missed opportunity for prevention? *American Journal of Emergency Medicine* 17:144–148.

Spielman, Seth E., Cynthia A. Golembeski, Mary E. Northridge, Roger D. Vaughan, Rachel Swaner, Betina Jean-Louis, et al. 2006. Interdisciplinary planning for healthier communities: Findings from the Harlem Children's Zone Asthma Initiative. *Journal of the American Planning Association* 72:100–108.

Stout, James W., Lisa C. White, LaTonya Rogers, Teresa McRorie, Barbara Morray, Marijo Miller-Ratcliffe, and Gregory J. Redding. 1998. The Asthma Outreach Project: A promising approach to comprehensive asthma management. *Journal of Asthma* 35:119–127.

Swider, Susan M. 2002. Outcome effectiveness of community health workers: An integrative literature review. *Public Health Nursing* 19(1):11–20.

Targonski, Paul V., Victoria.W. Persky, Peter Orris, and Whitney Addington. 1994. Trends in asthma mortality among African Americans and Whites in Chicago, 1968–1991. *American Journal of Public Health* 84:1830–1833.

Telleen, Sharon. 2000. Use of child health services by Latino families in Chicago. Final Report. Maternal and Child Health Bureau, HRSA Grant Number: MCJ 17080.

Thomas, Sandra D. and Steve Whitman. 1999. Asthma hospitalizations and mortality in Chicago: An epidemiologic overview. *Chest* 116(4S):135S–140S.

U.S. Department of Health and Human Services. 1990. Public Health Service. *Healthy People 2000: National Health Promotion and Disease Prevention Objectives.* DHHS Publication No. (PHS) 91-50212. Washington, DC: US Govt. Printing Office.

U.S. Department of Health and Human Services. 2000. Public Health Service. *Healthy People 2010: Understanding and Improving Health.* DHHS Publication No. 017-001-00543-6. Washington, DC: US Govt. Printing Office.

Weiss, Kevin B. Seasonal trends in US asthma hospitalizations and mortality. 1990. *Journal of the American Medical Association* 263:2323–2328.

Weiss Kevin B., Peter J. Gergen, and Diane K. Wagener. 1993. Breathing better or wheezing worse? The changing epidemiology of asthma morbidity and mortality. *Annual Review of Public Health* 14:491–513.

Weiss, Kevin B. and Diane K. Wagener. 1990. Changing patterns of asthma mortality: Identifying target populations at high risk. *Journal of the American Medical Association* 264:1683–1687.

West, Joseph and Charlene Gamboa. 2010. Working together to live tobacco free: Community-based smoking cessation in North Lawndale. In *Urban Health: Combating Disparities with Local Data*, eds. Steven Whitman, Ami M. Shah, and Maureen R. Benjamins. New York: Oxford University Press.

Whitman, Steve, Cynthia Williams, and Ami M. Shah. 2004. *Sinai's Community Health Survey: Report 1.* Chicago, IL: Sinai Health System.

Williams, Seymour G., Diana K. Schmidt, Stephen C. Redd, and William Storms. 2003. Centers for Disease Control and Prevention. Key clinical activities for quality asthma care: Recommendations of the National Asthma Education and Prevention Program. *Morbidity and Mortality Weekly Report* 52(RR06):1–8.

Willies-Jacobo, Lindia J., Joyce M. Denson-Lino, Angela Rosas, Richard D. O'Connor, and N. W. Wilson 1993. Socioeconomic status and allergy in children with asthma. *Journal of Allergy and Clinical Immunology* 92(4):630–632.

Wolf, Raoul L., Carolyn A. Berry, Trimina O'Connor, and Lenore Coover. 1996. Validation of the brief pediatric asthma screen. *Chest* 116(4 Suppl 1):224S–228S.

12

HUMBOLDT PARK: A COMMUNITY UNITED TO CHALLENGE ASTHMA

Molly Martin and Juana Ballesteros

Asthma Disparities in Puerto Rican Children Nationally and Locally: Defining the Problem

Puerto Rican children experience the highest asthma prevalence and morbidity rates of any racial/ethnic group (Centers for Disease Control and Prevention [CDC], 2002; CDC, 2004; Akinbami, Flores, and Morgenstern, 2006; Loyo-Berrios, Orengo, and Serrano-Rodriguez, 2006). Data from the National Health Interview Survey collected from 1997 to 2001 reported an overall prevalence rate of 26% in Puerto Rican children ages 2 to 17 years, compared to 16% in Black children, 13% in White children, and 10% in Mexican children (Akinbami, Flores, and Morgenstern, 2006). Asthma attack rates over the past 12 months showed a similar pattern: 12% for Puerto Rican children compared to 8% in Black children, 6% in White children, and 4% in Mexican children (Akinbami, Flores, and Morgenstern, 2006). Rates on the island of Puerto Rico appear to be even higher, with 46% of elementary school children reporting an asthma diagnosis and 32% reporting a wheezing attack requiring emergency room care (Loyo-Berrios, Orengo, and Serrano-Rodriguez, 2006).

The reasons for this disparity are not fully understood, although genetic and environmental factors play a role. Genetics determine individual asthma severity and atopy (Blumenthal and Blumenthall, 2002; Cookson, 2002). The genomic regions influencing asthma are slightly better understood for Blacks than for Latinos, but this remains an area of needed exploration for minority populations (Scirica and Celedón, 2007). Puerto Ricans and Mexicans are frequently combined into one group of "Hispanics"; however, their asthma prevalence rates vary dramatically, and differences have been shown in their responses to asthma medications (Stevenson et al., 2001) and in sensitivity to allergens (Celeón et al., 2004). This suggests differences in underlying genetics and severity between the two groups. Indoor environmental exposures, or "home asthma triggers," are related to asthma prevalence rates in Puerto Ricans (Celeón et al., 2004) and contribute to exacerbations (Huss et al., 1994; Freeman, Schneider, and McGarvey, 2003; Findley et al., 2004; Gruchalla et al., 2005). It is possible that an interaction of a genetic disposition with early life physical and social environmental exposures contributes as well (Lara et al., 1999). A recent study comparing clinical ratings of pediatric asthma severity in Island Puerto Ricans, Rhode Island Puerto Ricans, Rhode Island Dominicans, and Rhode Island Whites reported Island Puerto Rican children had significantly milder asthma than the other groups. However, Island Puerto Rican children had more emergency department visits than the other groups, which may be a function of health-care access on the island (Esteban et al., 2009).

Similar disparities have been documented in Chicago, which is home to one of the largest Puerto Rican populations in the mainland United States. Humboldt Park is the historic home of the Chicago Puerto Rican community. A rich and dynamic community with a long history of activism, Humboldt Park is racially and ethnically diverse, with Blacks, Mexicans, Puerto Ricans, and Whites living side-by-side. United States 2000 Census Data for Humboldt Park showed the population to be 48% Black (31,207) and 48% Latino (31,607), with 37% of Latinos claiming Puerto Rican heritage. When including the surrounding neighborhoods, the Puerto Rican population in 2000 was estimated at approximately 65,000. In addition, Humboldt Park is recognized for having some of the most robust community-based organizations anywhere in the city. There is an active communal life, and the community identity is reinforced by its own newspaper, its own radio station, and its own charter high school.

When selecting the community areas for the *Sinai's Improving Community Health Survey* (Sinai Survey), the diversity of Humboldt Park and its contiguous neighbor West Town were key factors in the decision to include these two community areas in the study. The details of the survey development are discussed in Chapter 3 (Shah and Whitman, 2010), and the specifics of the asthma portion are described in Chapter 11 (Margellos-Anast and Gutierrez, 2010). As shown in Figure 11-1 in Chapter 11 (Margellos-Anast and Gutierrez, 2010), the pediatric asthma prevalence rates were highest in Humboldt Park and West Town (17% and 28%, respectively). When broken down by ethnic groups (Fig. 11-2, Chapter 11, Margellos-Anast and Gutierrez, 2010), Puerto Rican children had the highest asthma prevalence rate of all

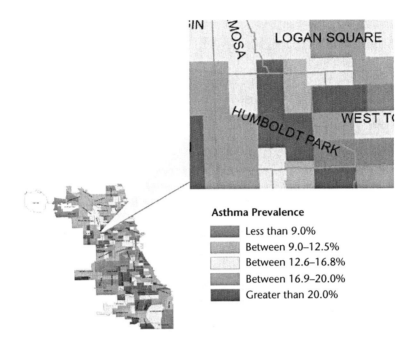

Figure 12-1   Pediatric Diagnosed Asthma Rates in Chicago and the Target Communities (Blown-Up Area)

Source: Gupta, Ruchi S. 2009. Unpublished data, Children's Memorial Hospital, Chicago, Illinois.

groups. Twenty-one percent of Puerto Rican children had diagnosed asthma and another 13% had a positive asthma screen for a potential total asthma burden of 34%. The asthma burdens for Black, White, and Mexican children were 25%, 20%, and 14%, respectively. These rates have subsequently been confirmed by another study that surveyed elementary school children and found dramatic variations in asthma prevalence by community boundaries (Fig. 12-1, Gupta et al., 2008).

Addressing Asthma Disparities for Puerto Rican Children Nationally

Despite clear evidence of the highest asthma morbidity and mortality of any racial or ethnic group in the United States, specific interventions that target Puerto Ricans are severely lacking. Only three intervention studies in this population could be found. Tatis and colleagues conducted a clinic-based asthma education intervention in a population of Latino adults in New York City (Tatis, Remache, and DeMango, 2005). Their intervention was associated with reduced emergency department and hospital utilization and improved asthma-related quality of life. However, the study had many limitations. Although the target community had a large Dominican and Puerto Rican population, ethnicity was not defined further than Latino. The study was not a randomized controlled trial; the control group consisted of non-responders. Outcomes were collected from emergency department records (Tatis, Remache, and DeMango, 2005). Cloutier and colleagues tested a clinic-based intervention for Black and Latino children in Connecticut, where the predominant Latino ethnicity was Puerto Rican. They reported the Latino children sought medical care more often and filled more prescriptions than the Black children. Their intervention appeared to reduce health-care utilization in both groups (Cloutier et al., 2008).

The most rigorous study to date with Puerto Rican children was conducted in Puerto Rico. The investigators used a randomized controlled trial to compare home education from asthma counselors to written education sent in the mail. The asthma counselor group had more symptom-free nights and less emergency room visits or hospitalizations. However, no difference was seen in symptom-free days, activity limitations, and medication use. Study limitations included a short intervention phase and self-reported outcomes (Canino et al., 2008). These studies, especially the third study in Puerto Rico, provide us with some preliminary evidence to inform dose and duration of future interventions with Puerto Rican children, but much more research is needed.

The Community Begins to Unite: The Greater Humboldt Park Community of Wellness Asthma Task Force

The Sinai Survey results intensified Humboldt Park leaders' focus on health. In particular, the Puerto Rican Agenda, an informal group of politicians, social service agency staff, community leaders, and residents concerned with the Humboldt Park Puerto Rican community decided to take on health as one of its focus issues in 2003. At the time the Sinai data were released, the New Communities Program (NCP) of the Local Initiatives Support Corporation/ Chicago supported community development in multiple Chicago neighborhoods, with intentions to include Humboldt Park. Their goal is to rejuvenate challenged communities, bolster those in danger of losing ground, and preserve diversity in the path of gentrification through the creation of a 5-year Quality-of-Life strategic plan. Many of the ideas of the Puerto Rican Agenda Health Committee were brought to and adopted by the NCP Healthcare Subcommittee. As a result, health was prioritized as an essential component of community development. In May 2005, the Humboldt Park NCP plan named seven strategies addressing education, wellness, families, land use, youth, safety, and job training. The Greater Humboldt Park Community of Wellness (GHPCW) was formed by members of the NCP Health Care Subcommittee and the Puerto Rican Agenda Health Committee to ensure implementation of the wellness strategy within a 5-year plan. The GHPCW gained strength when the Puerto Rican Cultural Center (a community-based organization that has served for more than 35 years as a catalyst for addressing some of the most important historical events of the Puerto Rican diaspora and Latino communities in Chicago) and the Sinai Urban Health Institute (SUHI) joined. They were further strengthened by the Near Northwest Neighborhood Network/Humboldt Park Empowerment Project's decision to rely on the GHPCW for health-oriented community-based partnerships.

The GHPCW defines itself as a grass-root, community-based health coalition serving the Chicago community areas of Humboldt Park and West Town. It takes a community-organizing, health promotion, preventive, collaborative, partnership-building, holistic, and community strengths-based approach at improving the community's health. GHPCW membership currently includes community members and more than 60 organizations, including health-care providers, human service agencies, advocacy groups, research institutions, schools, and institutions of higher education. The GHPCW organized its members into eight Task Forces, one for each prioritized disparity: asthma, mental health, oral health, HIV/AIDS, obesity, diabetes, school health, and health careers. Task Forces were charged with education, advocacy, service coordination, and project implementation as described in Table 12-1.

As the GHPCW grew and strengthened, it became known as the umbrella organization for community-wide, broad-based collaborative interventions impacting health in the greater Humboldt Park area. This caught the attention of some people outside of the community who wanted to come into the community and tap into its well-organized assets. For the most part, experiences and relationships with these individuals, including university-based researchers, were collaborative and mutually beneficial. However, there were occasions where researchers did not quite understand how to work with communities in equitable research relationships. This prompted the GHPCW to draft a document entitled "Values, Principles, and Protocols Guiding Research in the Greater Humboldt Park Community." The specific goals of these principles/protocols are to provide an agreed standard of research conduct that:

- clarifies, in advance, expectations of the research process and outcomes for everyone involved;
- fosters mutual exchange of information, ideas, skills, and appreciation; and
- builds a foundation for effective research relationships.

TABLE 12-1   Greater Humboldt Park Community of Wellness Task Force Activities

Task Forces
Asthma, Mental Health, Oral Health, HIV/AIDS, Obesity, Diabetes, School Health, Health Careers
Activities
1. Educate themselves and the community at large about each of these disparities. Educate regarding disease prevalence compared to other communities and across race and ethnicity within the community, regarding socio-economic contributors to health, and regarding disease prevention, self-care, medical screening diagnosis and treatment. For health careers, educate about health labor needs. Also prepare individuals for higher education and/or employment in health careers.
2. Advocate for changes in neighborhoods, and in city and state practices, policies and budgets, if these changes would improve the health status of our community.
3. Coordinate existing services among the numerous health and human service organizations. Service coordination crosses many sectors: public health departments and private non-profits; research institutions and community organizations; health, human services and advocacy organizations.
4. Implement community intervention projects to actually change the health, educational or employment status of individuals in our community. Projects are typically developed through collaborative processes. When a project is ready for funding and subsequent implementation, Community of Wellness staff assists with preparing grant applications, and fosters a collaborative approach to project implementation.

The GHPCW Asthma Task Force

The Asthma Task Force first convened in the summer of 2007. Initial members included parents, representatives from local community-based organizations such as Association House of Chicago (one of the oldest and largest of the original settlement houses in the city, providing social services to over 20,000 individuals annually), and West Town Leadership United (an organization that develops leadership, advocacy, and the organizing skills of local parents). Other initial members include the Respiratory Health Association of Metropolitan Chicago (a prominent lung health advocacy agency, formally the American Lung Association of Metropolitan Chicago) and two academic research centers (Rush University Medical Center and SUHI). The Task Force worked to strengthen existing collaborations, initiate a process to develop new collaborations, and secure funding to reduce asthma in the community.

Informed by research and the expertise of the members, the Task Force decided the most effective way to impact asthma was to focus on outreach and education. Specifically, the Task Force aimed to educate the community on the impact of asthma, disease self-management, and how to access medical care and pharmaceuticals. Efforts targeted the entire family, not just children with asthma. Furthermore, schools were identified as a potential focal point where asthma education could be centralized and most effectively reach many of the local asthma stakeholders (e.g., children, parents, teachers, administrators, community-based organizations, and local health-care providers). As the efforts of the Task Force strengthened and became more visible, its membership grew. The Task Force built strategic relationships with newer stakeholders, including a large academic research institution (Northwestern University) and the Chicago Public Schools Office of Specialized Services.

Since 2007, the Task Force members have worked together to leverage each other's strengths, capabilities, and expertise to meet a common goal—a reduction in the high prevalence and morbidity rates of asthma for children living in Humboldt Park and West Town. This has resulted in the successful implementation of two research initiatives to gather even more comprehensive data on cultural, social, and community factors impacting asthma, a CDC-funded community-wide asthma education project, and a National Institutes of Health (NIH)-funded intervention study for asthma (Table 12-2).

Looking ahead, the Task Force will be continuing its work with local schools as well as affordable housing developers to make the school and home environments asthma friendly. The Task Force will seek out funding and projects to educate tenants and landlords on integrated pest management, low allergen building options, and smoke-free buildings.

Community-Based Participatory Research Projects that Emerged

A Community–Academic Partnership for Asthma Control in Humboldt Park

Principal Investigators: Ruchi Gupta, MD (Children's Memorial Hospital), and Juana Ballesteros, RN BSN MPH (Greater Humboldt Park Community of Wellness)

The Sinai Survey provided preliminary data on asthma, but asthma prevalence and severity in the schools remained unclear. There was also minimal understanding of mediating community factors or the availability of asthma resources within the schools for children and families. A partnership to address these issues was created between the Asthma Task Force of the GHPCW and Dr. Ruchi Gupta, a pediatrician and researcher at Children's Memorial Hospital. Other key research team members included Maureen Damitz from the Respiratory Health Association of Metropolitan Chicago and Dr. Molly Martin from Rush University Medical Center. Funding was obtained from the Alliance for Research in Chicagoland Communities of the Northwestern University Clinical and Translational Sciences Institute.

TABLE 12-2 Summary of Asthma Research in Humboldt Park from 2005 to 2009

Title	Project Funding Source	Principal Investigator	Relevant other Investigators and Partners	Outcomes
A Community-Academic Partnership for Asthma Control in Humboldt Park	Alliance for Research in Chicagoland Communities of the Northwestern University Clinical and Translational Sciences Institute	Ruchi Gupta, MD* (Children's Memorial Hospital) and Juana Ballesteros, RN BSN MPH* (Greater Humboldt Park Community of Wellness)	Molly Martin, MD* (Rush University Medical Center), Maureen Damitz* (Respiratory Health Association of Metropolitan Chicago)	Asthma prevalence and control in schools. Violence and asthma.
The Impact of Community Factors on Childhood Asthma Severity	Robert Wood Johnson Foundation Physician Faculty Scholars Program	Ruchi Gupta, MD* (Children's Memorial Hospital)	Juana Ballesteros, RN BSN MPH* (Greater Humboldt Park Community of Wellness) and Maureen Damitz* (Respiratory Health Association of Metropolitan Chicago)	Violence and asthma. Intervention development.
Chicago Public Schools Asthma Management Project	Centers for Disease Control and Prevention	Project Manager: Lilliana De Santiago* (Chicago Public Schools)	Chicago Asthma Consortium and Juana Ballesteros, RN BSN MPH* (Greater Humboldt Park Community of Wellness), Respiratory Health Association of Metropolitan Chicago, Lenore Coover, Safer pest Control Project	Asthma prevalence in schools. Increased asthma training for school educators.

Project	Funder/Institution	Principal Investigator	Partners	Focus
The Chicagoland Asthma Network (CAN) Humboldt Park Town Hall Meeting	Chicago Asthma Consortium	Stephen Samuelson, MPA (Chicago Asthma Consortium)	Juana Ballesteros, RN BSN MPH* (Greater Humboldt Park Community of Wellness)	Community perceptions of asthma.
A Qualitative Exploration of Asthma Self-Management Beliefs and Practices in Puerto Rican Families	Rush University Department of Preventive Medicine	Molly Martin, MD* (Rush University Medical Center)		Puerto Rican families' perceptions of asthma.
La Comunidad Unida Retando el Asma/The Community United to Challenge Asthma	National Institutes of Health	Molly Martin, MD* (Rush University Medical Center)	Greater Humboldt Park Community of Wellness, Puerto Rican Cultural Center, Near Northwest Neighborhood Network, and Lilliana de Santiago* (Chicago Public Schools)	Intervention testing for Puerto Rican children.

Note: *Member of Greater Humboldt Park Community of Wellness Asthma Task Force.

A survey tool was developed, tested, and implemented in two area Chicago Public Schools. The two schools were selected because their student body was a good representation of school age children in Humboldt Park based on socio-economic, racial, and ethnic indicators. Almost 500 parents at two local Chicago Public Schools completed the survey tool to: *(1)* determine asthma prevalence and control; *(2)* understand community factors potentially contributing to asthma including issues of safety, pollution, and access to care; and *(3)* assess both the availability of resources for students with asthma and the degree of trust parents have in these resources.

The design of this research project utilized a Community-Based Participatory Research approach. Critical to the successful completion of 494 surveys was the trusted relationship between the GHPCW and the school administrators. This relationship did not develop during this project—it was brokered by a long-time, local resident who served as school organizer for the Near Northwest Neighborhood Network/Humboldt Park Empowerment Partnership (NNNN/HPEP). For the last 20 years, NNNN/HPEP has been organizing around the issues of affordable housing, church, employment, economic development, health, education, safety, and youth services. The NNNN/HPEP school organizer had worked for several years with local schools to organize and empower parents as well as to facilitate adult development opportunities for them. The trust parent leaders had in this school organizer made it easy to have them understand the importance of the project and gain their support. Also critical to the successful implementation of the surveys was the logistical, on-the-ground support offered by the Chicago Public Schools Health Assistants. These positions are unique to schools in Greater Humboldt Park as part of a pilot project, funded by the Otho S.A. Sprague Memorial Institute, to improve health services to Chicago Public School students. The Health Assistants' training was supported by a grant from the Centers for Disease Control and Prevention (*see* the Chicago Public Schools Asthma Management Project).

Although this was not a random survey of the city, results found that the prevalence of asthma in these two schools was 25%. This is very similar to the rate of 28% documented previously in the Sinai Survey. Smoking occurred in one of every four homes, 75% of respondents found motorized vehicles idling in their neighborhood on a regular basis, two of every three respondents noted feeling unsafe in their community, 80% reported feelings of nervousness or stress, and 60% of respondents prevented their children from playing outside because of neighborhood violence.

The dissemination of these findings occurred at several levels. They were included in another grant application that was subsequently funded by the Robert Wood Johnson Foundation (*see* next section). They will be published in an academic medical journal Gupta et al. 2010. Finally, findings have been taken back to the community. They have been presented at community forums and distributed in the schools to parents. Currently, the GHPCW is working with other community organizations to facilitate the formation of Wellness Councils within the schools, which are mandated by the No Child Left Behind Act of 2001. Their purpose is to oversee the implementation of the local school wellness policy, as well as to develop and implement an annual evaluation. Wellness Councils require representation of all school health stakeholders: school principal, key teachers, community-based organizations, No Child Left Behind Committee members, local school council member, bilingual committee members, school nurse, school counselor, food service representative, and students. Wellness Councils will offer the sustained infrastructure needed to effectively address the findings of the survey at the school level.

The Impact of Community Factors on Childhood Asthma Severity

Principal Investigator: Ruchi Gupta, MD (Children's Memorial Hospital)
    Using the methods and results of the "A Community-Academic Partnership for Asthma Control in Humboldt Park," Dr. Gupta applied for the Robert Wood Johnson Foundation Faculty Scholar Award. She received this award for the period from July 2009 to June 2012. She proposed to explore the contributions of socio-environmental factors in asthma health disparities. First, she will use an existing city-wide Chicago dataset to identify community factors influencing childhood asthma severity and disparities. Second, a survey will be developed and validated to assess the relevance in Humboldt Park of significant factors determined to impact asthma severity in Chicago. This survey will be administered to a minimum of 2000 residents. After completion of the survey, focus groups will be conducted with approximately 30 local residents to explore which potential strategies and resources are critical to address the community factors identified previously. Results will be used to identify potential strategies for a future community-based asthma intervention in Humboldt Park. She will partner with GHPCW and the Respiratory Health Association of Metropolitan Chicago to achieve these aims.

Chicago Public Schools Asthma Management Project

Recipient: Chicago Public Schools
    At the same time as the GHPCW and Dr. Gupta were beginning their survey of the Humboldt Park schools, the Chicago Public Schools received a larger grant to better address asthma in their schools. Chicago Public Schools was awarded the CDC "Improving Health and Educational Outcomes of Young People" Cooperative Agreement grant. Lilliana De Santiago leads this project and is also a member of the GHPCW Asthma Task Force. During

this grant cycle (2008–2013), Chicago Public Schools will focus efforts on creating district-wide sustainability through intensive asthma training for school nurses and district level personnel. Training will also be provided to all clinical personnel such as social workers, psychologists, occupational therapists, speech therapists, and physical therapists. Online trainings, educational materials, and resources are currently being developed and disseminated to reach all areas of the city and to provide ongoing capacity building to all school personnel and families of students with asthma.

A component of this project requires a more intensive approach to community outreach and education on asthma. Chicago Public Schools currently is working with 12 schools in the Greater Humboldt Park Community to provide continuing asthma management education to school staff, parents, and students with asthma. Data analysis on the prevalence of student's asthma at these schools is being closely monitored as well as student impact. As the project expands it will move into other areas of the city with a high prevalence of asthma.

The overall goals of the project are to:

1. Increase capacity through district-wide professional development on asthma management.
2. Increase capacity through education and outreach within targeted schools in communities with a high burden of asthma.
3. Educate schools on asthma-friendly environmental practices that reduce risk factors contributing to asthma episodes in students.

To date, the project has sponsored trainings for more than 200 school psychologists, 65 school nurses, 165 physical instruction teachers, more than 300 school personnel in the Greater Humboldt Park schools, and more than 300 students in the Greater Humboldt Park schools. In addition, 750 Chicago Public Schools and affiliated schools have received educational posters (e.g., Asthma First Aid, Help Your Child Breath Easier at School, and Please Help Me Breathe I Need My Inhaler).

The Chicagoland Asthma Network Humboldt Park Town Hall Meeting

The GHPCW organized and moderated two focus groups in the community to better understand perceptions of asthma. These focus groups—one in English and one in Spanish—were initiated by the Chicagoland Asthma Network (CAN), which is a Task Force of the Chicago Asthma Consortium. The focus groups were conducted in Humboldt Park during March 2009 with the goal of learning about the community's health-care experiences, communication with health-care providers, perspectives on asthma health-care disparities, and how they would like to receive information. CAN used this information to create a "Plan for Reducing Asthma in Chicago," a manageable list of tasks designed to reduce asthma disparities in the Chicagoland area.

When asked about barriers to obtaining good health care, participants first discussed money and insurance. They felt their care was limited by their financial resources and that the insurance process was difficult to navigate and understand. About half of participants were happy with the communication they had with their doctor. The others were not and said this was related to the quality of care they received. "They speak in 'doctor talk' that I can't understand." "They only write prescriptions." One person said, "I can't speak with my doctor on the phone; the receptionist will only take messages." Some participants described a lack of translation and how they felt this was disrespectful. Situations were described where families waited a long time for rushed, incomplete doctor visits. They expressed a need for more clinics and more specialized care, especially for asthma. Finally, they described transportation barriers—especially for those with disabilities—and a lack of understanding of how their insurance benefits may provide for transportation to medical appointments.

When asked where they would like to receive health information in addition to their doctor's office, participants said in their home, the church, local newspapers, fliers in the mail, and through the schools. They listed several ways to reduce health-care disparities. These included reducing pollution, pesticides, and cigarette smoking. The schools need to be involved addressing environmental issues therein. Finally, the political officials and all leaders in the community need to participate in the effort to reduce asthma disparities.

A Qualitative Exploration of Asthma Self-Management Beliefs and Practices in Puerto Rican Families

Principal Investigator: Molly Martin, MD (Rush University Medical Center)

Dr. Molly Martin, an investigator with specific interests in Latino health, asthma interventions, and community research, saw the Sinai Survey results on their release. Intrigued with the incredibly high prevalence, morbidity, and lack of interventions among Puerto Ricans, she met with the Sinai Study's leader, Dr. Steven Whitman, and a community leader in Humboldt Park to discuss possible research opportunities. The discussion resulted in two specific needs:

1. A need for asthma interventions specifically directed toward Puerto Rican children; and
2. A need to train and employ community members as health educators to build community capacity for asthma management and health education.

A qualitative study (Martin et al., 2010) and behavioral randomized controlled trial resulted directly from this discussion.

Several questions needed to be answered before an intervention could be finalized. The first question was to determine what specific asthma self-management behaviors were being performed by children, adolescents, and their caregivers. This information was essential to know who the intervention should target. Second, it was important to know the specific beliefs informing asthma self-management behaviors in Midwest Puerto Rican families. Asthma beliefs had been described for Puerto Ricans in the Northeast but never in the Midwest. An intervention would only be successful if it recognized and worked within the belief structure of the participants. Therefore, this structure needed to be described.

Dr. Martin presented the Sinai data and her literature review to the GHPCW Asthma Task Force on August 16, 2007. They agreed on the study design and questions and invited her to join the Task Force. Key informant interviews were conducted first to inform the topics and frame the questions. The key informants were recommended by local physicians and by GHPCW Asthma Task Force members. They included a local general pediatrician in private practice, a pediatrician from a mobile asthma van, two Puerto Rican parent educators from a community-based organization that is a member of the GHPCW (NNNN), and a Puerto Rican school organizer. Interviews were performed in the informants' language of choice (which was English) and were audio-recorded.

The questions framed by the interviews were then used to describe the focus group discussions. Three focus groups were conducted in the fall of 2007 in community schools. The first focus group consisted of Puerto Rican parents of children with asthma (13 participants). The second group contained Puerto Rican children with asthma in local elementary schools that run from kindergarten through eighth grade (three participants). Both groups were recruited by parent educators from NNNN. The third focus group of Puerto Rican adolescents with asthma was organized by the Puerto Rican Cultural Center (PRCC). The PRCC recruited nine participants who were students in their alternative high school. One of the parent coordinators from NNNN felt strongly that a separate elementary school in the neighborhood should be approached because this specific school did not receive as many programs as the other schools. Within this school, a local health-care system (Erie Family Health Care) ran a small clinic. Nursing staff from the school clinic contacted parents and recruited seven participants for a final elementary school group held in February 2008. All focus groups were conducted by a Puerto Rican bilingual moderator who was affiliated with the PRCC, with the exception of the final elementary school group that was moderated by Dr. Martin. The parent focus group was conducted in both English and Spanish, whereas the other groups were in English. Groups were audio-recorded, and participants were reimbursed $25 for their time.

Audio-recordings from the key informant interviews and focus groups were professionally transcribed and translated into English when appropriate. Transcriptions were analyzed using naturalistic inquiry methods that include an initial data review for topical coding and a second analysis for exploring relationships among the coding categories (Lincoln and Guba, 1985; Ryan and Bernard, 2000).

The first theme that emerged was asthma self-management behaviors of youth and caregivers. When participants were asked who actually managed the children's asthma and at what age, parents and informants agreed that children were assuming the management responsibilities for their asthma at younger ages than the parents ideally felt the children should. There were reasons for this. Parents felt that children needed to be able to care for themselves in case a parent could not be there. However, parents also stated that this was an unfair burden on young children. The adolescents discussed how developing asthma skills at a young age could be a good thing because it better prepared children for the future.

These parent and informant reports of behaviors were mirrored in the responses of the children. Each elementary and high school participant reported they typically self-administered their medication. The elementary school children received more assistance from their parents. The high school group described how their asthma had been better controlled when their parents helped them. Several stated they wanted more parental help now because their asthma was so uncontrolled. The key informants suggested that transitions into adulthood in this community could be difficult because parents often lacked resources to prepare their children to manage their asthma.

The second theme that emerged was related to beliefs influencing asthma self-management behaviors. Participants had extensive knowledge of asthma triggers. When attacks occurred, they preferred management techniques involving manipulation of the environment or emotions. Relaxation was the most discussed method for treatment of asthma attacks. Also discussed were changes in temperature, going inside, and wearing additional clothing when it was cold outside—all of which suggest attempts to repair imbalances. Participants generally tried to avoid all asthma medications mostly because of fears of overmedication and side effects.

Other themes emerged that helped to guide subsequent intervention design. All participants voiced a need for more education on asthma. They not only wanted education for the families and children with asthma but also for the community in general and for the schools. The purpose of this education was so that people without asthma could help create an asthma-friendly environment by reducing triggers, reducing stigmas, and providing emergency assistance when needed. Repeatedly mentioned was a specific need for education regarding cigarette smoke. Conversely, key informants and focus group participants identified multiple areas of strength and support in their community. The greatest assets identified by these groups were family and the schools.

The results of this qualitative study were presented to the GHPCW and at grand rounds for several local hospitals. The data are in publication and were incorporated into a grant to the National Institutes of Health which was subsequently funded. This study, Project CURA, is described next.

Project CURA

*La **C**omunidad **U**nida **R**etando el **A**sma/The Community United to Challenge Asthma*

Principal Investigator: Molly Martin, MD (Rush University Medical Center)

Project CURA began in the spring of 2009 and involves collaborations between Rush University Medical Center, PRCC, NNNN, the GHPCW, and the SUHI. Funding for this study comes from NIH. Project CURA is a behavioral randomized controlled trial of Puerto Rican children with asthma that tests two interventions to improve asthma self-management. Results of the intervention are not available because the study just began, but the following is a description of the study design.

The study contains two cohorts: one cohort of 50 elementary school children (grades K–8) and one cohort of 50 high school children. Half of the participants in each cohort will receive a community health worker (CHW) intervention, whereas half receive mailed information. A control group will receive written asthma education (but no individualized self-management training) on the same schedule as the CHW group. Primary outcomes include asthma medication adherence and home asthma triggers. Outcomes will be assessed in all participants pre-randomization, immediately after the 4-month active intervention phase, and 8 months after the active intervention phase completion to determine sustainability (*see* Fig. 12-2).

To ensure community representation in the project and an appropriate level of sensitivity to community values and beliefs, a community advisory board was assembled in collaboration with the community partners. Board members include representatives from each of the community partners (PRCC, NNNN, and GHPCW), a Puerto Rican adolescent physician, a pediatrician with asthma expertise, a representative of the Chicago Public Schools, and three Puerto Rican parents of children with asthma. The community advisory board facilitates planning of the project, community education and outreach, data interpretation, and proper dissemination of results. Board members meet in person every 3 months to discuss the progress of the study.

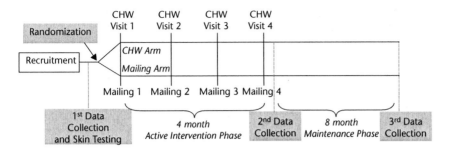

Figure 12-2   The Community United to Challenge Asthma (Project CURA) Study Design

To participate in the study, participants must be of self-identified Puerto Rican heritage, in school, and between ages 5 and 18 years; have persistent asthma; and have poorly controlled asthma. The CHW group will receive a home visit by a trained asthma CHW each month for 4 months. At the CHW home visits, the CHW will spend 1 to 2 hours with the family. The CHW will educate them on the core curriculum, which covers general asthma facts, controller medications, inhalers and spacers, symptom recognition, asthma triggers, and access to care. The CHW will tailor the education to the specific needs of each family and create behavior change plans that incorporate self-management techniques such as self-monitoring, environmental rearrangement, enlisting social support, and problem solving. The families in the mailings group will receive written materials in English and Spanish by mail once a month for 4 months. These materials will address the same core curriculum as the CHW home visits.

One of the project goals is to build community capacity for asthma. To achieve this goal, Project CURA began by training Puerto Rican asthma CHWs Advertisements for the training began in the summer of 2009 in a local newspaper and through the community partner list serves. Two initial training sessions were planned (12–15 hours each). These trainings were conducted by an experienced asthma educator from the Sinai Asthma Education Training Institute. The curriculum included information on asthma pathophysiology, symptoms, triggers, and environmental control, management, and medications. This training addressed how to approach families and keys to successful home visiting. The trainings also included a 1.5-hour lecture from Safer Pest Control, which is an organization that provides training on integrated pest management. Fifteen people attended some of either the weekday or weekend trainings, and 13 completed the training. Four people were selected from those who completed the initial training for subsequent training. Two would be CHWs on Project CURA, and two would be back-up CHWs. Another 12 hours of training were then conducted on asthma medications again, self-management skills, behavior change plans, and the research protocol. CHWs were evaluated for competency to perform the intervention at the end of this training using a standardized role play. The final two Project CURA CHWs then shadowed more experienced asthma CHWs from SUHI.

The two primary outcomes are medication adherence and home triggers. These are measured at baseline, immediately post-intervention (month 5), and after a maintenance phase (month 12). Other outcomes are collected as potential mediators of change. These are described in Table 12-3.

One of the main goals of this project is to build the community capacity in the area of health. This process is ongoing, but accomplishments include the training of the CHWs and the hiring of three research assistants. The research assistants are all Puerto Rican and have connections to the target community. The community partners participated fully in their selection.

TABLE 12-3 Data Collected in the Community United to Challenge Asthma (Project CURA) Study

---

1. Screener: Asthma control and severity
2. Skin test: Dust mite mix, cockroach mix, mold mix, cat, dog, mouse
3. Home data collection #1
   a. Demographics of child and caregiver: age, sex, race/ethnicity, place of birth, time lived in mainland US, education level, school lunch, marital status, home ownership, caregiver language acculturation
   b. Access to care: Child insurance and location for medical care
   c. Home triggers:
      i. Self-report of behaviors, smoking, animals, pests
      ii. Home inspection for pests, smoke, mold, dust, cleaning projects
      iii. Dust collection for dust mite, cockroach, cat, dog
      iv. Child saliva collection for cotinine
   d. Medicines
      i. Self-report and visual inspection
      ii. Medication administration observation
      iii. Adherence to inhaled corticosteroid over 3 weeks using Doser or counter
   e. Asthma symptoms and control
   f. Emergency care use: Hospital, emergency, urgent care, oral steroid bursts
   g. School absences
   h. Self-Efficacy: Caregiver and child
   i. Health Beliefs: Caregiver
   j. Life Stress: Caregiver and child
   k. Social Support: Caregiver and child
   l. Depression: Caregiver and high school participants
4. Telephone follow-up: every month except home visit months
   a. Emergency care use: Hospital, emergency, urgent care, oral steroid bursts
   b. School absences
5. Home data collection #2 (Month 5)
   a. Same as #1 except
      i. Remove demographics
      ii. Add acculturation of caregiver and child, violence/trauma for caregiver and high school participants
6. Home data collection #3 (Month 12)
   a. Same as #1 except remove demographics

The education and support provided to the research assistants and CHWs during the implementation of Project CURA will allow them better opportunities at the completion of the study. Currently, recruitment for the study involves all of the neighborhood schools, clinical sites, and service agencies, which helps to spread the word about asthma. Finally, at the completion of the study, results will be presented to all study partners and local agencies. They will be printed in the local Puerto Rican newspaper *La Voz*, which has a large distribution list. If indicated, discussions with community members will be conducted in open forums. Finally, the results will be used to generate more funding opportunities and programs for the community.

Lessons Learned in Humboldt Park

The asthma experience in Humboldt Park serves as a model of Community-Based Participatory Research. The GHPCW arose organically with the assistance of a community development program. The GHPCW Asthma Task Force was created as a direct result of the needs identified by the Sinai Study data. Because the GHPCW takes a collaborative approach in all that it does, it builds off of the already existing strong community assets, social capital, and community cohesion, and it takes a shared collective approach to the community's health and wellness. By leveraging these resources and assets, its efficacy as a health coalition becomes far greater than the sum of its parts.

The GHPCW wants to ensure that all research conducted in Greater Humboldt Park addresses the community's priorities, ensures that research does not harm community residents, offers job opportunities to residents, supports the local economy, and ensures proportional distribution of resources. As a result, the GHPCW has managed to position itself as the gatekeeper for health-related research in the community. Investigators wishing to work in Greater Humboldt Park must approach the GHPCW as collaborators on projects. This ensures an early understanding about how research should be conducted in and with the community. Academic institutions can attempt research in this community without going through the GHPCW, but recruitment and data collection would be very difficult without support from the community.

Besides ensuring the research conducted within its community is beneficial to and involves its community, the GHPCW serves another role— research coordinator. This role emerged naturally as multiple investigators from competing academic centers approached the community to conduct asthma research. Often in research, several separate teams work on the same research question. This can be beneficial in terms of replicability, but it can also be a waste of resources and a burden on participants. The GHPCW Asthma Task Force succeeded in bringing multiple competing researchers to the same table, where they planned research projects that were complementary and slightly overlapping but addressed different core areas of asthma disparities. All investigators now benefit from their own work and the work of the others. The community reaps the most benefit by receiving high-quality useful information, services, and opportunities from a wide variety of sources. The organization of the GHPCW has ensured that asthma research projects inform each other, complement each other, and build off of each other, making the most effective and efficient products possible.

Can this model of asthma research be replicated in other communities? The environment of Humboldt Park may be unique in several aspects. The community is very diverse in terms of race and ethnicity. The community income level is low, it is considered medically underserved, and it lacks sufficient health professionals. However, the community level of organization is very high. Leaders have been organizing around political issues for decades, resulting in the formation of multiple strong community-based organizations. These trusted organizations are linked by political and social justice ideologies. The establishment of the GHPCW was a natural extension of these organizations into the area of health and wellness. The subsequent success of research projects within this organizational structure is not surprising, despite the fact that community residents are not familiar with the research process. Trust in the community organizations is strong enough to overcome barriers of fear, economics, and discrimination. Another factor in the success of the research to date has been the high prevalence and morbidity of asthma within the community, and the community's awareness of this. Organizations and individuals, motivated by data from the Sinai Survey and by their own experiences with asthma, were very supportive of research on this issue.

Communities aiming to replicate this model should consider the importance of a strong community base. This is essential for building trust in populations that are unfamiliar with the research process and distrustful of academic institutions. Research should focus on disease areas that are identified by the community as being high-priority. Finally, community leaders and members should be involved in all stages of the research process. Their voices need to be heard, their ideas implemented, and their efforts compensated appropriately.

The GHPCW has established a research model that is not only successful but also sustainable. Leaders and investigators from all over Chicago are recognizing the strength of this community and this model. The current asthma projects are only the beginning. Future work is already being planned to potentially conduct more testing of asthma interventions, interventions aimed at co-morbid asthma and obesity, violence prevention and asthma, and the genetics of asthma. The structure of the GHPCW allows it to work with multiple partners and to implement projects on its own as well.

Asthma for children in Humboldt Park will improve. When that happens, it will be a result of the work done by many investigators. More importantly, it will also be the result of the work done by the residents themselves and their leaders.

> *Go to the people, live with them, love them, learn from them, work with them, start with what they have, build on what they know, and in the end when the work is done the people will say , we have done it ourselves.—Lao Tzu*

Acknowledgments

Significant contributions were made to this chapter by Maureen Damitz at the Respiratory Health Association of Metropolitan Chicago, Ruchi Gupta at Children's Memorial Hospital, Lilliana De Santiago from the Chicago Public Schools, and Stephen Samuelson, Joel Massel, and Amy Miller from the Chicago Asthma Consortium. Funding for the Community United to Challenge Asthma Study comes from National Institutes of Health. Specifically, 1R21 HL087769-01A1 from the National Heart Lung and Blood Institute, and 1R21HL087769-01A1 from the American Recovery and Reinvestment Act.

References

Blumenthal, Jacob Bryan and Malcolm N. Blumenthal. 2002. Genetics of asthma. *Medical Clinics of North America* 86:937–950.

Canino, Glorisa, Doryliz Vila, Sharon-Lise T. Normand, Edna Acosta-Pérez, Rafael Ramírez, Pedro García, and Cynthia Rand. 2008. Reducing asthma health disparities in poor Puerto Rican children: The effectiveness of a culturally tailored family intervention. *Journal of Allergy and Clinical Immunology* 121(3):665–670.

Celedón, Juan C., Diane Sredl, Scott T. Weiss, Marianne Pisarski, Dorothy Wakefield, and Michelle Cloutier. 2004. Ethnicity and skin test reactivity to aero allergens among asthma children in Connecticut. *Chest* 125:85–92.

Centers for Disease Control and Prevention. 2002. Surveillance for asthma—United States, 1980–1999. *Morbidity and Mortality Weekly Report* 51(No. SS-1):1–13.

Centers for Disease Control and Prevention. 2004. Asthma prevalence and control characteristics by race/ethnicity—United States, 2002. *Morbidity and Mortality Weekly Report* 53:145–148.

Cloutier, Michelle M.,Gloria A. Jones, Vanessa Hinckson, and Dorothy B. Wakefield. 2008. Effectiveness of an asthma management program in reducing disparities in care in urban children. *Annals of Allergy Asthma and Immunology* 100(6):545–550.

Esteban, Cynthia A., Robert B. Klein, Elizabeth L. McQuaid, Gregory K. Fritz, Ronald Seifer, Sheryl J. Kopel, et al. 2009. Conundrums in childhood asthma severity, control, and health care use: Puerto Rico versus Rhode Island. *Journal of Allergy and Clinical Immunology* 124(2):238–244.

Freeman, Natalie C. G. and Dona Schneider Patricia McGarvey. 2003. Household exposure factors, asthma, and school absenteeism in a predominantly Hispanic community. *Journal of Exposure Analysis and Environmental Epidemiology* 13:169–176.

Gruchalla, Rebecca S., Jacqueline Pongracic, Marshall Plaut, Richard Evans III, Cynthia M. Visness, Michelle Walter, et al. 2005. Inner City Asthma Study: Relationship among sensitivity, allergen exposure, and asthma morbidity. *Journal of Allergy and Clinical Immunology* 115:478–485.

Gupta, Ruchi S. 2009. Unpublished data, Children's Memorial Hospital, Chicago, IL.

Gupta RS, Ballesteros J, Springston EE, Smith B, Martin M, Damitz M. The State of Pediatric Asthma in Chicago's Humboldt Park: A Community- Based Study in Two Local Elementary Schools. BMC Pediatrics. Accepted for Publication June 1, 2010. In Press.

Huss, Karen, Cynthia S. Rand, Arlene M. Butz, Peyton A. Eggleston, Charles Murigande, Lera C. Thompson, Susan Schneider, Kathy Weeks, and Floyd J. Malveaux. 1994. Home environmental risk factors in urban minority asthmatic children. *Annals of Allergy* 72:173–177.

Lincoln, Yvonna S. and Egon G. Guba. 1985. *Naturalistic Inquiry.* Beverly Hills, CA: Sage.

Margellos-Anast, Helen and Melissa A. Gutierrez. 2010. Pediatric asthma in African American and Latino Chicago communities—local level data drives response. In: *Urban Health: Combating Disparities with Local Data*, eds. Steven Whitman, Ami M. Shah, and Maureen R. Benjamins, Chapter 11. New York, NY: Oxford University Press.

Marielena Lara, Hal Morgenstern, Naihua Duan, and Robert H. Brook. 1999. Elevated asthma morbidity in Puerto Rican children: A review of possible risk and prognostic factors. *Western Journal of Medicine* 170:75–84.

Marielena Lara, Lara Akinbami, Glenn Flores, and Hal Morgenstern. 2006. Heterogeneity of childhood asthma among Hispanic children: Puerto Rican children bear a disproportionate burden. *Pediatrics* 117:43–53.

Martin, Molly A., Jesse Beebe, Lolita, Lopez, and Sandra, Faux. 2010. A qualitative exploration of asthma self-management beliefs and practices in Puerto Rican families. *Journal of Health Care for the Poor and Underserved*. In press.

Nilsa I. Loyo-Berríos, Juan C. Orengo, and Ruby A. Serrano-Rodríguez. 2006. Childhood asthma prevalence in Northern Puerto Rico, the Rio Grande, and Loiza experience. *Journal of Asthma* 43:619–624.

Ryan, Gery W. and H. Russell Bernard. 2000. Data management and analysis methods. In: *Handbook of Qualitative Research*, 2nd ed., eds. Norman K. Denzin and Yvonna S. Lincoln. Thousand Oaks, CA: Sage, pp. 769–802.

Sally Findley, Katherine Lawler, Monisha Bindra, Linda Maggio, Madeline M. Penachio, and Christopher Maylahn. 2003. Elevated asthma and indoor environmental exposures among Puerto Rican children of East Harlem. *Journal of Asthma* 40:557–569.

Scirica, Christina V. and Juan C. Celedón. 2007. Genetics of asthma: Potential implications for reducing asthma disparities. *Chest* 132(5 Suppl):770S–781S.

Shah, Ami M. and Steven Whitman. 2010. Sinai Health System's Improving Community Health Survey: Methodology and key findings. In: *Urban Health: Combating Disparities with Local Data*, eds. Steven Whitman, Ami M. Shah, and Maureen R. Benjamins, Chapter 3. New York, NY: Oxford University Press.

Stevenson, Lori A., Peter J. Gergen, Donald R. Hoover, David Rosenstreich, David M. Mannino, and Thomas D. Matte. Sociodemographic correlates of indoor allergen sensitivity among United States children. *Journal of Allergy and Clinical Immunology* 108:747–752.

Tatis, Vianessa, Digna Remache, and Emily DiMango. 2005. Results of a culturally directed asthma intervention program in an inner-city Latino community. *Chest* 128:1163–1167.

William Osmond Charles Cookson. 2002. Asthma genetics. *Chest* 121:7S–13S.

Section 4

Implications

13

COMMUNITY-BASED HEALTH INTERVENTIONS: PAST, PRESENT, AND FUTURE

Leah H. Ansell

Introduction

Background

A community-based health intervention is theoretically an effective strategy to combat disease because it incorporates factors beyond the individual that contribute to disease manifestation. Unlike more reductionist research designs that focus on a single risk factor, this holistic view of disease encompasses the complex and often intangible disease determinants. The theoretical appeal of this study design, however, has not translated as well to real-life circumstances. Years of findings from studies using various elements of a community design have demonstrated inconsistent outcomes, with few successes and many failures. Despite these sobering results, many researchers remain convinced that a thoroughly planned and well-executed intervention truly based in the community is the best way to proceed to reign in the damage being done by many diseases.

A critical analysis of past community-based interventions is integral to the design of more effective interventions in the future. This is the purpose of this chapter. A number of community-based initiatives targeting different diseases and risk factors have been selected for this analysis, although it is not intended to be a complete review of all community-based health campaigns. Included are the five best-known community interventions for cardiovascular disease (CVD) as well as studies targeting HIV, obesity, smoking, and diabetes. These studies were selected for two major reasons. First, they were well-planned and executed and had sound study designs and analyses. Second was the extent and manner in which they engaged the community. The CVD studies will be a major focus of this chapter as they are the most prominent and comprehensive community-based prevention trials to date.

The chapter begins with a discussion of the definition of community interventions and how the community is conceptualized in the designs of various studies. Next is a comprehensive analysis of the rationale for community-based interventions. The following section offers a brief summary of the two pioneer CVD studies of the 1970s that served as the impetus for the three major trials that were carried out in the United States in the 1980s. These latter trials are summarized and explored in greater depth. What were the strengths and weaknesses of the interventions? To what extent was the community engaged? The following section is a review of other community-oriented trials in areas such as HIV, smoking, diabetes, and obesity. The chapter concludes by delineating the elements of community campaigns that seem to enhance intervention impact and facilitate sustainability of change. Finally, this information is assembled within the context of the current theories regarding community-based participatory research, with the hope that this information will allow interventionists to move community projects forward more effectively.

What Is a Community-Based Health Intervention?

Community-based health interventions are defined as "experiment[s] in which the unit of allocation to receive a preventive or therapeutic regimen is an entire community" (Last et al., 1995, pg. 34). Community-based intervention campaigns are designed to influence the knowledge, attitudes, and behaviors of a defined population by employing multiple interventions that integrate the organic social, cultural, and environmental dynamics that contribute to health (Wilcox and Knapp, 2000). A central tenet of community interventions is to imbed programs into the local, state, and national health promotion infrastructure to enhance sustainability (Elder et al., 1993; Mittelmark et al., 1993; Verheijden and Kok, 2005).

There are many terms used in the literature to describe community-based interventions, and the vocabulary can be confusing and problematic. In this chapter, various terms will be used interchangeably to describe community-based interventions, including "community-oriented campaigns/interventions/initiatives," "community-based campaigns/interventions/initiatives," and "community interventions." The emphasis in this chapter is not the semantics but rather distinguishing interventions from one another in regard to the nature of the intervention and the extent to which the community was engaged.

Thus, with the growing number of community-based interventions in the past 40 years, it is important to highlight the varying interpretations of what "community-based" signifies in a study's design. The five major CVD campaigns discussed in the upcoming sections employed multifaceted interventions in an entire community, and outcomes were measured at the community level. A key distinction is that such interventions were directed at an entire community rather than only those who were high-risk. Alternatively, many of the more recent community-oriented demonstration projects tended to focus on a single behavioral goal or disease or to deliver the intervention to specified population subgroups rather than the entire community. Although these latter interventions use elements of the community in their design (such as support groups, local health awareness campaigns, and the construction of parks or gyms to facilitate the adoption of healthy behaviors), they are not truly *based* in the community. In this sense, they do not address prevention in the same manner as the programs targeting entire communities.

Rationale of Community-Based Health Interventions

As was briefly discussed in the preceding section, community-based health interventions are considered to be a promising strategy to quell the growing prevalence of chronic disease in certain populations. What are the factors and observations that contribute to this theory? A major component of the rationale is that health behaviors and outcomes are the result of a complex amalgamation of factors. Nancy Krieger (1990, 1994, 2001, 2007) and others contend that disease may best be viewed within the context of one's biological make-up, individual behavior, environmental context, and broader societal forces such as discrimination, poverty, and disparity in the health-care system (Williams, 1990; Schooler et al., 1997; Jack et al., 1999; Smedley, Stitch, and Nelso, 2003; Mechanic, 2005; Williams and Jackson, 2005; Israel et al., 2006; Shaya, Gu, and Saunders, 2006). Although community-wide interventions cannot address the physiological processes of disease, they can influence the environmental, social, and behavioral patterns that contribute to the manifestation of disease. Below is a summary of the chief reasons why community-oriented health campaigns are considered to be a promising mechanism of health intervention:

- Health behavior is influenced by the familial, social, and cultural environment in which one lives (Aiken and Mott, 1970; Warren, 1972; McLeroy et al., 1988; Andersson, 2003).
- The diffusion of health information is enhanced when all sectors of the community are involved (Farquhar, 1978; Shea and Basch, *Part I*, 1990).

- Community interventions are a cost-effective and feasible strategy to disseminate health information to a large, diverse population (Farquhar, 1978; Hancock et al., 1997).
- Community interventions enable individuals to learn practical methods for modifying behaviors within the context of the stresses of their everyday lives (Farquhar, 1978).
- Targeting an entire community rather than a small number of high-risk individuals can have a greater impact on reducing a disease's prevalence on the population level (Rose, 1981, 1992).
- Results of community interventions can be better generalized to a diverse population than those of more controlled clinical trials (Farquhar, 1978; Sorensen et al., 1998; Glasgow, Vogt, and Boles, 1999).
- Primary prevention efforts are essential to diminishing the rate at which new individuals become high-risk (Smedley and Syme, 2001; Syme, 2004).

These observations offer compelling reasons to employ community-oriented research projects as an intervention strategy to combat disease.

The First and Second Generation CVD Community-Based Intervention Trials

The Major CVD Trials of the 1970s and 1980s

The first generation of community-based health promotion campaigns were conceptualized in the 1960s with the intention to reduce the growing rates of CVD at the population level. The pervasiveness of CVD in the United States, the many etiologic risk factors, and their well-established relationship to individual and social behaviors made CVD an ideal focus for these first community-based interventions (Rose, 1981; Lefebvre, Harden, and Zompa, 1988; Shea and Basch, *Part I*, 1990; Parker and Assaf, 2005). Based in part on evidence presented by prominent epidemiologist Geoffrey Rose (1992) as well as concepts from social ecology theory (Bandura, 1969 and 1971; Kotler and Zaltman, 1971), it was hypothesized that by targeting the entire community, widespread sustainable health changes could be achieved.

The very first programs of the 1960s followed almost exclusively a medical framework, which emphasized targeting high-risk individuals only (Blackburn, 1983). The strategy evolved during the 1970s and 1980s, in part because of the seminal Framingham Heart Study (initiated in 1948) that presented epidemiological surveillance data demonstrating that individual behaviors were associated with coronary heart disease (Dawler, 1980). The new approach shifted the target of such programs from high-risk individuals to entire communities, with the strategy of modifying both individual behaviors and also the social environment in which behaviors develop.

The two major pioneer community-based CVD campaigns were conducted in the early 1970s in North Karelia, Finland, and three small communities near Stanford University in California. Both studies employed multifaceted interventions to address the behavioral and social risk factors for CVD and were successful in reducing the CVD burden in the intervention communities.

The North Karelia Project (NKP) delivered an intervention to citizens in North Karelia whose residents were, on average, of low SES and had one of the highest rates of CVD mortality in the world. This region was compared to a matched reference community. The campaign was initiated at the request of community members who were concerned about the high rates of CVD in their province. Central campaign features included a mass media education program, risk factor testing, tracking and follow-up, as well as integrating the intervention community programs with primary medical care (Salonen, Puska, and Mustaniemi, 1978; Tuomilehto et al., 1980; Puska et al., 1998; N. Record et al., 2000; Parker and Assaf, 2005). Significant sustained reductions were found in smoking prevalence, cholesterol levels, blood pressure, and CVD morbidity and mortality rates as compared to a matched reference community (Puska et al., 1983; Shea and Basch, *Part II*, 1990; Schooler et al., 1997; Vartiainen et al., 2000).

The Stanford Three-Community Project (STCP), which was conceptualized and implemented concurrently with the NKP, also had a significant impact on intervention community members' health-related behavior. The aims and interventions were similar to those of the NKP, with the exception of primary medical care integration, which was not a focus of the STCP (Farquhar et al., 1977). Instead, the major thrust was a rigorous mass media campaign, reaching the entire community through radio, television, billboards, and mail. The STCP compared two intervention communities (both of which included the media campaign and one that additionally received individual and group counseling) to a reference community, which received neither intervention. Significant favorable changes were observed for smoking rates, blood pressure, cholesterol, CVD knowledge, saturated fat intake, and CVD risk (Farquhar et al., 1977; Fortmann et al., 1981; Shea and Basch, *Part II*, 1990).

The two projects demonstrated that natural entities within a community, including health professionals, political leaders, local institutions, and citizens, could work together to shift the trajectory of unhealthy trends. These studies provided the impetus and basic framework for the three other major community-based CVD campaigns that were conducted in the United States in the early 1980s. The Stanford Five-City Project (SFCP), the Pawtucket Healthy Heart Program (PHHP), and the Minnesota Healthy Heart Program (MHHP), all of which were funded by the National Heart, Lung, and Blood Institute, incorporated many strategies from the first generation of studies (NKP and STCP) to test their effectiveness within larger, diverse U.S. populations. These are described below.

Theoretical Basis, Methodology, and Design

The SFCP, PHHP, and MHHP methods, design, and results are summarized briefly below, as they have been described extensively elsewhere (Carlaw et al., 1984; Farquhar et al., 1985; Fortmann et al., 1986; Assaf et al., 1987; Carleton et al., 1987; Lasater, Lefebvre, and Carleton, 1988; Luepker et al., 1994; Carleton et al., 1995; Murray, 1995; Luepker et al., 1996; Winkleby, 1996). The studies used concepts from social ecology theory to guide program development and implementation. This broad theory integrates several multidisciplinary perspectives to address the interactive biological, individual, and environmental factors that influence health. It is beyond the scope of this chapter to review these theoretical foundations. Several references are listed below for those seeking more extensive background (Bandura, 1969, 1971; Kotler and Zaltman, 1971; Lefebvre et al., 1987; Flora and Farquhar, 1988; Shea and Basch, *Part I*, 1990).

The studies shared many organizational similarities (Table 13-1). Each utilized a quasi-experimental design because randomized city selection was precluded by constraints concerning independent media outlets and the need for cities to share similar demographic characteristics. Outcomes were measured using data from a longitudinal cohort study, independent samples, and epidemiologic surveillance of CVD morbidity and mortality.

The studies also shared similar objectives. Each primarily sought to achieve a lasting reduction in the prevalence of CVD health behavioral risk factors and a significant decline in CVD morbidity and mortality. The interventions addressed many of the risk factors known to contribute to CVD, including poor nutrition, sedentary lifestyle, cigarette smoking, elevated serum cholesterol levels, and hypertension. All involved the following health promotion intervention strategies to varying degrees: education through mass media (print and/or electronic media), groups, schools, worksites, and medical settings; weight loss or smoking contests, and restaurant and grocery store menu/shelf labeling (Lefebvre, Harden, and Zompa, 1988; Hunt et al., 1990; Shea and Basch, *Part II*, 1990).

The studies differed, however, in the emphasis of intervention programs, process measures, and maintenance efforts. In regard to program emphasis, the SFCP intervention utilized electronic and print media to deliver the

TABLE 13-1 Comparison of the Study Characteristics of the Stanford Five City Project, the Pawtucket Healthy Heart Program, and the Minnesota Healthy Heart Program

Study Characteristic	Trial		
	Stanford Five City Project[a]	Pawtucket Healthy Heart Program[b]	Minnesota Healthy Heart Program[c]
Participant selection	Random selection of eligible participants (12–74 years old who live in household for at least 6 months of year) through city directories of households	Random selection of eligible participants (18–64 years old) through city directory of households and city street lists in comparison city	Random selection of eligible participants (25–74 years old) through census-identified blocks. Further randomization included the selection of geographically adjacent groups of five households
Location	Northern California; Intervention: Salinas and Monterey; Reference: San Luis Obispo, Modesto, Santa Maria	New England; Intervention: Pawtucket, Rhode Island; Reference: unnamed New England community	Upper Midwest; Intervention: Mankato, Minnesota; Fargo-Moorhead, North Dakota/Minnesota; Bloomington, Minnesota; Reference: Winona, Minnesota; Sioux Falls, South Dakota; Roseville, Minnesota
Community type	Small towns	Mid-sized blue-collar towns	Isolated towns, mid-sized cities, and suburban areas
Population	Salinas: 80,000; Monterey: 45,000; San Luis Obispo: 34,000; Modesto: 130,000; Santa Maria: 40,000	Pawtucket: 70,000; Reference: 100,000	Isolated towns: 30,000; Suburban areas: 80,000; Cities: 110,000
Racial/ethnic makeup	Intervention: 88% non-Hispanic White; Reference: 80% non-Hispanic White	Pawtucket: 1.4% Black; Reference: 2.7% Black	Not Available
Education level	Intervention: 11.8–14 years; Reference: 12.5–14 years	Pawtucket: 50% had graduated from high school; Reference: 38%	Intervention: 64% had graduated from high school; Reference: 53%

(Continued)

TABLE 13-1 *(Continued)*

Study Characteristic	Trial		
	Stanford Five City Project[a]	Pawtucket Healthy Heart Program[b]	Minnesota Healthy Heart Program[c]
Average income	Intervention: 43% of families made <$20,000/year; Reference: 51.4%	Pawtucket: $16,000; Reference: $14,000	Not Available
Years of study	1978–1992	1980–1993	1980–1991
Years of intervention	1980–1986	1982–1990	1981–1989

Sources: [a]Farquhar et al., 1985; Fortmann, Taylor, and Winkleby, 1993; Winkleby, Feldman, and Murray, 1997; Fortmann and Varady, 2000.
[b]Weisbrod et al., 1991; Carleton et al., 1995.
[c]Lefebvre et al., 1987; Luepker et al., 1994; Weisbrod, Pirie, and Bracht, 1992.

majority of the campaign's educational messages. These strategies served a smaller role in PHHP and MHHP; the media were used instead to increase awareness about CVD and provide information about available programs and opportunities for involvement (Mittelmark et al., 1986). Unlike the SFCP, systematic risk factor screening programs, referrals for medical care, and individual counseling were central features of the PHHP and MHHP (Lasater, Lefebvre, and Carleton, 1988). The PHHP was distinctive in that churches served as a major modality of campaign information and programs. Additionally, although all three campaigns used lay volunteers to deliver segments of the intervention, this was a major emphasis of the PHHP. Unique features of the MHHP included risk-factor tracking and participant follow-up. The MHHP also devoted the majority of their efforts to face-to-face interaction (Schooler et al., 1997).

Process measures were organized, monitored, and evaluated for each study to ensure the fidelity of the interventions and that the programs were delivered appropriately (Wolff, 2001). Each study had distinct methods to evaluate the effectiveness and reach of their programs. This ongoing assessment provided feedback to the study investigators to modify a specific program's strategy or delivery when it was needed. Pirie and colleagues (1994) outlined a typology of several process measures employed in community-oriented health promotion interventions. This schema has been adapted to pertain to the specific objectives of this chapter.

- *Formative evaluation*: assessing the specific characteristics and needs of the target population in the design stages of the study to ensure that program messages are appropriate, understandable, and applicable
- *Quality assurance*: monitoring program implementation to ensure that the programs are meeting their intended purpose and to examine study participants' satisfaction
- *Assessment of delivered intervention dose*: quantifying the number of programs or program messages disseminated in the intervention community
- *Assessment of received intervention dose*: quantifying the number of programs or program messages *actually* received by the target and comparison communities; this includes programs or messages coming from sources unaffiliated with the campaign
- *Impact of intervention subcomponent*: assessing whether subsets of the multifaceted interventions are having their anticipated impact and how they are contributing to the overall program results
- *Community impact*: determining how community organizational units perceived the intervention impact on the community

Table 13-2, also adapted from Pirie et al., 1994, presents a summary of some of the process measures used by the three studies as they fit into the categories listed above.

Investigators of all three campaigns recognized the importance of intervention monitoring systems to evaluate the progress and reach of the individual programs. However, because community-based programs followed a synergistic approach, it was extremely difficult to determine the contribution of individual programs to the overall results (Mittelmark et al., 1993). As a result, investigators relied on various methods to ensure the programs were serving their intended purpose. Formative evaluation was integral to the design of the campaigns' interventions. The PHHP developed the most elaborate participant-tracking system, which enabled investigators to identify the strengths and weaknesses of programs and to adapt and rapidly implement necessary changes. The SFCP and the MHHP used more informal methods to ascertain this information.

Outcome Measure Results

Throughout and after the completion of the studies, substantial literature emerged deconstructing the successes and failures of the CVD trials. By examining many of these articles, it became evident that investigators often arrived at remarkably different conclusions, although virtually all of the literature post-study completion concluded that no substantial health improvements had occurred. Much of the discrepancy between investigators' analyses stems from the data used for evaluation. Data were collected at several intervals during and after each study. Additionally, data were collected for both longitudinal cohorts and cross-sectional samples. Researchers, thus, had several options of data sets from which to choose. The results of a paper that used data comparing the "peak intervention" to baseline, for example, may have differed greatly from a paper that compared "post-intervention" data to the baseline. As emphasized earlier, one of the principal goals of community-based interventions is to achieve sustainability of the programs and, as a result, longevity of behavioral and health change. Thus, the outcomes of most interest are those that were evaluated *after* the interventions had ended. These findings are elucidated in the subsequent paragraphs and tables.

The major goals of the SFCP were to achieve a lasting reduction in the prevalence of CVD risk factors and a significant decline in CVD morbidity and mortality (Winkleby et al., 1996). However, the results of the study indicated that despite the multifaceted interventions employed, the intervention showed limited, variable, and often insignificant impact in engendering these changes. Table 13-3 presents these.

TABLE 13-2 Comparison of the SFCP, PHHP, and PHHP Evaluation Methods

Process Measure	Trial		
	Stanford Five City Project[a]	Pawtucket Healthy Heart Program[b]	Minnesota Healthy Heart Program[c]
Formative Evaluation	Focus groups, interviews, surveys, pilot tests, in-depth analysis of baseline risk factor data	Focus groups, interviews with community agencies, analysis of baseline risk factor data	Focus groups, interviews, pilot tests, community analysis to assess resources
Quality Assurance	Informal system of interviews with program participants and community members	Follow-up telephone surveys of participants	Exit interviews, follow-up phone calls, telephone surveys of participants and those who declined to participate
Assessment of Delivered Dose	Tabulated the number of face-to-face and media messages delivered, media ratings for television programs, content analysis of newspapers in treatment and reference cities, Community Education Monitoring System	Database tracked participants' contacts through contact cards to determine the number and nature of participants, local newspaper content tracking for health-related articles	Tabulated attendance at program events and audience characteristics, evaluation studies of randomly selected population samples, Community Education Monitoring System
Assessment of Received Dose	Telephone surveys of entire community to assess program and message awareness, content analysis of newspapers in intervention and reference cities	Telephone surveys to assess program and message awareness, newspaper content analysis for health related articles and cigarette advertisements,	Telephone surveys of entire community to assess program and message awareness

(Continued)

TABLE 13-2 (Continued)

Process Measure	Trial		
	Stanford Five City Project[a]	Pawtucket Healthy Heart Program[b]	Minnesota Healthy Heart Program[c]
		interviews with health agencies to document secular trends for CVD interventions carried out by other agencies	
Impact of Intervention Sub-component	Experimental and quasi-experimental studies of individual programs	Experimental and quasi-experimental studies of individual programs	Experimental and quasi experimental studies of individual programs
Community Impact	Institutional changes were evaluated through interviews with key individuals regarding alterations in organization structure and policies	Surveys of physicians, assessment of changes of food availability in supermarkets and restaurants, newspaper content analysis	Telephone surveys of providers of health promotion programs in communities and worksites, restaurant managers, and physicians

Sources: [a]Flora et al., 1993; Fortmann et al., 1993; Schooler, Flora, and Farquhar, 1993; Schooler, Sundar, and Flora, 1996.
[b]Assaf et al., 1987; Lefebvre et al., 1987; Lefebvre et al., 1988; Carleton et al., 1995; Carleton, Lasater, and Assaf, 1995.
[c]Shea and Basch, Part II.

TABLE 13-3   The Stanford Five City Project Major Objectives and Results

Objectives	Results
Significant decline in CVD morbidity and mortality rates	CVD morbidity and mortality rates declined uniformly; three-year follow-up revealed that CVD morbidity and mortality rates were maintained or improved in treatment cities while they leveled out or rebounded in reference cities. However, differences were not significant except in coronary heart disease risk for women in intervention cities
Decline in Body Mass Index (BMI)	BMI rose uniformly. The increase was significantly smaller in the treatment communities in the cross-sectional surveys, but not in the cohort. Three-year follow-up revealed no significant between-city difference among women and a significant difference in men, favoring control cities
2% decline in relative weight	Weight increased uniformly; no significant between-city differences
Increase in physical activity	No significant between-city difference
9% decrease in smoking frequency	Significant declines in intervention cities in the cohort by study's end; none noted in the independent samples. Three-year follow-up revealed that rates leveled or increased in treatment cities, while declines in control cities continued. Between-city differences were not significant
Decline in alcohol consumption	Alcohol consumption declined uniformly; rates were not maintained at three-year follow-up
Increased CVD knowledge	Treatment cities had significantly greater net improvements in CVD knowledge as compared to reference cities in the independent samples. At three-year follow-up, CVD knowledge had improved uniformly, but the improvements were significantly greater in the reference cities
4 % decline in cholesterol levels	Significant intervention improvements in the cohort up to the third survey; effect dissipated by the fourth survey. No significant between-city difference in cholesterol levels at three-year follow-up
7% reduction in blood pressure (BP)	Blood pressure declined uniformly; significant difference noted only in cohort. Three-year follow-up revealed that improvements were maintained in the intervention cities only. Significant between-city differences were observed among men only

Sources: Farquhar et al., 1990; Fortmann et al., 1990; Taylor et al., 1991; Fortmann, Taylor, and Jatulis, 1993; Young et al., 1993; Winkelby, 1994; Winkelby et al., 1996; Young et al., 1996; Parker and Assaf, 2005; Verheijden and Kok, 2005.

Results from the 3-year follow-up revealed that there were, for the most part, no significant differences in CVD morbidity and mortality between treatment and reference communities (Winkleby et al., 1996). Although there were declines in sodium intake, smoking frequency, alcohol consumption, cholesterol levels, and blood pressure (BP) in the intervention communities, these trends were also evident in the reference communities, and the between-city differences were not significant. During the intervention, treatment cities in the independent samples had significantly greater net improvements in CVD knowledge than control cities. After the follow-up, however, the improvements shifted and were significantly greater in the reference cities. Maintained significant differences were observed in a few cases, such as a decline in BP among men in treatment cities. School-based interventions, although not depicted in the table, had notable success at 1-year follow-up. Among the students in intervention classes, significant changes were observed in healthy behaviors and health knowledge (Fortmann et al., 1993; Mittelmark et al., 1993). Like the SFCP, the PHHP aimed to reduce the prevalence of CVD risk factors and thus CVD morbidity and mortality rates (Carleton et al., 1987). The data presented in Table 13-4, most of which were collected 3 years after the program ended, similarly demonstrate very limited support for achieving these goals.

No sustained statistically significant between-city differences were observed in physical activity, smoking prevalence, CVD knowledge, cholesterol levels, or BP in the PHHP. Although at-peak intervention CVD morbidity and mortality rates were significantly lower in the intervention community, the difference had disappeared in 3-year post-intervention. The projected CVD risk declined in each city, but the difference was not significant. The same trends were evident in the cohort data. BMI was the only risk factor for which the between-city difference was significant. Although BMI rose among all individuals in both communities, the increase was significantly smaller in Pawtucket. However, this result was limited to males, younger persons, and individuals with lower education levels. Positive treatment effects were noted among those who participated in the church-based education component of the intervention compared to baseline. Significant improvements were observed in dietary behaviors and practices as compared to baseline levels.

The MHHP results largely mirror those of the SFCP and the PHHP. These are presented in Table 13-5. Consistent with the findings of the two aforementioned studies, very few statistically significant between-city differences were observed in the MHHP. Improvements were noted in smoking prevalence among women and those who received school-based interventions and also physical activity (Perry et al., 1992).

TABLE 13-4   The Pawtucket Healthy Heart Program Major Objectives and Results

Objectives	Results
15% reduction in total fatal and non-fatal CVD event rates	CVD risk declined uniformly. A small but significant between-city difference was noted during peak intervention, but this effect dissipated by the three-year follow-up
2% reduction in BMI	BMI increased uniformly. There was a statistically significant relative change between cities in independent samples post-intervention among males, young-persons, and those with less education
Increased physical activity	No significant between-city difference
30% reduction in proportion of active smokers	Prevalence declined uniformly; the between-city difference was not significant
Increased CVD knowledge	CVD knowledge increased uniformly; the between-city difference was not significant
6% reduction in cholesterol levels	Mean cholesterol levels fell uniformly; there was no significant between-city difference
6 mmHg reduction in blood pressure	No significant between-city difference

Sources: Carleton et al., 1995; Derby et al., 1998; Eaton et al., 1999; Gans et al., 1999; Verheijden and Kok, 2005.

TABLE 13-5   The Minnesota Healthy Heart Program Major Objectives and Results

Objectives	Results
15% decline in CVD morbidity and mortality rates	CVD mortality declined uniformly; no significant between-city differences
Decline in BMI	Increased uniformly; no significant between-city difference
50 kcal/day increase in physical activity	Small variable differences noted in intervention communities; no significant between-city differences
3% decline in smoking prevalence	Uniform decline among men; no significant between-city difference. Small significant decline in women in independent samples of intervention cities, but limited evidence of an intervention impact in the cohort
7 mg/dL reduction in cholesterol levels	Mean cholesterol levels fell uniformly; levels were lower in intervention communities during the first three yrs. but higher in final 2 years. None of the between-city differences were significant
2 mmHg decline in blood pressure	No significant between-city differences

Sources: Luepker et al., 1994; Lando et al., 1995; Luepker et al., 1996; Schooler et al., 1997.

323

TABLE 13-6   A Comparison of Intervention Impact and Penetration in the Stanford Five City Project, the Pawtucket Healthy Heart Program, and the Minnesota Healthy Heart Program

Trial		
Stanford Five City Project[a]	Pawtucket Healthy Heart Program[b]	Minnesota Healthy Heart Program[c]
• 59% recalled seeing televised public service announcement • 21% recalled television programs • 40%–60% recalled various print education materials • Each resident was exposed to ~5 hours/year of the study's educational messages	• 42,000 individuals (59%) participated in one or more programs • 55% received screening services only • 10.6% participated in exercise programs	• 60% of adults participated in screening and education programs • 30% received face-to-face interventions • 4.1% of smokers participated in smoking cessation programs compared to 3.1% in comparison areas

Sources: [a]Farquhar et al., 1990; Flora et al., 1993; Fortmann et al., 1995; Parker and Assaf, 2005.
[b]Eaton et al., 1999; Merzel and D'Afflitti, 2003.
[c]Luepker et al., 1994; Murray, 1995; Schooler et al., 1997.

Finally, Table 13-6 presents information regarding the reach of the interventions within the targeted communities. Under the circumstances of most health-related controlled clinical studies, it is relatively simple to tabulate the "dose" of intervention a participant receives (Flora et al., 1993). A multicomponent community intervention, on the other hand, involves many intangible elements such as electronic delivery of the campaigns' programs or educational messages or even person-to-person communication. However, the developers of the SFCP, the PHHP, and the MHHP implemented several measures to evaluate the penetration and reach of their efforts.

It was difficult to recruit and engage a large proportion of the targeted populations for each study. For the SFCP, electronic media was the major thrust of information dissemination, but less than 60% of the population recalled seeing the televised public service announcements and only 21% recalled seeing the educational television programs. Although each resident was exposed to an average of 5 hours of the study's educational messages per year, this number pales in comparison to the inundation of the television advertisements individuals view yearly, estimated at that time to be approximately 292 hours (Farquhar et al., 1990; Fortmann et al., 1995).

The PHHP and the MHHP closely tracked the number of individuals participating in the campaign's events. The emphasis of the interventions for these campaigns was on direct education and group programs. Participation rates for each were relatively well-documented. Nearly 60% of Pawtucket residents participated in one or more of the campaign's events; just over half received screening services only. Similarly, 60% of adults in the MHHP participated in the screening and education programs, and 30% received face-to-face interventions.

The intervention programs had difficulties permeating the deeply entrenched social, cultural, and environmental fabric of the communities. Less than 60% of targeted populations in the SFCP and the PHHP recalled campaign educational messages or participated in any one of the campaigns' programs. The penetration data present the fundamental difficulty of these community interventions: their inability to demonstrate an active engagement with the target population.

Comparing the First and Second Generation CVD Campaigns

The paucity of significant findings in the second generation of CVD interventions (the SFCP, the PHHP, and the MHHP) stands in contrast to the successes of the first generation (the NKP and the STCP) interventions of the 1970s. How can this discrepancy be explained? In the exploration of the pertinent literature, many investigators have found it instructive to consider the unique contexts and circumstances, such as the target population, setting, and timing in which the studies took place (Blackburn, 1983; Schooler et al., 1997; Lindholm and Rosén, 2000; McLaren et al., 2007). First, there were notable differences between the populations targeted in the earlier and later trials. The NKP, for example, was conducted in a region of Finland where the prevalence of CVD risk factors and the risk of coronary heart disease was one of the highest in the world (McAlister et al., 1982; Luepker et al., 1996). The targeted populations of the second generation trials (the SFCP, the PHHP, and the MHHP), conversely, were generally at or below the average risk for CVD (Winkleby, Fortmann, and Rockhill, 1992; Carleton et al., 1995; Fortmann and Varady, 2000). Although there were secular downward trends for CVD risk in the earlier and later studies, individuals in the studies of the 1970s (whose CVD risk was much higher to begin with) had more potential for detectable improvement, as it may have been more feasible to move from very high-risk to high- or moderate-risk as opposed to moving from moderate-risk to low-risk (Luepker et al., 1996).

Similarly, differences also existed between the earlier and later populations regarding nutritional practices. For example, in the first generation studies, declines in saturated fat intake could be achieved through relatively simple behavioral changes, such as substituting low-fat milk with whole milk and replacing butter with healthier oils. By the onset of the second generation studies, many individuals had already implemented these behavioral changes. The later campaigns' nutritional programs advocated behavior changes that may have been more difficult to adopt, such as reducing meat and cheese intake, drinking only non-fat milk, and encouraging vegetarianism (Fortmann et al., 1993).

Second, it is important to consider the setting in which the studies were conducted. The governmental regulation of medical services in Finland may have engendered an environment in which citizens were more receptive to programs endorsed by the government (McAlister et al., 1982; Elder et al., 1993; Schooler et al., 1997). Thus, large-scale policy changes may have been more feasible. One example of governmental involvement was the offering of economic incentives to food producers and distributors in North Karelia to produce and distribute low-fat dairy products to the population. The universal health-care system of Finland may have also been a more conducive environment for implementing successful community-wide campaigns and achieving long-term health improvements.

A third consideration is the contextual circumstances of the studies. Although the second generation studies began only 10 years after the initiation of the NK and STC projects, by the onset of the later studies, CVD had become a much greater concern in the public sphere. National and local health organizations and the media had begun campaigns to promote awareness about the risks of CVD-associated behaviors. Many communities in the second generation of studies had already been exposed to CVD-related education programs. Some cities even had institutionalized programs aimed at reducing CVD behavioral risks, such as the control of smoking in public places (Elder et al., 1993; Mittelmark et al., 1993; Winkleby, Feldman, and Murray, 1997; Merzel and D'Afflitti, 2003). As a result, the second generation CVD prevention trials' educational messages may have lost their novelty and prominence, as they could not overcome the synchronized efforts and messages of external campaigns aimed at the same issues.

Despite these noted differences, there were fundamental problems that the first and second generation of CVD trials shared. These include methodological constraints, lack of community involvement, and the confounding influence of secular trends. However, despite the similarities of the constraints in the first and second generation of CVD trials studies, the unique circumstances during which the first generation studies were conducted may have enabled the detection of significant changes in outcomes between intervention and reference communities.

Why did the Second Generation of U.S. Community Intervention Studies Fail?

The notable successes of the NKP and the STCP trials compared to lack of findings in the second generation trials raises two major questions: What specific factors contributed to the failures of these campaigns? More importantly, given the disappointing outcomes, how do interventionists proceed in the future with community-based prevention interventions?

With regard to the failures of the second generation trials, many explanations have been proposed. The four most prominent explanations include: design and methodological constraints, the limited scope of the interventions, the presence of powerful secular trends, and the lack of community input and integration (Fortmann, Flora, Winkleby, 1995; Winkelby, Feldman, and Murray, 1997; Merzel and D'Afflitti, 2003; Parker and Assaf, 2005).

Design and Methodological Constraints

Fundamental limitations of all observational studies include the difficulty of establishing satisfactory control and analysis measures (Murray et al., 1994). As previously mentioned, the need to identify comparable demographically matched intervention and reference communities renders a randomized controlled trial, considered to be the gold standard of interventional research, nearly impossible (Farquhar, 1978; Berkowitz, 2001). Thus, despite covariate analyses to control for confounding variables, if differences were present between the two groups, the conclusion that the difference was the result of the intervention's efforts cannot exclude the possibility that the changes resulted from factors beyond the intervention.

It has also been suggested that using morbidity and mortality as the major outcome measures in community prevention trials is not an appropriate endpoint. Lindholm and Rosén (2000) claim that various impediments inherent to community-based studies, such as reference group contamination, population mobility bias, and time-lag bias (the period of time needed for risk factor reduction to have full impact), limit the potential to detect significant differences in hard end-points such as morbidity and mortality. Similarly, Berkowitz (2001) contends that traditional research evaluation methods may be too indiscriminate to detect such differences.

Intervention Limitations

A second criticism of the second generation trials' designs was that the interventions may have been too broad and not sufficiently intensive. These interventions were not generally refined or tailored to the diverse subgroups of the target population and thus unlikely to be effective. The interventions may have raised awareness about CVD issues in general but had a limited impact in inducing changes in deeply ingrained behavior among a heterogeneous population (Merzel and D'Afflitti, 2003). For example, although the SFCP developers were cognizant of the large Hispanic population in the treatment communities and designed Spanish education materials for them, they may have overlooked the need to tailor the delivery and content of their messages to this culturally distinct subgroup of the population.

Additionally, certain segments of the population may be more receptive to change than others, and it is important to recognize this distinction when developing interventions (Winkleby, Flora, and Kraemer, 1994; Ribisl et al., 1998). For example, research consistently indicates that there is a disparity in CVD mortality rates, with those who are White, educated, and of higher SES less likely to die from cardiovascular diseases compared to minority groups with lower education and SES levels (Smedley, Stith, and Nelso, 2003; Shaya, Gu, and Saunders, 2006). Pearson et al. (2001) contend that the populations at highest risk for CVD tend to be more resistant to change, underscoring the need to tailor health interventions to specific subpopulations within a broader community-wide intervention. The broad interventions of the second generation CVD trials, which targeted large, diverse populations, may have had more success had they identified population subgroups and designed specific intervention programs for them.

Building upon Pearson and his colleagues' postulation, Winkleby, Flora, and Kraemer (1994) decided to explore this issue of tailoring for the SFCP. They stratified individuals from the intervention communities into four distinct groups based on changes in their CVD risk factor score, comparing those who exhibited the most positive change to those who exhibited the least. Group I consisted of older adults who had the highest baseline BP and cholesterol levels. This group was found to be the most motivated and responsive to the campaign's interventions. Groups II and III were comprised mostly of younger individuals with moderate levels of responsiveness and receptivity to programs put forth by the campaign. Group IV was 40% Hispanic and had the lowest education levels, SES, and baseline CVD knowledge. This group also had the highest smoking rates and was at highest risk for CVD. Individuals in this group were found to be the "most resistant" to change.

It is essential to explore and understand why certain high-risk groups are least receptive to change to develop strategies to reduce the health burdens that disproportionally afflict them. Several variables may contribute to this disparity, including lack of leisure time, inadequate resources, and competing priorities besides CVD reduction. For example, although CVD may be the leading cause of death in a community, if residents live in an area with a high crime rate or high unemployment, they may perceive these threats to be greater than that of CVD (Elder et al., 1993; Stokols, 1996; Hancock et al., 1997).

Secular Trends

It is widely acknowledged that strong secular health trends may have eclipsed the potential intervention effects in the community-oriented interventions of the 1980s (Murray, 1995; Susser, 1995; Winkleby, Feldman, and Murray, 1997; Merzel and D'Afflitti, 2003; Parker and Assaf, 2005). The second generation of CVD interventions were implemented during a period when health-related issues such as smoking, diet, and exercise at the forefront of the public health movement in the United States. The same social forces that led to the concept of population-wide health interventions during the 1970s also stimulated independent public health campaigns across the United States, targeting many of the same health issues promoted by the CVD trials. Although all three second generation CVD trials observed declines in CVD morbidity and mortality and cigarette smoking and saw increases in CVD knowledge in the experimental communities, the same trends were observed in the control communities, reflecting a broader national improvement in CVD-related attitudes and behaviors. The concomitant efforts of the campaigns' interventions and the secular effect of systemic changes experienced in U.S. society during the same time period may have nullified or concealed any of the campaigns' true intervention effects.

Modest Community Engagement

A fundamental difficulty in population-wide health promotion interventions is genuinely engaging the community in the design, implementation, and maintenance stages of the programs. Comprehensive collaboration with community members should encompass their active participation in all stages of the campaign and engender a sense of ownership. The achievement of a true sense of community ownership of public health campaigns has been an elusive challenge, however, as organizations external to the community generally select the health concern to be targeted as well as the intervention strategies (Jackson et al., 1994; Green, Daniel, and Novick, 2001). This can be especially problematic because community residents and local leaders, rather than external program developers, know and understand the characteristics and needs of their own community. Community stakeholders are best suited to select effective interventions and targets because of this innate knowledge. Additionally, when a community is empowered and motivated to confront an issue affecting their population, as was observed for CVD in the NKP, community members and local organizations seem to be more receptive to the intervention programs.

To illustrate varying degrees of community engagement in the SFCP, the PHHP, and the MHHP, Table 13-7 compares aspects of engagement, including the presence of a community board, community involvement in issue selection, program development, implementation, and maintenance.

TABLE 13-7 A Comparison of the Level of Community Engagement in the Stanford Five City Project, the Pawtucket Healthy Heart Program, and the Minnesota Healthy Heart Program

	Trial		
	Stanford Five City Project[a]	Pawtucket Healthy Heart Program[b]	Minnesota Healthy Heart Program[c]
Community Board	A Community Board, comprised of local leaders and residents representing various segments of the population, was responsible for advisory, directory, and gate-keeping roles	A Church Advisory Board (CAB), comprised of church leaders, provided resources to parishes that wanted to participate in heart health programming	A Community Advisory Board, comprised of community leaders who were identified through formative analysis, coordinated education activities and formed smaller task forces to help develop program activities
Community Involvement in Issue Selection	No	No	No
Community Involvement in Program Development	No	Yes	Yes
Community Involvement in Implementation	Local organizations delivered the majority of the campaign's messages	Volunteers and local organizations, with a strong emphasis on churches, were responsible for carrying out many of the programs	Volunteers carried out many of the programs. Additionally, project staff worked with physicians and health care professionals to alter practice in the healthcare settings

| Community Involvement in Program Maintenance | The "Community Health Promotion Program of Monterey County" was established to continue the campaign's programs after the study ended, but dissolved three-years after. The Monterey County Health Department took over at this point. | Program maintenance was an established objective; specific details were not enumerated about the extent of the maintenance phase beyond the continuance of certain program elements through the local Parks and Recreation Department | Three years post-research phase, 61% of MHHP programs were operated by local providers |

Sources: [a]Shea and Basch, *Part II*, 1990; Jackson et al., 1994; Schooler et al., 1997.
[b]Carleton et al., 1987; Lefebvre et al., 1987; Shea and Basch, *Part II*, 1990.
[c]Blackburn, 1983; Bracht, 1988; Shea and Basch, *Part II*, 1990; Weisbrod, Pirie, and Bracht, 1992; Bracht et al., 1994; Jeffery et al., 1995.

All three campaigns established community advisory boards to help with different aspects of the intervention programs. Each board served a distinct function. The SFCP board, for example, was used for general advisory purposes. The PHHP board, on the other hand, was comprised of church leaders who helped to allocate campaign materials and deliver educational programs. The MHHP advisory committee was formed through extensive formative analysis of the community, in which leaders in the community were identified and asked to sit on the committee. The board was active in coordinating activities and forming smaller task forces to address different components of the intervention campaign.

Despite efforts to facilitate community engagement in all phases of the campaigns, a recurring problem was that often, the partnerships between local entities and the study investigators were externally imposed and devoid of real community input and direction. This resulted in the campaign researchers selecting the intervention targets and methods of delivery rather than the community itself. Over time, the investigators did attempt to incorporate the community in other dimensions, such as certain aspects of program development (PHHP and MHHP) and the implementation of intervention programs. The PHHP, in particular, was responsive to data it received from its tracking system. The PHHP leadership found that there was a slow rate of organizational involvement, group participation, and volunteer recruitment, in addition to minimal penetration of the program's efforts into the greater community during the initial phases of the study. This feedback helped shape the next phase of the study, which focused on community-wide programming in addition to the organization-based efforts (Lefebvre et al., 1988).

All campaigns included in their design a maintenance phase to shift the CVD intervention programs from the study designers to local resources. This transition proved to be a complicated undertaking, as members of the transition team encountered various barriers that impeded a smooth shift of responsibilities. According to Jackson and her colleagues (1994), for the SFCP in particular, these barriers included interagency competition for limited resources, insufficient time and resources for the established agencies to raise funds and organize program continuance, and conflicts with agencies' established programs and objectives that were often dictated by state and national organizations. Still, local organizations continued to carry out a number of campaign programs after the formal intervention concluded.

The engagement of the community in the planning stages of the intervention, throughout the campaign and after the intervention ends, may lead to more positive results. As discussed above, although the second generation CVD interventions incorporated the community in several aspects of the interventions, each also had gaps in fundamental areas, most strikingly in the selection of issues and the method of delivery of campaign programs.

Community Trials Beyond CVD: HIV, Smoking, Diabetes, and Obesity

It is instructive to examine community-based trials that address health issues beyond CVD. Although not an exhaustive review of the literature, the hope is that by illuminating some of the successes and failures of these campaigns, strategies for improving community-wide interventions can be developed for many public health concerns. It is important to reiterate that although the projects that will be discussed in the subsequent paragraphs followed a general community intervention framework, many differ from the CVD studies of the 1970s and 1980s in that they target high-risk groups only or individuals already presenting with the disease or risk factor.

HIV Campaigns

Community-oriented efforts to curtail the mounting prevalence of HIV were first implemented in the early 1990s. The results of a small number of comprehensive community-based studies conducted across the United States demonstrated that these interventions were often successful in modifying high-risk behaviors such as sexual practices and/or injection-related drug use (Kelly et al., 1991; Kelly et al., 1992; Holtgrave et al., 1995; *AIDS Community Demonstration Projects*, 1996; Kegeles, Hays, and Coates, 1996; Kelly et al., 1997). These findings, which provide evidence for the potential of community-wide prevention programs to bring about changes in health-related behaviors, stand in contrast to the CVD prevention campaigns of the 1980s discussed in the previous sections.

Interestingly, the HIV and CVD studies shared many structural and organizational similarities. These included similar theoretical approaches that served as the basis of the quasi-experimental study design, intervention strategies, data collection and analysis, and minimal emphasis on policy changes (Janz et al., 1996; Merzel and D'Afflitti, 2003). Moreover, large favorable secular trends were present in both the CVD and HIV studies.

What elements of the HIV-focused prevention efforts distinguish it from the CVD campaigns and what can be gained from their experiences? An excellent analysis by Merzel and D'Afflitti (2003) addresses these questions. Their main observations are summarized below. It is important to note that there are inherent differences between the nature of the diseases and the targeted populations, which may render HIV a more promising target of community interventions. First, HIV is communicable and can be contracted through relatively few incidents of high-risk behavior; even a small lapse can have dire consequences. CVD, conversely, is characterized by a complex interaction of risk factors, multiple risk factor etiology, and a substantial time delay between risk factor exposure and disease manifestation. Thus, because HIV poses a more "immediate" threat and can generally be avoided through concrete behavior changes such as condom use, there may be a greater motivation for modifying behavior and adopting safer practices.

A second notable difference between HIV and CVD campaigns is the target population. Unlike the CVD campaigns that delivered interventions to a large, diverse community, the HIV campaigns targeted relatively small homogenous population subgroups. As a result, HIV interventions were designed specifically for those subgroups most at risk of becoming infected with HIV.

Despite these fundamental differences, important lessons can be gained from the experiences of the HIV campaigns. First, a major feature of HIV community programs was the extensive use of formative research in the initial stages of the studies. Such analyses enabled researchers to define discrete population subgroups that were most in need of interventions as well as to identify key leaders and community members to help promote and disseminate the campaigns' messages (Higgins et al., 1996). With the help of the community members and leaders, the researchers were able to develop highly tailored interventions that addressed the specific needs and the social environment of the targeted populations. This strategy may be useful for future CVD studies. As discussed earlier, it may also be beneficial to identify distinct subgroups of the population and design targeted strategies to get them engaged in addition to the generalized population-wide interventions.

A second distinction is the emphasis of HIV campaigns on altering the normative practices and social milieu in which behaviors are shaped. A number of researchers sought to modify attitudes and behavior by designing interventions that involved "peer role models" from the target population in the implementation and endorsement of the risk-modifying programs (Simons et al., 1996; Kelly, 1999). An assessment of 37 HIV prevention campaigns found that the use of trained community peer role models whose life circumstances and characteristics reflected those of the target population was one of the most important factors influencing the acceptance of health messages (Janz et al., 1996). Although the second generation CVD interventions also used community volunteers to deliver many of the campaign programs and messages, the HIV campaigns had a strong emphasis on identifying and training trustworthy community role models to provide education on health information and behavioral change techniques. The shared experience that these peer educators had with the target group might have contributed to their success.

The success community HIV prevention campaigns have had in modifying behaviors and norms and curtailing high-risk behaviors reveals the potential for community-wide interventions to bring about health improvements at the population level. Major lessons from the HIV campaigns include the need to identify distinct subgroups of the target population and to understand the ways in which they can be actively engaged. Additionally, such studies show the promise of using community peers or "role models" to deliver the programs in all stages of the campaign and to help modify social attitudes and norms.

Smoking Campaigns

Community-based prevention programs that targeted cigarette smoking have also been attempted with variable results. Gnich (2004) conducted a comprehensive literature review of community initiatives in which smoking cessation was a component or the chief target of the intervention. She found that although a majority of studies demonstrated significant behavioral outcomes in at least one area, the magnitude of the impact was minimal and smaller than anticipated.

For example, the well-known COMMIT trial had mixed outcomes. The study was a randomized, controlled, community- based effort that sought to increase the "quit rate" among heavy cigarette smokers as well as to reduce smoking prevalence in 11 intervention communities (*COMMIT I and II*, 1995). The intervention included education through the media and community events, cessation efforts, and involvement of health-care providers, work sites, and local organizations. Results of the 4-year effort indicated that the intervention did not significantly alter quit rates among heavy smokers. A modest but significant intervention effect was noted, however, among light-to-moderate smokers, particularly among the least educated subgroup, suggesting that an exclusive focus on smoking reduction may have promise in this dimension.

Another study, the "Neighbors for a Smoke Free North Side," sought to reduce smoking prevalence in three low-income, predominantly Black neighborhoods in St. Louis (Fisher et al., 1998). The 2-year intervention involved smoking cessation classes, door-to-door efforts, community programs, and the media. Smoking prevalence declined significantly in intervention communities as compared to reference neighborhoods. The results suggest promise in targeting more homogenous city neighborhoods and refining strategies that meet the needs of area residents.

However, the drastic 50% reduction in smoking prevalence over the last 50 years, when nearly half of the U.S. population smoked, did not occur because smokers enrolled in cessation classes or participated in smaller-scale smoking reduction campaigns, such as those mentioned in the preceding paragraphs. Rather, the reduction was the cumulative effect of broad public health and public policy changes that have been implemented over many years. These have drastically altered the social environment and thus the public perception of smoking (Syme, 2004, 2007). Such large-scale policy efforts were initiated in response to a growing literature that documented the harmful effects of tobacco use. The public health policies and environmental constraints include bans on smoking in public places, targeting the dangers of secondhand smoke, a rise in cigarette prices and taxes, anti-tobacco advertising, restrictions on tobacco advertising, and lawsuits against tobacco companies (Smedley and Syme, 2001; McLeroy et al., 2003; Brownson, Haire-Joshu, and Luke, 2006).

The widespread systemic changes that occurred over the past 60 years were instrumental in altering the perception of tobacco use and thus greatly reducing the number of smokers in the United States. The successes highlight two important lessons. First, large-scale efforts that address complex behaviors and deeply embedded social norms may require a longer period of time for large-scale changes to be observed. Second, widespread policy changes may be necessary to alter the normative environment in which behaviors are developed.

Diabetes Campaigns

Community-based health initiatives have also been carried out for Type 2 diabetes. These studies have served as a guide in the design of the Sinai Urban Health Institute (SUHI) Type 2 Diabetes Prevention project (Whitman et al., 2010). A major distinction will be the role of the community in the projects' designs. The diabetes studies delineated below generally targeted and recruited individuals already exhibiting Type 2 diabetes, rather than entire communities or high-risk groups. Despite this difference, there are lessons to be learned from their efforts. Of particular interest is the fact that the diabetes studies demonstrated greater success in modifying some of the same unhealthy behaviors that were targeted in the CVD studies of the 1970s. What strategies were employed that seemed to facilitate the favorable changes?

Satterfield et al. (2003) conducted a systematic literature review of community-based interventions conducted from 1990 to 2001 in which the aim was to reduce diabetes onset and complications associated with the disease. Their search revealed a sparse collection of studies in this domain, particularly in areas of primary prevention. This review illuminated the need for further research, given the growing burden of Type 2 diabetes, particularly among minority groups and low-income individuals who are disproportionately affected (Smedley, Stith, and Nelso, 2003; Marshall, 2005).

Since 2001, when the Satterfield et al. review was conducted, several interesting studies were carried out that targeted minority populations with diabetes. These studies demonstrated appreciable success in ameliorating behavioral risk factors associated with diabetes. Two examples are diabetes campaigns conducted in Detroit and Charlotte. Racial and Ethnic Approaches to Community Health 2010 (REACH), an initiative through the Centers for Disease Control and Prevention (CDC) in which the aim was to eliminate racial and ethnic disparities in health, implemented successful diabetes programs in these cities (DeBate et al., 2004; Two Feathers et al., 2005; Kieffer et al., 2006; Plescia, Herrick, and Chavis, 2008). The REACH Detroit partnership employed a multifaceted community-based approach to target Black and Latinos in low-income neighborhoods of Detroit. Although participants were recruited through hospitals and community clinics, the intervention was based on the major principles of community-based participatory research. A steering committee was established that was comprised of health leaders, health-care providers, researchers, and REACH Detroit staff. Extensive focus groups were conducted with community residents to guide all aspects of the intervention. The central strategic feature was using community support groups to educate and teach techniques for healthy diabetes-related behaviors. The vast majority of the selected participants participated in at least one of the intervention programs. Significant differences between intervention and reference groups were found in diabetes-related knowledge (e.g., dietary behavior vegetable and whole-grain bread consumption, cooking practices and soda consumption) and HbA1c levels.

The Charlotte REACH program, which targeted an area that was 90% Black, also had favorable results. Significant declines in physical inactivity and tobacco use among women and middle-aged adults were observed by study's end (DeBate, 2004; Prescia, 2008).

The results of both REACH 2010 studies suggest that a culturally sensitive, community-wide health campaign delivered by local residents can significantly improve glycemic control and improve risk factors associated with diabetes. The positive outcomes may partly result from the cultural tailoring of the intervention materials for the targeted Black and Latino communities, the use of local community members in all stages of the campaign, and the frequency and nature of the intervention's educational classes.

Another intervention with similar methods of the REACH studies, known as the Starr County Border Health Initiative (Brown and Hanis, 1999; Brown et al., 2002), targeted Mexican-Americans in a community bordering Texas and Mexico. The emphasis of the intervention included weekly educational sessions in addition to support groups. Peer role models with Type 2 diabetes were utilized to advocate in support the campaign for behavioral modification strategies.

The experimental group had significantly lower HbA1c and fasting blood glucose levels at 6 and 12 months in addition to higher diabetes knowledge scores when compared to a reference group. The study demonstrates the effectiveness of a culturally sensitive campaign on improving diabetes outcomes of Mexican-Americans.

Another campaign targeting a largely Hispanic population with diabetes was the Hispanic Chronic Disease Self-Management Initiative, a 6-week randomized community-oriented trial (Lorig, Ritter, and Gonzalez, 2003). Trained community health workers delivered support groups in Spanish at local settings, discussing the disease and offering techniques for maintaining a healthier lifestyle. A 4-month post-intervention follow-up revealed improvements in health behaviors, health status, and self-efficacy in addition to reductions in health-care utilization. After 1 year, improvements were maintained or improved.

Like Blacks and Hispanics in the United States, Native Americans also suffer disproportionately from Type 2 diabetes. The "Strong in Body and Spirit" campaign was designed for Native-American adults with diabetes living in New Mexico (Gilliland et al., 2002). The intervention integrated both clinical care and community participatory principles. A major focus of the intervention was incorporating traditional Native-American values and foods. By the end of the study, participants in the intervention group had better glycemic control and less weight gain than those in the control group.

A final study of note conducted in a low-income urban community in Norway is distinguished from the diabetes campaigns above because it incorporated the community to a greater degree in its design (Jenum et al., 2006). The campaign promoted physical activity as a means to reduce diabetes complications. The intervention included exercise classes, culturally sensitive health counseling, walking groups, and education programs. Broader environmental changes included new signage and development of walking trails and improved street lighting to increase accessibility to and feasibility of exercise. Individuals in the experimental arm of the study significantly improved on the frequency of physical activity, cholesterol levels, and blood pressure and glucose levels in men.

These studies, with a focus on diabetes and behavioral change across a number of diverse communities, underscore the idea that individuals and communities who are disproportionately burdened with a disease can be effectively targeted and their health outcomes improved.

Obesity Campaigns

Obesity has also been a target for community-based campaigns, as its onset is largely determined by behavior. Similarly to the previously mentioned health campaigns, the degree of community engagement has varied from study to study. One recent study stands out because it involved genuine community engagement and collaboration and had remarkably positive outcomes. A 12-year campaign was carried out in two communities in northern France with the aim to curtail the country's overweight and obesity epidemic in children (Westley, 2007; Levi, Segal, and Juliano, 2008; Romon et al., 2008; Katan, 2009). By involving every sector of the small intervention community, including the mayor and the local government, shop owners, school teachers, doctors, nutritionists, caterers, restaurant owners, sports associations, and the media, substantial benefits were observed. Five years into the study, the prevalence of overweight in children in the intervention town had fallen to 8.8%, whereas it had risen to 17.8% in the neighboring reference towns, reflecting the greater national trend. Intensive efforts by the intervention communities included building new sports facilities and playgrounds, training teachers to deliver school-based nutrition classes, offering healthy cooking classes and individual counseling to families, mapping out and highlighting walking paths, hiring sports instructors, and instituting a comprehensive referral and feedback system. This approach, known as the EPODE Study, is currently being employed in 200 towns across Europe.

The results suggest that a multifaceted community-based intervention targeting a single risk factor, conducted over a long period of time, and genuinely owned by the community can significantly improve population health outcomes.

Future of Community Interventions

The modest results of the community-based CVD campaigns of the 1980s raise questions about the future of broad public health targeted interventions to combat chronic disease. One interpretation would simply be that community-based health campaigns are ineffectual forms of interventions. However, the results of the health campaigns discussed in the preceding section seem to indicate the potential viability of this design for certain outcomes. Such community-based interventions should not be abandoned but must be modified to encompass recommendations from recent studies and address modern circumstances.

A community health promotion campaign is a valuable strategy for reducing the burden of disease because it incorporates the inextricably bound elements that contribute to disease, including one's environment and social interactions. Unlike more reductionist-controlled clinical trials that generally involve a homogenous group of participants, community-wide campaigns target representative populations within their natural social and cultural setting (Glasgow, Vogt, and Boles, 1999; Minkler, 1999). If interventionists can move beyond their focus on the individual and acknowledge the complex mediating forces that shape behavior and health, then future researchers may have more success involving the community as an "empowered partner" to improve health outcomes (Syme, 2004).

This chapter's examination of the CVD trials and health promotion interventions targeting HIV, smoking, diabetes, and obesity has helped to illuminate elements that have contributed to the successes and failures of these public health campaigns. Enumerated in the succeeding section are four major recommendation areas based on the lessons learned from the studies reviewed.

Recommendation 1: Select the Target Condition to Foster Improved Health

The modification of deeply ingrained habits and behaviors requires voluntary sustained effort on the part of the individual. Based on the outcomes of the community-based trials reviewed, enduring favorable health and behavioral changes were facilitated by the presence of two inherent characteristics: the "urgency of behavior change" and the presence of a feedback system.

The "urgency of behavior change" characterizes the immediacy of the threat. The redeeming health benefits or the "pay-off" for modifying behavior to avoid certain diseases or risk factors may take years to manifest or may produce negligible perceptible improvements in a person's lifetime. An instructive analogy is the situation of anti-hypertensive medications used to lower one's blood pressure. Although the long-term physiological benefits of the medications, such as stroke and cardiac arrest risk reduction, are significant, the associated side effects (frequent urination, erectile dysfunction, persistent cough, etc.) or lack of perceptible improvements may prevent one from taking the medication regularly. Thus, the deleterious consequences of CVD and other chronic diseases may be sufficiently remote and delayed such that individuals place greater value on the short-term satisfaction of engaging in their deeply entrenched behaviors.

Another consideration in the selection of a target condition is whether a feedback system is in place or can be developed. A feedback system is a useful component in interventions because it provides participants with immediate information regarding their behavioral changes. With diabetes, for example, the post-meal feedback from blood glucose tests enables individuals to see how the food they ingest affects their glucose levels. Accordingly, they can alter their food intake based on this number. A feedback system can be established in other ways as well. The Franklin Cardiovascular Health Program, a small-scale community-based intervention (initiated in 1974) conducted in towns throughout Maine, demonstrated positive outcomes for CVD over 20 years (N. Record et al., 2000). A unique feature of this program was an emphasis on physician and nurse involvement. In addition to genuine community-wide education efforts, frequent individual clinic visits with nurses provided participants with risk factor screening and tracking, counseling, referrals for medical care, and active client follow-up. The study authors cite this intensive feedback system as a contributor to the demonstrated enduring health changes.

Future investigators may want to consider these elements when selecting a disease or risk factor to target when employing a community-based research approach.

Recommendation 2: Conduct Formative Research and Design Refined Interventions for Target Population Subgroups

The segmentation of a diverse population into more distinct subgroups has been shown to enhance program impact on attitudes and behavior (Slater and Flora, 1991; Schooler et al., 1997). Thus, extensive formative research to assess the make-up and needs of the community should be a focus of future interventions. For example, individuals with low education levels and SES, many of whom are racial or ethnic minorities, are at high risk for developing and dying from heart disease, yet these individuals are often the hardest to reach (Winkleby, Flora, and Kraemer, 1994). When population subgroups at high risk for developing disease are identified, they must be targeted specifically.

Recommendation 3: Emphasize Primary Prevention and Focus on the Social Determinants of Health

Reversing poor health trends requires effective primary prevention programs. A major feature of future interventions should be to develop better preventive measures and proactive strategies to reduce population-wide risk of disease. Even if interventionists could successfully mitigate the health problems plaguing individuals already exhibiting disease risk factors, this would not necessarily diminish the rate at which new individuals become "high-risk," thus propagating the cycle (Smedley and Syme, 2001; Syme, 2004). Instead of focusing exclusively on individual risk factors and secondary prevention, interventionists should seek to address the underlying forces that cause and perpetuate disease.

In addition, it may be important to consider strategies that incorporate both community-oriented health promotion principles to address the social and behavioral determinants of health as well as local primary medical practice. Diseases such as CVD that are characterized by complex etiologies may require this amalgam of approaches. The NKP and the previously mentioned

Franklin CVD Campaign in Maine demonstrated notable success following such an integrated strategy.

Recommendation 4: Multifaceted Intervention Strategies for Sustained Change

The success of future campaigns may depend on a synergistic approach that utilizes various channels within the community to promote the intervention's messages once the research phase ends. Communities are diverse entities and each resident responds differently to the intervention's programs (Winkleby, 1994). Therefore, multiple strategies should be employed to ensure broad reach and longevity of behavior change.

Additionally, many of the CVD campaigns demonstrated favorable behavioral health trends during the apex of the intervention, but the effect often dissipated in sync with the gradual conclusion of the study. Thus, sustained interventions that become integrated into standard practice of the community are likely an essential ingredient of successful community campaigns. This was demonstrated in the community-wide pediatric obesity study in France; the community itself was empowered to continue the nutritional- and physical activity-centered programs endorsed by the campaign.

It has been widely argued that a facilitating factor to achieve such sustainability is the inclusion of structural, policy, and environmental change strategies (Schwartz et al., 1993; Jeffery et al., 1995; Stokols, 1996; Israel et al., 1998; Glasgow, Vogt, and Boles, 1999; Green, Daniel, and Novick, 2001; Smedley and Syme, 2001; Brownson, Haire-Joshu, and Luke, 2006; Doyle, Furey, and Flowers, 2006). These strategies have the capacity to benefit all individuals exposed without requiring much active and voluntary effort on their part. The NKP and the tobacco initiatives of the past 50 years have revealed the potential for policy interventions to facilitate change in the social environment in which behaviors are formed.

Although the universities and institutions that carry out community research are not necessarily in the position to influence broad policy changes, there is promise for this dimension to be explored and developed. One such example, mentioned previously, is The Border Health Strategic Initiative, a community-based effort to curtail the growth of diabetes among Hispanics living in Arizona–Mexico border communities (Cohen, Meister, and de Zapien, 2004; Meister and de Zapien, 2005; Hill et al., 2007). A major feature of this campaign was the establishment of special action groups (SAGs) whose purpose was to advocate for policy and infrastructure change in their communities. SAG leaders were employed to influence policy by mobilizing large numbers of residents to attend city council or board of supervisors meetings. They successfully facilitated policy change in the communities,

TABLE 13-8   Summary of Facilitating Factors in Successful Community Based Campaigns

- Selecting a target condition for which there is great personal motivation and relative ease of instituting changes
- Presence of a feedback system within the intervention as well as on the individual level
- Segmenting a diverse target population into more homogenous subgroups and design distinct interventions that address their individual characteristics and needs
- Emphasis on primary prevention
- Selecting appropriate start and end points to assess physical and behavioral change
- Effective integration of social and cultural interventions with primary medical care
- History of positive working relationship between research organization and community (including local organizations, government, business owners, and community members)
- Identifying and employing trustworthy community peer role models to endorse the behavioral changes of the intervention and deliver segments of the intervention
- Major emphasis on planning and facilitating a transfer of responsibilities from campaign designers to local organizations
- Including in the design a sub-committee to work towards achieving broader policy and environmental changes within the community

which led to the development of parks and walking trails and the creation of healthier food options at local grocery stores.

Thus, embedding an intervention's messages within the social and environmental fabric of the community may be a major facilitating factor needed to sustain efforts through time and to ensure lasting change.

The four major recommendation areas delineated in the preceding paragraphs may point a way forward as interventionists embark on genuine community-based endeavors in the future. To enhance the planning and design of such campaigns, a concise summary of 10 facilitating factors exhibited in successful campaigns is presented below (Table 13-8).

Conclusion: Community-Based Participatory Research, Engagement, and Translational Science

In recent years, health promotion research campaigns utilizing community-based participatory research (CBPR) approaches have gained support and acceptance in the field of public health. A major feature that distinguishes participatory research from other public health community efforts is the notion that the community is viewed not as the setting in which an intervention is carried out but rather as an active partner throughout the research process (Higgins and Metzler, 2001; Metzler et al., 2003). This collaborative partnership is enhanced when there is a history of prior positive relationships between the "external" organization leading the project and the community itself (Schooler et al., 1997; Israel et al., 1998; Lantz et al., 2001; Israel et al., 2006).

And although CBPR may be considered an idealized or perhaps a romanticized model of public health research, it is important to consider how the theoretical underpinnings are translated into practical intervention strategies and "real-life" circumstances. This chapter's examination of studies employing participatory approaches has revealed that although interventionists may have recognized the importance of involving the community in all phases of the campaign, most were unable to achieve genuine community engagement.

Given the rising incidence of disease with significant social etiological components in recent years, strategies directed at cure alone will be inadequate to stem their rapid trajectory. This observation is the basis for much of Geoffrey Rose's research. The thesis of his seminal book "The Strategy of Preventive Medicine" (1992), a culmination of much of his earlier work is that health interventions are most effective if they focus on communities rather than individuals. His main points are summarized below:

1. In general health conditions exist on a continuum in a population;
2. Medicine or health care pays most attention to a "disease" that is defined as existing beyond a cut-point of the distribution in an extreme tail (e.g., glucose tolerance test > 140 → diabetes or blood pressure > 140/90 mm Hg → hypertension, etc.). Rose referred to this as the "individual approach" or the "high-risk strategy";
3. Paying most (or all) of our attention to this extreme part of the distribution does not allow us to work with the remainder of the population to help improve its health and to truly prevent disease. Rose referred to working with the entire distribution of people as the "population approach" and urged us to consider the "continuum of risk"; and
4. Rose's conclusion is that preventive medicine must embrace both of these approaches but argues that "of the two, power resides with the population strategy."

Thus, the path is available for improved health for all people. As often as possible, it should employ a community-based approach, and whenever possible, it should regard the community as agent in pursuing and creating its own health and destiny. One must regard the failed community-based interventions around cardiovascular disease outcomes as one might view a failed treatment for a disease, not as a clarion call to abandon community interventions but, rather, a time to redouble efforts to design more effective community participatory-based interventions—ones that truly engage with the community in their own improvement efforts. The lesson from Rose's work is that population based interventions have to be the major focus of disease reduction strategies. The lesson from the literature review on CBPR is that for these population based public health efforts to be effective they need to engage the community in a meaningful manner. The path to meaningful public health improvement in the United States can best be achieved by applying Rose's strategies with true CBPR efforts.

Acknowledgments

I would like to acknowledge Dr. Steve Whitman and the Sinai Urban Health Institute team for their support and feedback in making this chapter possible. It was an honor working with and learning from them.

References

Aiken, Michael and Paul Mott. 1970. *The structure of community power.* New York: Random House.

Andersson, Camilla, Gunilla Bjaras, Per Tillgren, and Claes-Goran Ostenson. 2003. Health promotion activities in annual reports of local governments. *European Journal of Public Health* 13: 235–239.

Assaf, AnnLouise, Stephen Banspach, Thomas Lasater, Sonja McKinlay, and Richard Carleton. 1987. The Pawtucket Heart Health Program II: evaluation strategies. *Rhode Island Medical Journal* 70: 541–546.

Bandura, Albert. 1969. *Principles of behavior modification.* New York: Rinehart and Winston.

Bandura, Albert. 1971. *Social learning theory.* Morristown, New Jersey: General Learning Press.

Berkowitz, Bill. 2001. Studying the outcomes of community-based coalitions. *American Journal of Community Psychology* 29(2): 213–227.

Blackburn, Henry. 1983. Research and demonstration projects in community cardiovascular disease prevention. *Journal of Public Health Policy* 4(4): 398–421.

Bracht, Neil. 1988. Use of community analysis methods in community-wide intervention programs. *Scandinavian Journal of Primary Health Care* Suppl. 1: 23–30.

Bracht, N., J. Finnegan, C. Rissel, R. Weisbrod, Julie Gleason, Julia Corbett, et al.1994. Community ownership and program continuation following a health demonstration project. *Health Education Research* 9: 243–255.

Brown, Sharon, Alexandra Garcia, Kamiar Kouzekanani, and Craig Hanis. 2002. Culturally competent diabetes self-management education for Mexican Americans. *Diabetes Care* 25 (2): 259–268.

Brown, Sharon and Craig Hanis. 1999. Culturally competent diabetes education for Mexican Americans: the Starr County Study. *The Diabetes Educator* 25 (2): 226–236.

Brownson, Ross, Debra Haire-Joshu, and Douglas Luke. 2006. Shaping the context of health: A review of environmental and policy approaches in the prevention of chronic diseases. *Annual Review of Public Health* 27: 341–370.

Carlaw, Raymond, Maurice Mittlemark, Neil Bracht, and Russel Luepker. 1984. Organization for a community cardiovascular health program: experiences from the Minnesota Heart Health Program. *Health Education & Behavior* 11: 243–252.

Carleton, Richard, Thomas M. Laseter, R. Craig Lefebvre, and Sonja M. McKinlay. 1987. The Pawtucket Heart Health Program I: An experiment in population-based disease prevention. *Rhode Island Medical Journal* 70: 533–538.

Carleton, Richard, Thomas Lasater, Annlouise Assaf, Henry Feldman, and Sonja McKinlay. 1995. The Pawtucket Heart Health Program: Community changes in cardiovascular risk factors and projected disease risk. *American Journal of Public Health* 85: 777–785.

Carleton, Richard, Thomas Lasater, and Annlouise Assaf. 1995. The Pawtucket Heart Health Program: progress in promoting health. *Rhode Island Medical Journal* 78: 74–77.

Cohen, Stuart, Joel Meister, and Jill DeZapien. 2004. Special action groups for policy change and infrastructure support to foster healthier communities on the Arizona-Mexico border. *Public Health Reports* 119: 40–47.

Centers for Disease Control and Prevention. 1996. Community-level prevention of human immunodeficiency virus infection among high-risk populations: The AIDS community demonstration projects. *Morbidity and Mortality Weekly Report 45(RR-6)*: 1–24.

Dawler, T.R. 1980. *The Framingham Study--the epidemiology of atherosclerotic disease.* Cambridge: Harvard University Press.

DeBate, Rita, Marcus Plescia, Dennis Joyner, and LaPronda Spann. 2004. A qualitative assessment of Charlotte REACH: An ecological perspective for decreasing CVD and diabetes among African Americans. *Ethnicity and Disease* 14(Supp. 1): S77–S82.

Derby, Carol, Henry Feldman, Linda Bausserman, Donna Parker, Kim Gans, and Richard Carleton. 1998. HDL cholesterol: trends in two southeastern New England communities, 1981-1993. *Annals of Epidemiology* 8 (2): 84–91.

Doyle, Y.G., A. Furey, and J. Flowers. 2000. Sick individuals and sick populations: 20 years later. *Journal of Epidemiology and Community Health* 60: 396–398.

Eaton, Charles, Kate Lapane, Carol Garber, Kim Gans, Thomas Lasater, and Richard Carleton. 1999. Effects of a community-based intervention on physical activity: The Pawtucket Heart Health Program. *American Journal of Public Health* 89(11): 1741–1744.

Elder, John, Sarah McGraw, David Abrams, Andrea Ferreira, Thomas Lasater, Helene Longpre, et al.1986. Organizational and community approaches to community-wide prevention of heart disease: The first two years of the Pawtucket Heart Health Program. *Preventive Medicine* 15: 107–117.

Elder, John, Thomas Schmid, Phyllis Dower, and Sonja Hedlund. 1993. Community heart health programs: Components, rationale, and strategies for effective interventions. *Journal of Public Health Policy* 14 (4): 463–479.

Farquhar, John. 1978. The community-based model of life style intervention trials. *American Journal of Epidemiology* 108 (2):103–111.

Farquhar, John, Peter Wood, Henry Breitrose, William Haskell, Anthony Meyer, Nathan Maccoby, et al. 1977. Community education for cardiovascular health. *The Lancet*: 1192–1195.

Farquhar, John, Stephen Fortmann, June Flora, C. Barr Taylor, William Haskell, Paul Williams, et al. 1990. Effects of communitywide education on cardiovascular disease risk factors. *Journal of the American Medical Association* 264(3): 359–365.

Farquhar, John, Stephen Fortmann, Nathan Maccoby, William Haskell, Paul Williams, June Flora, et al.1985. The Stanford Five-City Project: Design and methods. *American Journal of Epidemiology* 122: 323–334.

Fisher, Edwin, Wendy Auslander, Janice Munro, Cynthia Arfken, Ross Brownson, and Nancy Owens. 1998. Neighbors for a smoke free north side: Evaluation of a community organization approach to promoting smoking cessation among African Americans. *American Journal of Public Health* 88 (11): 1658–1663.

Flora, June, and John Farquhar. 1988. Methods of message design: Experiences from the Stanford Five City Project. *Scandinavian Journal of Primary Health Care* Suppl. 1: 39–47.

Flora, June, R. Craig Lefebvre, David Murray, Elaine Stone, Annlouise Assaf, Maurice Mittelmark, et al. 1993. A community education monitoring system: Methods from the Stanford Five-City Project, the Minnesota Heart Health Program and the Pawtucket Heart Health Program. *Health Education Research* 8 (1): 81–95.

Fortmann, Stephen and Ann Varady. 2000. Effects of a community-wide health education program on cardiovascular disease morbidity and mortality. *American Journal of Epidemiology* 152 (4): 316–323.

Fortmann, Stephen, C. Barr Taylor, and Darius Jatulis. 1993. Changes in adult cigarette smoking prevalence after 5 years of community health education: The Stanford Five-City Project. *American Journal of Epidemiology* 137: 82–96.

Fortmann, Stephen, C. Barr Taylor, June Flora, and Marilyn Winkleby. 1993. Effect of community health education on plasma cholesterol levels and diet: The Stanford Five-City Project. *American Journal of Epidemiology* 137 (10): 1039–1055.

Fortmann, Stephen, June Flora, Marilyn Winkleby, Caroline Schooler, C.Barr Taylor, and John Farquhar. 1995. Community intervention trials: Reflections on the Stanford Five-City Project experience. *American Journal of Epidemiology* 142(6): 576–586.

Fortmann, Stephen, Marilyn Winkleby, June Flora, William Haskell, and C. Barr Taylor. 1990. Effect of long-term community health education on blood pressure and hypertension control. *American Journal of Epidemiology* 132 (4): 629–646.

Fortmann, Stephen, Paul Williams, Stephen Hulley, William Haskell, and John Farquhar. 1981. Effect of health education on dietary behavior: The Stanford Three Community Study. *The American Journal of Clinical Nutrition* 34: 2030–2038.

Fortmann, Stephen, William Haskell, Paul Williams, Ann Varady, Stephen Hulley, and John Farquhar. 1986. Community surveillance of cardiovascular diseases in the Stanford Five-City Project. *American Journal of Epidemiology* 123: 656–669.

Gans, Kim, Susan Assmann, Anthony Sallar, and Thomas Lasater. 1999. Knowledge of cardiovascular disease prevention: An analysis from two New England communities. *Preventive Medicine* 29: 229–237.

Gilliland, Susan, Stanley Azen, Georgia Perez, and Janette Carter. 2002. Strong in body and spirit: Lifestyle intervention for Native American adults with diabetes in New Mexico. *Diabetes Care* 25: 78–83.

Glasgow, Russel, Thomas Vogt, and Shawn Boles. 1999. Evaluating the public health impact of health promotion interventions: The RE-AIM framework. *American Journal of Public Health* 89 (9): 1322–1327.

Gnish, Wendy. 2004. *Community-based interventions to promote non-smoking: A systematic review.* Edinburgh: University of Edinburgh.

Green, Lawrence, Mark Daniel, and Lloyd Novick. 2001. Partnerships and coalitions for community-based research. *Public Health Reports* 116(Suppl. 1): 20–31.

Hancock, Lynne, Rob Sanson-Fisher, Alexander Reid, Margot Schofield, Tony Tripodi, Raoul Walsh, et al. 1997. Community action for health promotion: A review of methods and outcomes 1990-1995. *American Journal of Preventive Medicine* 13(4): 229–239.

Higgins, Donna, Kevin O'Reilly, Nathaniel Tashima, Cathleen Crain, Carolyn Beeker, Gary Goldbaum, et al. 1996. Using formative research to lay the foundation for community level HIV prevention efforts: An example from the AIDS community demonstration projects. *Public Health Reports* 111(Suppl. 1): 28–35.

Higgins, Donna and Marilyn Metzler. 2001. Implementing community-based participatory research centers in diverse urban settings. *Journal of Urban Health: Bulletin of the New York Academy of Medicine* 78(3): 488–494.

Hill, Anne, Jill Guernsey De Zapien, Joel Meister, Lisa Staten, Deborah Jean McClelland, Rebecca Garza, et al. 2007. From program to policy: Expanding the role of community coalitions. *Preventing Chronic Disease* 4(4): 1–12. Online. Available: http://www.cdc.gov/pcd/issues/2007/oct/07_0112.htm. Accessed: December 18, 2009.

Holtgrave, David, Noreen Qualls, James Curran, Ronald Valdiserri, Mary Guinan, and William Parra. 1995. An overview of the effectiveness and efficiency of HIV prevention programs. *Public Health Reports* 110(2): 134–146.

Hunt, Mary, R. Craig Lefebvre, Mary Lynne Hixson, Stephen Banspach, Annlouise Assaf, and Richard Carleton. 1990. Pawtucket Heart Health Program point-of-purchase nutrition education programs in supermarkets. *American Journal of Public Health* 80(6): 730–732.

Israel, Barbara, Amy Schulz, Edith Parker, and Adam Becker. 1998. Review of community-based research: Assessing partnership approaches to improve public health. *Annual Review of Public Health* 19: 173–202.

Israel, Barbara, Amy Schulz, Lorena Estrada-Martinez, Shannon Senk, Edna Viruell-Fuentes, Antonia Villarruel, et al. 2006. Engaging urban residents in assessing neighborhood environments and their implications for health. *Journal of Urban Health: Bulletin of the New York Academy of Medicine* 83(3): 523–539.

Israel, Barbara, James Krieger, Gary Tang, David Vlahov, Sandra Ciske, Mary Foley, et al. 2006. Challenges and facilitating factors in sustaining community-based participatory research partnerships: Lessons learned from the Detroit, New York City and Seattle urban research centers. *Journal of Urban Health: Bulletin of the New York Academy of Medicine* 83(6): 1022–1040.

Jack, Leonard, Leandris Liburd, Frank Vinicor, Gene Brody, and Velma McBride Murry. 1999. Influence of the environmental context on diabetes self-management: A rationale for developing a new research paradigm in diabetes education. *The Diabetes Educator* 25(5): 775–790.

Jackson, Christine, Stephen Fortmann, June Flora, Robert Melton, John Snider, and Diane Littlefield. 1994. The capacity-building approach to intervention maintenance implemented by the Stanford Five City Project. *Health Education Research* 9(3): 385–396.

Janz, Nancy, Marc Zimmerman, Patricia Wren, Barbara Israel, Nicholas Freudenberg, and Rosalind Carter. 1996. Evaluation of 37 AIDS prevention projects: successful approaches and barriers to program effectiveness. *Health Education & Behavior* 23(1): 80–97.

Jeffery, Robert, Clif Gray, Simone French, Wendy Hellerstedt, David Murray, Russel Luepker,et al.1995. Evaluation of weight reduction in a community intervention for cardiovascular disease risk: Changes in body mass index in the Minnesota Heart Health Program. *International Journal of Obesity* 19: 30–39.

Jenum, Anne, Sigmund Anderssen, Kare Birkeland, Ingar Holme, Sidsel Graff-Iversen, Catherine Lorentzen, et al. 2006. Promoting physical activity in a low-income multiethnic district: Effects of a community intervention study to reduce risk factors for type 2 diabetes and cardiovascular disease. *Diabetes Care* 29 (7): 1605–1612.

Katan, Martijn. 2009. Weight-loss diets for the prevention and treatment of obesity. *The New England Journal of Medicine* 360 (9): 923–925.

Kegeles, Susan, Robert Hays, and Thomas Coates. 1996. The MPowerment project: A community level HIV prevention intervention for young gay men. *American Journal of Public Health* 86: 1129–1136.

Kelly, Jeffrey. 1999. Community-level interventions are needed to prevent new HIV infections. *American Journal of Public Health* 89 (3): 299–301.

Kelly, Jeffrey, Debra Murphy, Kathleen Sikkema, Timothy McAuliffe, Roger Roffman, Laura Solomon, et al. 1997. Randomised, controlled, community-level HIV-prevention intervention for sexual-risk behavior among homosexual men in US cities. *The Lancet* 350: 1500–1505.

Kelly, Jeffrey, Janet St. Lawrence, Yolanda Diaz, L. Yvonne Stevenson, Allan Hauth, Ted Brasfield, Seth Kalichman, Joseph Smith, and Michael Andrew. 1991. HIV risk reduction following intervention with key opinion leaders: an experimental analysis. *American Journal of Public Health* 81: 168–171.

Kelly, Jeffrey, Janet St. Lawrence, Yvonne Stevenson, Allan Hauth, Seth Kalichman, Yolanda Diaz, Ted Brasfield, et al.1992. Community AIDS/HIV risk reduction: The effects of endorsements by popular people in three cities. *American Journal of Public Health* 82: 1483–1489.

Kieffer, Edith, Brandy Sinco, Ann Rafferty, Michael Spencer, Gloria Balmisano, Earl Watt, et al. 2006. Chronic disease-related behaviors and health among African Americans and Hispanics in the REACH Detroit 2010 communities, Michigan, and the United States. *Health Promotion Practice* 7(3): 256S–264S.

Kotler, Philip and Gerald Zaltman. 1971. Social marketing: An approach to planned social change. *The Journal of Marketing* 35 (3): 3–12.

Krieger, Nancy. 1990. Racial and gender discrimination: Risk factors for high blood pressure? *Social Science & Medicine* 30 (12): 1173–1181.

Krieger, Nancy. 1994. Epidemiology and the web of causation: Has anyone seen the spider? *Social Science & Medicine* 39 (7): 887–903.

Krieger, Nancy. 2001. Theories for social epidemiology in the 21st century: An ecosocial perspective. *International Journal of Epidemiology* 30: 668–677.

Krieger, Nancy. 2007. Why epidemiologists cannot afford to ignore poverty. *Epidemiology* 18 (6): 658–663.

Lando, Harry, Terry Pechacek, Phyllis Pirie, David Murray, Maurice Mittelmark, Edward Lichtenstein, et al. 1995. Changes in adult cigarette smoking in the Minnesota Heart Health Program. *American Journal of Public Health* 85 (2): 201–208.

Lantz, Paula, Edna Viruell-Fuentes, Barbara Israel, Donald Softley, and Ricardo Guzman. 2001. Can communities and academia work together on public health research? Evaluation results from a community-based participatory research partnership in Detroit. *Journal of Urban Health: Bulletin of the New York Academy of Medicine* 78: 495–507.

Lasater, Thomas, R. Craig Lefebvre, and Richard Carleton. 1988. The Pawtucket Heart Health Program IV: Community level programming for heart health. *Rhode Island Medical Journal* 71: 31–34.

Lasater, Thomas, Richard Carleton, and R. Craig Lefebvre. 1988. The Pawtucket Heart Health Program V: Utilizing community resources for primary prevention. *Rhode Island Medical Journal* 71: 63–67.

Last, John, J. Abramson, Gary Friedman, Miquel Porta, Robert Spasoff, and Michel Thuriaux, eds. 1995. *A Dictionary of Epidemiology.* New York: Oxford University Press.

Lefebvre, R. Craig, Elizabeth Harden, and Barbara Zompa. 1988. The Pawtucket Heart Health Program III: Social marketing to promote community health. *Rhode Island Medical Journal* 71: 27–30.

Lefebvre, R. Craig, Thomas Lasater, Annlouise Assaf, and Richard Carleton. 1988. Pawtucket Heart Health Program: The process of stimulating community change. *Scandinavian Journal of Health Care* Suppl. 1: 31–37.

Lefebvre, R. Craig, Thomas Lasater, Richard Carleton, and Gussie Peterson. 1987. Theory and delivery of health programming in the community: The Pawtucket Heart Health Program. *Preventive Medicine* 16: 80–95.

Levi, Jeffrey, Laura Segal, and Chrissie Juliano. 2008. Prevention for a healthier America: Investments in disease prevention yield significant savings, stronger communities. Washington DC: *Trust for America's Health.*

Lindholm, L. and M. Rosén. 2000. What is the 'golden standard' for assessing population-based interventions?--problems of dilution bias. *Journal of Epidemiology and Community Health* 54: 617–622.

Lorig, Kate, Phillip Ritter, and Virgina Gonzalez. 2003. Hispanic chronic disease self-management. *Nursing Research* 52 (6): 361–369.

Luepker, Russel, David Murray, Richard Grimm, Peter Hannan, Robert Jeffrey, Harry Lando, et al. 1994. Community education for cardiovascular disease prevention: Risk factor changes in the Minnesota Heart Health Program. *American Journal of Public Health* 84: 1383–1393.

Luepker, Russel, Lennart Rastam, Maurice Mittelmark, Henry Blackburn, Peter Hannan, David Murray, et al. 1996. Community education for cardiovascular disease prevention: Morbidity and mortality results from the Minnesota Heart Health program. *American Journal of Epidemiology* 144: 351–362.

Marshall, Merville C. Jr. 2005. Diabetes in African Americans. *Postgraduate Medical Journal* 81: 734–740.

McAlister, Alfred, Pekka Puska, Jukka Salonen, Jackko Tuomilehto, and Kaj Koskela. 1982. Theory and action for health promotion: Illustrations from the North Karelia Project. *American Journal of Public Health* 72 (1): 43–50.

McLaren, Lindsay, Laura Ghali, Diane Lorenzetti, and Melanie Rock. 2007. Out of context? Translating evidence from the North Karelia project over place and time. *Health Education Research* 22 (3): 414–424.

McLeroy, Kenneth, Barbara Norton, Michelle Kegler, James Burdine, and Ciro Sumaya. 2003. Community-based interventions. *American Journal of Public Health* 93 (4): 529–533.

McLeroy, Kenneth, Daniel Bibeau, Allan Steckler, and Karen Glanz. 1988. An ecological perspective on health promotion programs. *Health Education & Behavior* 15 (4): 351–377.

Mechanic, David. 2005. Policy challenges in addressing racial disparities and improving population health. *Health Affairs* 24 (2): 335–338.

Meister, Joel and Jill Guernsey de Zapien. 2005. Bringing health policy issues front and center in the community: Expanding the role of community health coalitions. *Preventing Chronic Disease* 2 (1): 1–7. Online. Available: http://www.cdc.gov/pcd/issues/2005/jan/04_0080.htm. Accessed: December 18, 2009.

Merzel, Cheryl and Joanna D'Afflitti. 2003. Reconsidering community-based health promotion: Promise, performance, and potential. *American Journal of Public Health* 93 (4): 557–574.

Metzler, Marilyn, Donna Higgins, Donald Softley, Carolyn Beeker, Nicholas Freudenberg, Paula Lantz, et al. 2003. Addressing urban health in Detroit, New York City, and Seattle through community-based participatory research partnerships. *American Journal of Public Health* 93 (5): 803–811.

Minkler, Meredith. 1999. Personal responsibility for health? A review of the arguments and the evidence at century's end. *Health Education and Behavior* 26 (1): 121–140.

Mittelmark, Maurice, Mary Hunt, Gregory Heath, and Thomas Schmid. 1993. Realistic outcomes: lessons from community-based research and demonstration programs for the prevention of cardiovascular diseases. *Journal of Public Health Policy* Winter 14 (4): 437–460.

Mittelmark, Maurice, Russel Luepker, Rebecca Mullis, David Murray, Terry Pechacek, Cheryl Perry, et al. 1986. Community-wide prevention of cardiovascular disease: education strategies of the Minnesota Heart Health Program. *Preventive Medicine* 15 : 1–17.

Murray, David. 1995. Design and analysis of community trials: lessons from the Minnesota Heart Health Program. *American Journal of Epidemiology* 142 (6): 569–575.

Murray, David, Peter Hannan, David Jacobs, Paul McGovern, Linda Schmid, William Baker, et al. 1994. Assessing intervention effects in the Minnesota Heart Health Program. *American Journal of Epidemiology* 139 (1): 91–103.

Parker, Donna and Annlouise Assaf. 2005. Community interventions for cardiovascular disease. *Primary care: Clinics in office practice* 32: 865–881.

Pearson, Thomas C. Lewis, Stig Wall, P.L. Jenkins, Anne Nafziger, and L. Weinhall. 2001. Dissecting the 'black box' of community intervention: Lessons from community-wide cardiovascular disease prevention programs in the US and Sweden. *Scandinavian Journal of Public Health* 29 (Suppl. 56): 69–78.

Perry, Cheryl, Steven Kelder, David Murray, and Knut-Inge Klepp. 1992. Communitywide smoking prevention: Long-term outcomes of the Minnesota Heart Health Program and the class of 1989 study. *American Journal of Public Health* 82 (9): 1210–1216.

Pirie, Phyllis, Elaine Stone, Annlouise Assaf, June Flora, and Ulrike Maschewsky-Schneider. 1994. Program Evaluation strategies for community-based health promotion programs: Perspective from the cardiovascular disease community research and demonstration studies. *Health Education Research* 9 (1): 23–26.

Plescia, Marcus, Harry Herrick, and LaTonya Chavis. 2008. Improving health behaviors in an African American community: The Charlotte Racial and Ethnic Approaches to Community Health Project. *American Journal of Pubic Health* 98 (9): 1678–1684.

Puska, Pekka, Jukka Salonen, Aulikki Nissinen, Jaakko Tuomilehto, Erkki Vartiainen, Heikki Korhonen, et al. 1983. Change in risk factors for coronary heart disease during 10 years of a community intervention programme (North Karelia project). *The British Medical Journal* 287: 1840–1844.

Puska, Pekka., Erkki Vartiainen, Jaakko Tuomilehto, Veikko Salomaa, and Aulikki Nissinen. 1998. Changes in premature deaths in Finland: Successful long-term prevention of cardiovascular diseases. *Bulletin of the World Health Organization* 76 (4): 419–425.

Record, N. Burgess, David Harris, Sandra Record, Jane Gilbert-Arcari, Michael DeSisto, and Sheena Bunnell. 2000. Mortality impact of an integrated community cardiovascular health program. *American Journal of Preventive Medicine* 19 (1): 30–38.

Ribisl, Kurt, Marilyn Winkleby, Stephen Fortmann, and June Flora. 1998. The interplay of socioeconomic status and ethnicity on Hispanic and White men's cardiovascular disease risk and health communication patterns. *Health Education Research* 13 (3): 407–417.

Romon, Monique, Agnes Lommez, Muriel Tafflet, Arnaud Basdevant, Jean Michel Oppert, Jean Jouis Bresson, et al. 2009. Downward trends in the prevalence of childhood overweight in the setting of 12-year school- and community-based programmes. *Public Health Nutrition* 12 (10):1735–1742.

Rose, Geoffrey. 1981. Strategy of prevention: lessons from cardiovascular disease. *British Medical Journal* 282: 1847–1851.

Rose, Geoffrey. 1985. Sick individuals and sick populations. *International Journal of Epidemiology* 14: 32–38.

Rose, Geoffrey. 1992. *Rose's strategy of preventive medicine*. New York: Oxford University Press.

Salonen, Jukka, Pekka Puska, and Harri Mustaniemi. 1979. Changes in morbidity and mortality during comprehensive community programme to control cardiovascular diseases during 1972-7 in North Karelia. *British Medical Journal* 2: 1178–1183.

Satterfield, Dawn, Michele Volansky, Carl Caspersen, Michael Engelgau, Barbara Bowman, Ed Gregg, et al. 2003. Community-based lifestyle interventions to prevent type 2 diabetes. *Diabetes Care* 26: 2643–2652.

Schooler, Caroline, John Farquhar, Stephen Fortmann, and June Flora. 1997. Synthesis of findings and issues from community prevention trials. *Annals of Epidemiology* 7 (57): S54–S68.

Schooler, Caroline, June Flora, and John Farquhar. 1993. Moving toward synergy: media supplementation in the Stanford Five-City Project. *Communication Research* 20 (4): 587–610.

Schooler, Caroline, S. Shyam Sundar, and June Flora. 1996. Effects of the Stanford Five-City project media advocacy program. *Health Education & Behavior* 23 (3): 346–364.

Schwartz, Randy, Carol Smith, Marjorie Speers, Linda Dusenbury, Frank Bright, Sonja Hedlund, et al. 1993. Capacity building and resource needs of state health agencies to implement community-based cardiovascular disease programs. *Journal of Public Health Policy* 14: 480–494.

Shaya, Fadia, Ana Gu, and Elijah Saunders. 2006. Addressing cardiovascular disparities through community interventions. *Ethnicity and Disease* 16: 138–144.

Shea, Steven and Charles Basch. 1990. A review of five major community-based cardiovascular disease prevention programs. Part I: Rationale, design, and theoretical framework. *American Journal of Health Promotion* 4: 203–210.

Shea, Steven and Charles Basch. 1990. A review of five major community-based cardiovascular disease prevention programs. Part II: Intervention strategies, evaluation methods, and results. *American Journal of Health Promotion* 4: 279–286.

Simons, Paul, Cornelis Rietmeijer, Steven Kane, Carolyn Guenther-Grey, Donna Higgins, and David Cohn. 1996. Building a peer network for a community level HIV prevention program among injecting drug users in Denver. *Public Health Reports* 111 (Suppl. 1): 50–53.

Slater, Michael and June Flora. 1991. Health lifestyles: Audience segmentation for public health interventions. *Health Education Quarterly* 18: 221–234.

Smedley, Brian, Adrienne Stith, and Alan Nelso. 2003. *Unequal treatment: Confronting racial and ethnic disparities in healthcare.* Washington, DC: National Academies Press.

Smedley, Brian and S. Leonard Syme. 2001. Promoting health: Intervention strategies from social and behavioral research. *American Journal of Health Promotion* 15 (3): 149–166.

Sorensen, Glorian, Karen Emmons, Mary Kay Hunt, and Douglas Johnston. 1998. Implications of the results of community intervention trials. *Annual Review of Public Health* 19: 379–416.

Stokols, Daniel. 1996. Translating social ecological theory into guidelines for community health promotion. *American Journal of Health Promotion* 10 (4): 282–298.

Susser, Mervyn. 1995. Editorial: The tribulations of trials--interventions in communities. *American Journal of Public Health* 85 (2): 156–158.

Syme, S. Leonard. 2004. Social determinants of health: The community as an empowered partner. *Public Health Research, Practice, and Policy* 1, 1: 1–5. Online. Available: http://www.cdc.gov/pcd/issues/2004/jan/03_0001.htm. Accessed: December 18, 2009.

Syme, S. Leonard. 2007. The prevention of disease and promotion of health: The need for a new approach. *European Journal of Public Health* 17(4): 329–330.

Taylor, C. Barr, Stephen Fortmann, June Flora, Susan Kayman, Donald Barrett, Darius Jatulis, et al. 1991. Effect of long-term community health education on body mass index. *American Journal of Epidemiology* 134 (3): 235–249.

The COMMIT Research Group. 1995. Community intervention trial for smoking cessation (COMMIT): I. Cohort Results from a four-year community intervention. *American Journal of Public Health* 85: 183–192.

The COMMIT Research Group. 1995. Community intervention trial for smoking cessation (COMMIT): II. Changes in adult cigarette smoking prevalence. *American Journal of Public Health* 85: 193–200.

Tuomilehto, Jaakko, Jukka Salonen, Aulikki Nissinen, and Thomas Kottke. 1980. Community programme for control of hypertension in North Karelia, Finland. *Lancet* October 25; 2(8200): 900–904.

Two Feathers, Jacqueline, Edith Kieffer, Kiberlydawn Wisdom, Sherman James, Gloria Palmisano, Mike Anderson, et al. 2005. Racial and ethnic approaches to community health (REACH) Detroit partnership: Improving diabetes-related outcomes among African American and Latino adults. *American Journal of Public Health* 95(9): 1552–1560.

Vartiainen, Erkki, Pekka Jousilahti, Georg Alfthan, Jouko Sundvall, Pirjo Pietinen, and Pekka Puska. 2000. Cardiovascular risk factor changes in Finland, 1972-1997. *International Journal of Epidemiology* 29: 49–56.

Verheijden, Marieke and Frans Kok. 2005. Public health impact of community-based nutrition and lifestyle interventions. *European Journal of Clinical Nutrition* 59(Suppl. 1): S66–S76.

Warren, Roland. 1972. *The community in America.* Chicago, IL: Rand McNally.

Weisbrod, Rita, Neil Bracht, Phyllis Pirie, and Sara Veblen-Mortenson.1991. Current status of health promotion in four midwest cities. *Public Health Reports* 106(3): 310–317.

Weisbrod, Rita, Phyllis Pirie, and Neil Bracht. 1992. Impact of a community health promotion program on existing organizations: The Minnesota Heart Health Program. *Social Science & Medicine* 34 (6): 639–648.

Westley, Hannah. 2007. Thin living. *British Medical Journal* 335: 1236–1237.

Whitman Steven, Jose E. Lopez, Steven K. Rothschild, Jaime Delgado. 2010. Disproportionate impact of diabetes in a Puerto Rican Community of Chicago. In *Urban health: Combating health disparities with local data.* eds. Steven Whitman, Ami M. Shah, and Maureen R. Benjamins. New York, NY: Oxford University Press.

Wilcox, Robin and Alexa Knapp. 2000. Building communities that create health. *Public Health Reports* 115: 139–143.

Williams, David. 1990. Socioeconomic differentials in health: A review and redirection. *Social Psychology Quarterly* 53(2): 81–99.

Williams, David and Pamela Jackson. 2005. Social sources of racial disparities in health. *Health Affairs* 24(2): 325–334.

Winkleby, Marilyn. 1994. Editorial: The future of community-based cardiovascular disease intervention studies. *American Journal of Public Health* 84(9): 1369–1372.

Winkleby, Marilyn, C. Barr Taylor, Darius Jatulis, and Stephen Fortmann. 1996. The long-term effects of a cardiovascular disease prevention trial: The Stanford Five-City Project. *American Journal of Public Health* 86(12): 1773–1779.

Winkleby, Marilyn, Henry Feldman, and David Murray. 1997. Joint analysis of three U.S. community intervention trials for reduction of cardiovascular disease risk. *Journal of Clinical Epidemiology* 50(6): 645–658.

Winkleby, Marilyn, June Flora, and Helena Kraemer. 1994. A community-based heart disease intervention: Predictors of change. *American Journal of Public Health* 84 (5): 767–772.

Winkleby, Marilyn, Stephen Fortmann, and Beverly Rockhill. 1992. Trends in cardiovascular disease risk factors by educational level: The Stanford Five-City Project. *Preventive Medicine* 21: 592–601.

Wolff, Thomas. 2001. Community coalition building--contemporary practice and research: Introduction. *American Journal of Community Psychology* 29(2): 165–172.

Young, Deborah Rohm, William Haskell, C. Barr Taylor, and Stephen Fortmann. 1996. Effect of community health education on physical activity knowledge, attitudes, and behavior. *American Journal of Epidemiology* 144(3): 264–274.

Young, Deborah Rohm, William Haskell, Darius Jatulis, and Stephen Fortmann. 1993. Associations between changes in physical activity and risk factors for coronary heart disease in a community-based sample of men and women: The Stanford Five-City Project. *American Journal of Epidemiology* 138(4): 205–216.

14

THE FUTURE HOLDS PROMISE

Steven Whitman, Ami M. Shah, and
Maureen R. Benjamins

Introduction

Although this book is finished, more remains to be said. Much writing about
science, epidemiology, and public health takes place in journals. This publishing process is well-defined and understood by those tens of thousands
of individuals who regularly read and write for such journals, which almost
always specify the length of the articles they will accept (often as short as
5–10 pages). As a result of this limitation, writers of these articles learn
quickly what must be omitted to save room. There is thus rarely space to
explain how the idea of an article emerged, who took part in the conversations, how many false steps were taken until the idea was shaped, how
considerations of funding were involved, and a great deal more. These are
essential concepts for many involved in research; thus, not being able to put
these issues on display for colleagues is a serious limitation in how this publishing process works.

As the various successes (and failures) in the wake of *Sinai's Improving
Community Health Survey* (Sinai Survey) emerged, the question of how to best
tell the full story became a prominent one. We started our dissemination efforts,
as one usually does, by publishing several reports and articles describing the
work. These have been referenced frequently in the previous chapters and will
not be repeated here. However, as these publications emerged, the full story and
the lessons did not. In addition to the issues listed above, the inter-relationships
of the various articles often were unexamined. Perhaps most importantly, the

interventions that were implemented found only little place in these journal articles. We thus thought that a book would allow us to tell the more complete story, which we hoped (and still expect) will help others who want to be part of the efforts to improve health in vulnerable communities.

Ironically, now that the book is complete, 13 chapters later, there is still much that needs to be said to portray the full richness of the events surrounding the Sinai Model so that we can optimally move ahead. This concluding chapter is an attempt to include some additional dimensions to the story the authors of the chapters in this book have tried to convey.

The Goal of the "Sinai Model"

The Sinai Model, described in the Introduction (Whitman, Shah, Benjamins, 2010), presents a strategy for gathering meaningful data, which in turn can help structure interventions and attract resources in an effort to improve health for vulnerable communities and reduce health disparities. In Chapter 2, Dell and Whitman (2010) noted that disparities in health are more than differences. They are inequities that could be avoided. These disparities occur for many reasons, but at their core, they reflect omnipresent inequities in power and resources. These are variously referred to as fundamental causes (Link and Phelan, 1995) or distal factors (Krieger, 2008). It is bad enough to structure a society so that some people can afford flat screen televisions and automobiles while others cannot, but when the structure of a society systematically limits the health, well-being, and life span of entire groups of people, that should be seen as intolerable and unacceptable (Whitman, 2001).

Mount Sinai Hospital, where the editors of this book work, is located in one of the poorest communities in Chicago. Although Chicago is a very diverse city of 3 million people, that diversity is restrained by an enormously segregated community structure, resulting in a city that has been labeled as "hyper-segregated" (Massey and Denton, 1993). Notably, Mount Sinai Hospital sits on a corner between a Black community area (North Lawndale) and a Mexican community area (South Lawndale). Both communities are very poor, and thus so is Mount Sinai. Many residents of these communities have no insurance (Shah and Whitman, 2010), and far too many will not even live long enough to be eligible for Medicare. Many of their lives are too short and too filled with debilitating illness.

This is the problem that confronted us as we tried to think of a strategy to improve health for these (and other) vulnerable communities. It was hoped that if community-level data could be acquired, these data could guide efforts to improve health. The Sinai Survey produced such data and improvement efforts are very much underway, as detailed by the six case studies in Section 3.

Successes and Challenges

The successes that have occurred thus far are initial ones. Several are described in preceding chapters, and some others have not yet been discussed:

1. The first survey of six community areas was replicated in a Jewish Community and three Asian communities, bringing the total of diverse surveyed communities to 10.
2. More communities in Chicago—notably the Laotian, Indian, and Pakistani communities—have expressed interest in trying to raise funds to also replicate the survey.
3. Perhaps most importantly, many interventions have been funded as a result of the survey. These involve issues such as smoking, diabetes, obesity, and pediatric asthma. Each one of these is impressive. Taken together, they present an affirmation of the Sinai Model and all of its possibilities.
4. As a direct result of the survey, many other grants and initiatives have been pursued by local foundations, health clinics, churches, and community organizations. These include areas such as arthritis, pediatric obesity, and cancer screening.
5. A diabetes intervention for a very poor Black community (North Lawndale) has just recently been funded, modeled on the one for mostly Hispanic Humboldt Park (Whitman et al., 2010). The establishment of this intervention and the receipt of funding have been important events. Now, substantial efforts to prevent diabetes are underway in two very poor Chicago communities and both have emanated directly from the Sinai Survey data.
6. The Greater Humboldt Park Community of Wellness (Martin and Ballesteros, 2010) was shaped around the Sinai Survey findings and now is widely seen as the pre-eminent community-based health organization in Chicago. In fact, as this book goes to press, the National Institutes of Health has just issued a call for proposals for "Building Sustainable Community-Linked Infrastructure to Enable Health Science Research," and the Community of Wellness is being consulted frequently by groups eager to submit a proposal and to replicate its success.

7. Multiple Chicago health foundations have told us that numerous proposals they have received are based on the Sinai, Jewish, and Asian Survey findings.

8. It is common now for community-based organizations and universities to mount health surveys in Chicago communities, an occurrence that was relatively rare just a few years ago.

9. Various medical center projects have been taken to task by community groups that established themselves in the context of the survey data. These challenges have been substantial, and ideology is beginning to shift about how one regards community interaction, indirect costs, and other related areas.

10. Many presentations have been made about survey findings. In fact, they number more than 150 and still counting. For example, the authors organized a panel workshop at the 2006 annual meeting of the American Public Health Association on the topic of local data. Speaking at the panel were representatives of New York City, Los Angeles, the Centers for Disease Control and Prevention (CDC), and Chicago.

11. Groups in other cities, counties, and states have approached us for copies of our materials and advice on how to mount replications of the Sinai Survey. These include the Philadelphia Health Management Corporation, Winnebago County Department of Public Health in Rockford (IL), Los Angeles County Department of Public Health, Sullivan County Regional Health Department in Tennessee, Minnesota Department of Public Health, Morehouse School of Medicine, and Delaware Department of Public Health, to name a few.

12. The Sinai Urban Health Institute participated in various surveys that were assembling an inventory of cities that have gathered local area surveys on health issues. For example, we corresponded with prominent researchers from Rand, Inc. for the Primary Prevention Project in Washington D.C. and with the Canadian Alliance for Regional Risk Factor Surveillance network that was administering a survey on local-level chronic disease risk factor surveillance systems.

Although it is early in the process, there have thus far been important areas where the Sinai Survey and its sequellae have suggested that some important opportunities have not been brought to fruition. These challenges include the following:

1. Some of the 10 surveyed communities have not yet been able to mount any interventions related to the survey findings. In some cases, there are no strong community-based organizations (CBOs) to lead this effort; in one community, there are too many CBOs and they have not been

able to coordinate efforts; and, in two cases relatively strong CBOs that work in other areas have not been able to include health as a focus, even in the face of likely funding.

2. The widely acknowledged challenge of sustainability has already confronted several initiatives. For example, the smoking prevention effort in North Lawndale (see Chapter 7), implemented in the face of one of the highest smoking rates documented in recent decades, lost its state funding two years into a five-year project when the current economic crisis hit Illinois and additional resources could not be located to continue. Other interventions described in Section 3 will certainly face issues of sustainability in the near future.

3. We have no way of knowing how health changes in a community over time. For example, did some measures improve while others grew worse? Did all improve or grow worse? Thus, replicating the survey after 10 years would be an invaluable event. If we are able to accomplish this, then this item will move dramatically from the challenges category where it now sits to the success category above.

Meeting the Need for Local Health Data Elsewhere

The effort described in this book to gather local level data and to assess the health of communities is, of course, not the only one of its kind. There are a growing number of agencies that are gathering such data in an effort to improve health (Simon et al., 2001; Fielding and Frieden, 2004; Frieden, 2004).

At the national level, there are efforts to examine the health of smaller geographic areas. For example, the CDC, which conducts state-based health surveys (BRFSS), designed the Selected Metropolitan/Micropolitan Area Risk Trends Project to mathematically estimate health-related prevalence proportions in smaller geographic areas (CDC, 2009). These data have been studied at selected metropolitan and micropolitan statistical areas. In addition, there is the Community Health Status Indicators Project, developed by the Department of Health and Human Services (U.S. Department of Health and Human Services, 2009). This includes a health profile of over 3,000 counties in the United States and allows for a comprehensive and systematic measurement of health across counties. This is an important effort for performance monitoring and comparisons. Although these data are most useful to compare health outcomes from BRFSS for different regions within the United States, the utility of these data in guiding plans and policies at the local community or neighborhood level is unknown.

Efforts put forth by the state of California are also noteworthy. UCLA's Center for Health Policy and Research in collaboration with the California Department of Public Health, the Department of Health Care Services, and the Public Health Institute conducts the nation's largest state health survey: the California Health Interview Survey (CHIS). It is conducted and funded by various state and federal agencies along with several private foundations. CHIS is an invaluable data resource used by researchers, advocates, public health professionals, and others to understand the health of residents in smaller geographic areas within the state at the county and health services planning area. In addition, analyses of data for diverse populations by race/ethnicity (Kagawa-Singer et al., 2007; Meng et al., 2007; Holtby et al., 2008), age (Chen et al., 2005; Wallace, Lee, and Aydin, 2008), or immigration status (Ortega et al., 2007; Wallace, Mendez-Luck, and Castañeda, 2009) are also available in numerous reports, journal articles, policy briefs, and other publications (UCLA Center for Health Policy Research, 2009). Results are used to guide local, state, and national health policies, and impact at the policy level is most notable (UCLA Center for Health Policy Research, 2009). In addition, efforts to utilize data as a tool for community-level change have been exemplary. For example, data are available about Los Angeles County's Service Planning Areas and regional areas within the county and are used to direct programs and resources to communities most in need through formation of planning councils. In addition, there are other public health programs, such as the Building Healthy Communities Program funded by the California Endowment, that are organizing local communities to create healthy environments and increase access to needed health programs and services to address disparities in certain geographic regions and ethnic groups.

Another example comes from Seattle. Seattle's King County Department of Public Health conducts a health survey every 3 years (http://communities-count.org/) and analyzes data by region and Health Planning Areas, which were defined in consultation with Department of Neighborhoods (Communities Count, 2008). Results from these surveys have been used to guide planning and community-based programs for improved health, such as Seattle Partners for Healthy Communities and the Eastside Human Services.

In addition, sound work is taking place in New York City where they are gathering local level health information and documenting disparities. The NYC Department of Health and Mental Hygiene, Division of Epidemiology, Bureau of Epidemiology Services conducts city-level health surveys (e.g., NYC Community Health Surveys and NYHANES) and provides data on the health of New Yorkers, including neighborhoods within boroughs and city-wide estimates on chronic disease and behavioral risk factors. In addition to city-wide surveys, another local health survey conducted in Harlem found that the smoking prevalence there (42%) was notably different from the rate in New York State as a whole (25%) and even the rate among non-Hispanic Blacks residing in the state (25%) (Northridge et al., 1998). In this instance, racial and ethnic smoking data at the state level did not reveal any differences, but locally there were serious disparities. These surveys allow us to document disparities, which in turn enables local communities to take action to improve matters.

Community-Based Interventions

A very important issue not discussed much in this book, but about which we have learned a fair amount while participating in the projects described in Section 3, is how to select the interventions that offer the most potential. This is a topic we pursue now, finding helpful formulations in the work of Geoffrey Rose.

In the 1970s and 1980s, several major community-based interventions for improved cardiovascular health were put into place in the United States. They are referred to as "community-based" because the goal was to alter morbidity and mortality for the entire targeted communities rather than just for sick or high-risk people. McLeroy and his colleagues present a helpful delineation of the various definitions of "community-based" (McLeroy et al., 2003). These projects were very well-funded and led by some of the best epidemiologists and interventionists. Yet they failed rather substantially (Susser, 1995; Merzel and D'Afflitti, 2003; Hawe, Shiell, and Riley, 2009). Ansell (2010) summarizes these trials and the huge resulting literature that emerged in the wake of these efforts. For quite a long time, such community-based efforts were shunned but are now gradually making a comeback and are growing in different areas, such as diabetes and HIV (Merzel and D'Afflitti, 2003). This comeback is a positive development.

Geoffrey Rose: "Sick Individuals and Sick Populations"

Geoffrey Rose's seminal work is a book entitled *The Strategy of Preventive Medicine* (1992) and is a culmination of much of his earlier work (Rose, 1985; Rose and Day, 1990). The central point of the book, that interventions are often most effective if they focus on communities rather than individuals, emerges from these basic observations:

1. In general, health conditions exist on a continuum in a population.
2. Medicine or health care pays most attention to a "disease" that is defined as existing beyond a cut-point of the distribution in an extreme

tail (e.g., a fasting blood sugar level over 125 mg/dL indicates diabetes, or a blood pressure level over 90/140 mm Hg indicates hypertension). Rose referred to this as the "individual approach" or the "high-risk strategy."

3. Paying most (or all) of our attention to this extreme part of the distribution does not allow us to work with the remainder of the population to help improve its health and to truly prevent disease. Rose referred to working with the entire distribution of people as the "population approach" and urged consideration of the "continuum of risk." This theme was examined in one of his earlier papers entitled "Sick individuals and sick populations" (Rose, 1985).

4. Rose's conclusion is that preventive medicine must embrace both of these approaches that are each effective in different ways "... but, of the two, power resides with the population strategy."

There is very substantial literature discussing these formulations of Rose (e.g., Charleton, 1995; Ebrahim and Lau, 2001; Schwartz and Diez-Roux, 2001; Weed, 2001; Doyle, Furey, and Flowers, 2006; Harper, 2009). Some of these critiques agree with Rose, pointing us toward the "population strategy," and some disagree, favoring the "high-risk strategy." These calibrations of an optimal strategy, as absolutely essential as they are, nonetheless miss the recurring theme of political necessity that courses through Rose's book. This theme is well worth pursuing.

Shifting Ideology

When trying to help improve the health of people in the community, we believe that THE key task is to facilitate a shift from the community as object (which doctors and public health professionals can act upon) to the community as subject (which acts on its own behalf). The community will only be genuinely engaged when this process is facilitated. Thus, for example, if a community decides that it is interested in diabetes, as Humboldt Park did (Whitman et al., 2010), or even if a community can be convinced that it is in its best interest to focus its attention on diabetes, then the role of public health professionals should be to offer technical assistance (e.g., medical or epidemiological) but to otherwise turn the issue over to the community.

The goal here would be to arrange matters so that people in the community talk to their family members and neighbors about diabetes much the same way they always do about assorted other issues like the presidential election, the death of Michael Jackson, or the fire that burned down a house on the block. These discussions might involve, for example, diabetes-friendly cooking, the best way to be active, or how to check your blood sugar level in the least painful way. We see this as a shift in ideology because members of this vulnerable community, so often oppressed or acted upon, can now be active participants in pursuing and shaping their own health. This shift will allow such "subject communities" to organize themselves in a manner that will be able to mitigate risk factors, broadly defined, for morbidity and mortality.

Thus, the community must be a genuine partner, preferably even the leader, in such efforts. This, we believe, is the essence of effective community-based work for improved community health. Further, we believe failure to understand this is the main reason that the cardiovascular interventions in the 1970s and 1980s failed. They simply did not, in any meaningful manner, engage the communities in which they were intervening. They communicated with the community, they used some community institutions, and they distributed messages to the community, but in the end they regarded the community as an object rather than the subject, and thus these massive projects failed. This, by the way, remains the leading dynamic to this day at many medical centers across the country that aim to engage the community (because that is required by multimillion-dollar translational research grants) but more often only succeed in enraging the community.

In addition to helping improve health, such a shift in ideology will likely work to improve other aspects of the community. For example, a community organized for better health will also be able to use that empowerment to fight for better housing or education, for example. Some view this as idealistic, noting that such a view "... hinges on a romanticised view of certain communities that, far from exhibiting potential for networks, exist on the edge of regular conflict" (Doyle, Furey, and Flowers, 2006). We do not believe the ability to empower vulnerable communities is "romanticized." In fact, we believe it is possible and necessary for improved health as well as for overall well-being. Notably, this notion of shifting ideology and empowerment is fully consonant with the concept of *conscientization* and genuine education put forward by Freire and his colleagues (1976). This brings us back to Rose.

Rose and the Politics of Community Engagement

Rose finds his idea of the relationship of the "population strategy" to be interconnected in many ways with the political dynamics of the community. These ideas are stated with such clarity and eloquence that we quote Rose extensively rather than paraphrasing him. The page numbers next to the quotes are from the recently re-issued edition with commentary by Kay-Tee Khaw and Michael Marmot (Rose, 2008).

1. "The visible tip of the iceberg of a disease can be neither understood nor properly controlled if it is thought to constitute the entire problem" (p. 45).
2. "...in order to grasp the principles of public health one must understand that society is not merely a collection of individuals but is also a collectivity, and the behavior and health of its individual members are profoundly influenced by its collective characteristics and social norms" (p. 96).
3. "Yet in truth the deviants are simply the tail of the population's own distribution; they belong to each other and society is one, whether it likes it or not" (p. 99).
4. "This position [that individuals are solely responsible for their health and their fate] conveniently exonerates the majority from any blame for the deviants, and the remedy can then be to extend charity towards them or to provide special services. This is much less demanding than to admit a need for general or socioeconomic change" (p. 130).

In the end, Rose provides two overarching observations that we believe to be essential:

1. "The aim of all of these endeavors is to help a vulnerable minority of individuals. A rescue operation of this nature may be highly appropriate, but it can no more solve the problem of mass diseases than famine relief can solve the problem of hunger in the Third World. The strategy is symptomatic, not radical. The radical strategy is to identify and if possible to remedy the underlying causes of our major health problems" (Preface to the original edition, Rose, 1992).
2. Rose closes his book with these words: "The primary determinants of disease are mainly economic and social, and therefore its remedies must also be economic and social. Medicine and politics cannot and should not be kept apart" (Rose, 1992, p. 161).

One reason why Rose's political analyses are infrequently discussed (Weed, 2001, being a prominent exception) may have to do with the following quote of his:

"This prevalent view [that the majority has no responsibility for the deviants – ed] may be convenient but it is based on a false assumption, as well as being manifestly ineffective. As illustrated earlier in previous chapters, the 'deviant tail of trouble makers' belongs to the parent population. The problem groups do not arise independently... These are facts, and they imply that the occurrence of deviance and its associated distress reflect population-wide characteristics, and hence that prevention calls for acceptance of collective responsibility. As Dostoevsky wrote, 'We are all responsible for all.' The implications are unwelcome and most people reject them. The population strategy of prevention involves an unpopular moral choice" (Rose, 1992, p. 120).

Rose also begins his book with this quote from Dostoevsky, which clearly has great meaning for him. Our main community partner in the work that takes place in Humboldt Park (Whitman et al., 2010; Becker et al., 2010; Martin and Ballesteros, 2010) is the Puerto Rican Cultural Center. Its members are energetic in quoting the Puerto Rican national heroine, Dona Consuelo Corretjer, as saying that one's task is not "to live and let live" but rather "to live and help to live." What an interesting path it is that runs from London to San Juan, from epidemiology to community activism.

Community Engagement

This, then, is the reason we find Rose's theory so compelling, a theory that can instruct us how to improve population health. Indeed, as Rose notes, it is a radical approach, not a symptomatic one. It can lead us to the root of the problem, and this is the direction in which our community colleagues have led us. It is rather straightforward ("convenient," Rose says) to treat individuals in our office, to abstract them from the community setting into a medical center. And clearly there are many times when this is necessary and useful. But it is not prevention. Prevention in the community requires the community and will work best when it asks all to be responsible for all.

Making Things Better

There are any number of well-known quotations that call for action to improve society, including those cited above of Dostoevsky (from *The Brothers Karamazov*) and Corretjer. In this context, there have been widespread discussions about whether it should be the goal of epidemiologists to help to make things better by means beyond research, such as activism and/or involvement in more general public health efforts (Rothman and Poole, 1985; Weed, 1999; Savitz, Poole, and Miller, 1999; Marks, 2009; Kreiger, 1999). This is an important question for the field to debate. However, the larger question is not so much whether the task should be left to epidemiologists, public health workers, or others but rather how can we get it done. Consistent with this larger discussion is one of Karl Marx's best-known theses, that "The philosophers have only interpreted the world, in various ways; the point, however, is to change it," (Marx, 1845, re-published in 1959).

Changing the world, in however small a manner, was our goal when we initiated *Sinai's Improving Community Health Survey*. Our expectation was that the data we gathered would be able to guide us through the morass that is poor health caused by racism and poverty in many of Chicago's communities. It was not a secret that large disparities exist. We only had to look out our windows (Whitman, 2001) or analyze life expectancy data for different groups to appreciate this reality. We also had no interest in implementing still one more study that would produce many more papers and reports with no discernible impact on the lives of the people we wish to serve.

Thus, once data were collected we knew that we had to gather resources in an effort to make actual improvements. Out of this emerged the Sinai Model, a model that has at its essence the dictums of Dostoevsky, Corretjer, and Marx, a model that holds improved health as its goal. Thus far, our pursuit has gone quite well. As the results from the interventions described in Section 3 emerge, some efforts appear to be changing important processes, some appear to be changing important outcomes, and some appear to be ineffective.

Whether all of these interventions succeed or not, we are convinced that the Sinai Model is an effective way to improve health in vulnerable communities and thus to reduce disparities, a proclaimed overarching goal of the United States. We believe that the future holds promise, that the potential is there if we pursue it. We also believe that looking away and walking away from the problem will not make anything better. The problem has to be confronted with energy and resources.

We hope this book has helped elucidate the issues of disparity and health inequity as well as demonstrate a model that, if pursued in genuine partnership with community, might eventually lead to a long and healthy life for all.

References

Ansell, Leah. 2010. Community-Based Health Interventions: Past, Present, and Future. In *Urban Health: Combating Disparities with Local Data,* ed. Steven Whitman, Ami M. Shah, and Maureen R. Benjamins. New York: Oxford University Press.

Becker, Adam B., Kathy Kaufer Christoffel, Miguel Morales, José Luis Rodriguez, José E. Lopez, and Matt Longjohn. 2010. Combating childhood obesity through a neighborhood coalition: Community Organizing for Obesity Prevention in Humboldt Park. In *Urban Health: Combating Disparities with Local Data,* ed. Steven Whitman, Ami M. Shah, and Maureen R. Benjamins. New York: Oxford University Press.

Centers for Disease Control and Prevention. 2009. *Behavioral Risk Factor Surveillance System (BRFSS): Turning Information into Health.* November 17, 2009. Online. Available: http://www.cdc.gov/brfss/. Accessed December 16, 2009.

Charleton, Bruce G. 1995. A critique of Geoffrey Rose's 'population strategy' for preventive medicine. *Journal of the Royal Society of Medicine* 88:607–610.

Chen, Judy Y., Allison Diamant, Nadereh Pourat, and Marjorie Kagawa-Singer. 2005. Racial/ethnic disparities in the use of preventive services among the elderly. *American Journal of Preventive Medicine* 29(5):388–395.

Communities Count. 2008. *A Report on the Strength of King County's Communities: Social and Health Indicators across King County.* 2008. Online. Available: http://www.communitiescount.org/uploads/pdf/archives/2008%20Report/CC08%20Report-logos%20removed.pdf. Accessed December 17, 2009.

Dell, Jade, and Steven Whitman. 2010. A history of the movement to address health disparities. In *Urban Health: Combating Disparities with Local Data,* ed. Steven Whitman, Ami M. Shah, and Maureen R. Benjamins. New York: Oxford University Press.

Doyle, Y. G., A. Furey, and J. Flowers. 2006. Sick individuals and sick populations: 20 years later. *Journal of Epidemiology and Community Health* 60:396–398.

Ebrahim, Shah, and Lau Edith. 2001. Commentary: Sick populations and sick individuals. *International Journal of Epidemiology* 30; 433–434.

Fielding, Jonathan E., and Thomas R. Frieden. 2004. Local knowledge to enable local action. *American Journal of Preventive Medicine* 27(2):183–184.

Freire, Paulo. 1976. *Pedagogy of the Oppressed.* New York: Continuum Press.

Friedan, Thomas R. 2004. Asleep at the switch: Local public health and chronic disease. *American Journal of Public Health* 94(12):2059–2061.

Harper, Sam. 2009. Essay review: Rose's strategy of preventive medicine. *International Journal of Epidemiology* 38:1743–1745.

Hawe, Penelope, Shiell Alan, and Riley Therese. 2009. Theorizing interventions as events in systems. *American Journal of Community Psychology* 43:267–276.

Holtby, Sue, Elaine Zahnd, Jenny Chia, Nicole Lordi, David Grant, and Mirabai Rao. 2008. *Health of California's Adults, Adolescents and Children: Findings from CHIS 2005 and CHIS 2003.* UCLA Center for Health Policy Research, September 2008. Online. Available: http://www.healthpolicy.ucla.edu/pubs/files/Hlth_CAs_RT_090908.pdf. Accessed December 16, 2009.

Kagawa-Singer, Marjorie, Nadereh Pourat, Nancy Breen, Steven Coughlin, Teresa Abend McLean, Timothy S. McNeel, et al. 2007. Breast and cervical cancer screening rates of subgroups of Asian American women in California. *Medical Care Research and Review* 64(6):706–730.

Krieger, Nancy. 1999. Questioning epidemiology: Objectivity, advocacy, and socially responsible science. *American Journal of Public Health* 89:1151–1153.

Krieger, Nancy. 2008. Proximal, distal, and the politics if causation: What's level got to do with it? *American Journal of Public Health* 98:221–230.

Link, Bruce.G., and Phelan Jo. 1995. Social conditions as fundamental causes of disease. *Journal of Health and Social Behavior* 80–94, Extra Issue.

Marks, James S. 2009. Epidemiology, public health, and public policy. *Preventing Chronic Disease* 6(4). Online. Available: http://www.cdc.gov/pcd/issues/2009/oct/09_0110.htm. Accessed December 17, 2009.

Martin, Molly, and Juana Ballesteros. 2010. Humboldt Park: A community united to challenge asthma. In *Urban Health: Combating Disparities with Local Data,* ed. Steven Whitman, Ami M. Shah, and Maureen R. Benjamins. New York: Oxford University Press.

Marx, Karl. 1959. 1845 Theses on Feuerbach. In *Marx & Engels: Basic Writings on Politics and Philosophy*, ed. Lewis S. Feuer. New York City: Anchor Press.

Massey, Douglas. S., and Denton Nancy A. 1993. *American Apartheid: Segregation and the Making of the Underclass*. Cambridge, MA: Harvard University Press.

McLeroy, Kenneth R., Barbara L. Norton, Michelle C. Kegler, James N. Burdine, and Ciro V. Sumaya. 2003. Editorial: Community-based interventions. *American Journal of Public Health* 93(4):529–533.

Meng, Ying-Ying, Susan H. Babey, Theresa A. Hastert, and Richard Brown. 2007. California's racial and ethnic minorities more affected by asthma (Health Policy Research Brief). Los Angeles: Center for Health Policy Research, 2007.

Merzel, Cheryl, and Joanna D'.Afflitti. 2003. Reconsidering community-based health promotion: Promise, performance, and potential. *American Journal of Public Health* 93(4):557–574.

Ortega, Alexander N., Hai Fang, Victor H. Perez, John A. Rizzo, Olivia Carter-Pokras, Steven Wallace, et al. 2007. Health care access, use of services, and experiences among undocumented Mexicans and other Latinos. *Archives of Internal Medicine* 167(21):2354–2360.

Rose, Geoffrey. 1985. Sick individuals and sick populations. *International Journal of Epidemiology* 14:32–38.

Rose, Geoffrey. 1992. *The Strategy of Preventive Medicine*. New York: Oxford University Press.

Rose, Geoffrey, and S. Day. 1990. The population mean predicts the number of deviant individuals. *British Medical Journal* 301:1031–1034.

Rose, Geoffrey, with commentary by Kay-Tee Khaw and Michael Marmot. 2008. *Rose's Strategy of Preventive Medicine*. New York: Oxford University Press.

Rothman, Kenneth J., and Poole Charles. 1985. Science and policy making. *American Journal of Public Health* 75:40–41.

Savitz, David. A., Poole Charles, and Miller William C. 1999. Reassessing the role of epidemiology in public health. *American Journal of Public Health* 89:1158–1161.

Schwartz, Sharon, and Diez-Roux Ana. 2001. Commentary: Causes of Incidence and causes of cases—a Durkheimian perspective on Rose. *International Journal of Epidemiology* 30:435–439.

Shah, Ami M., and Whitman Steven. 2010. Sinai's Improving Community Health Survey: Methodology and key findings. In *Urban Health: Combating Disparities with Local Data,* ed. Steven Whitman, Ami M. Shah, and Maureen R. Benjamins. New York: Oxford University Press.

Simon, Paul A., Cheryl M. Wold, Michael R. Cousineau, and Jonathan E. Fielding. 2001. Meeting the data needs of a local health department: The Los Angeles County Health Survey. *American Journal of Public Health* 91(12):1950–1952.

Susser, Merwyn. 1995. Editorial: The tribulations of trials—interventions in communities. *American Journal of Public Health* 85(2a):156–158.

U.S. Department of Health and Human Services. 2009. *Community Health Status Indicators (CHIS)*. Online. Available: http://www.communityhealth.hhs.gov/homepage.aspx?j=1. Accessed December 16, 2009.

UCLA Center for Health Policy Research. 2009. *CHIS Making an Impact*. Online. Available: http://www.chis.ucla.edu/pdf/chis_making_impact.pdf. Accessed December 16, 2009.

UCLA Center for Health Policy Research. 2009. *Publications and Data Overview.* Online. Available: http://www.healthpolicy.ucla.edu/Pub_Overview.aspx. Accessed December 16, 2009.

Wallace, Steven, Jennifer Lee, and May Jawad Aydin. 2008. *Trends in the Health of Older Californians: Data from the 2001, 2003 and 2005 California Health Interview Surveys.* November 2008. Online. Available: http://www.healthpolicy.ucla.edu/pubs/files/Trends_Older_CAs_RT_111708.pdf. Accessed December 15, 2009.

Wallace, Steven P., Carolyn A. Mendez-Luck, and Xóchitl Castañeda. 2009. Heading south: Why Mexican immigrants in California seek health services in Mexico. *Medical Care* 47(6):662–669.

Weed, Douglas L. 1999. Towards a philosophy of public health. *Journal of Epidemiology and Public Health* 53:99–104.

Weed, Douglas L. 2001. Commentary: A radical future for public health. *International Journal of Epidemiology* 30:440–441.

Whitman, Steven. 2001. Racial disparities in health: taking it personally. *Public Health Reports* 116(5):387–389.

Whitman, Steven, Ami M. Shah, and Maureen R. Benjamins. 2010. Introducing the Sinai Model for reducing health disparities and improving health. In *Urban Health: Combating Disparities with Local Data,* ed. Steven Whitman, Ami M. Shah, and Maureen R. Benjamins. New York: Oxford University Press.

Whitman, Steven, Jose E. Lopez, Steven K. Rothschild, and Jaime Delgado. 2010. Disproportionate impact of diabetes in a Puerto Rican community of Chicago. In *Urban Health: Combating Disparities with Local Data,* ed. Steven Whitman, Ami M. Shah, and Maureen R. Benjamins. New York: Oxford University Press.

INDEX